T0227151

Adolescent Medicine

Editor

BENJAMIN SILVERBERG

PRIMARY CARE:
CLINICS IN OFFICE PRACTICE

www.primarycare.theclinics.com

Consulting Editor
JOEL J. HEIDELBAUGH

June 2020 • Volume 47 • Number 2

ELSEVIER

1600 John F. Kennedy Boulevard • Suite 1800 • Philadelphia, Pennsylvania, 19103-2899

http://www.theclinics.com

PRIMARY CARE: CLINICS IN OFFICE PRACTICE Volume 47, Number 2
June 2020 ISSN 0095-4543, ISBN-13: 978-0-323-71151-7

Editor: Katerina Heidhausen
Developmental Editor: Laura Fisher

Primary Care: Clinics in Office Practice (ISSN: 0095-4543) is published quarterly by Elsevier Inc., 360 Park Avenue South, New York, NY 10010-1710. Months of issue are March, June, September, and December. Periodicals postage paid at New York, NY and additional mailing offices. Subscription prices are $253.00 per year (US individuals), $538.00 (US institutions), $100.00 (US students), $303.00 (Canadian individuals), $609.00 (Canadian institutions), $100.00 (Canadian students), $357.00 (international individuals), $609.00 (international institutions), and $175.00 (international students). Foreign air speed delivery is included in all *Clinics* subscription prices. All prices are subject to change without notice. POSTMASTER: Send address changes to *Primary Care: Clinics in Office Practice*, Elsevier Periodicals Customer Service, 11830 Westline Industrial Drive, St. Louis, MO 63146. Customer Service Health Sciences Division, Subscription Customer Service, 3251 Riverport Lane, Maryland Heights, MO 63043. **Customer Service: 1-800-654-2452 (U.S. and Canada); 314-447-8871 (outside U.S. and Canada). Fax: 314-447-8029. E-mail: journalscustomerservice-usa@elsevier.com (for print support); journalsonlinesupport-usa@elsevier.com (for online support).**

Reprints. For copies of 100 or more, of articles in this publication, please contact the Commercial Reprints Department, Elsevier Inc., 360 Park Avenue South, New York, NY 10010-1710. Tel. 212-633-3874; Fax: 212-633-3820; E-mail: reprints@elsevier.com.

Primary Care: Clinics in Office Practice is covered in *MEDLINE/PubMed (Index Medicus)* and *EMBASE/ Excerpta Medica, Current Contents/Clinical Medicine,* and *ISI/BIOMED.*

Contributors

CONSULTING EDITOR

JOEL J. HEIDELBAUGH, MD, FAAFP, FACG
Clinical Professor, Departments of Family Medicine and Urology, University of Michigan
Medical School, Ann Arbor, Michigan; Ypsilanti Health Center, Ypsilanti, Michigan

EDITOR

BENJAMIN SILVERBERG, MD, MSc, FAAFP
Assistant Professor, Departments of Emergency Medicine and Family Medicine, WVU
Medicine; Medical Director, Division of Physician Assistant Studies, Department of Human
Performance, West Virginia University School of Medicine, Morgantown, West Virginia,
USA

AUTHORS

MEGAN ADELMAN, PharmD, BCPS, BCGP
Clinical Assistant Professor, Department of Clinical Pharmacy, West Virginia University
School of Pharmacy, Morgantown, West Virginia

MARTHA R. ARDEN, MD
Assistant Professor of Pediatrics, Icahn School of Medicine at Mount Sinai, New York,
New York

AMIE M. ASHCRAFT, PhD, MPH
Research Assistant Professor, Department of Family Medicine, West Virginia University,
Morgantown, West Virginia

CHRISTINE BANVARD-FOX, MD, FAAP
Assistant Professor, Departments of Pediatrics and Adolescent Medicine, West Virginia
University, Morgantown, West Virginia, USA

ASHLEIGH L. BARRICKMAN, PharmD, BCACP
Clinical Assistant Professor, Department of Clinical Pharmacy, West Virginia University
School of Pharmacy, Morgantown, West Virginia

KEVIN BERNSTEIN, MD, MMS, CAQSM, FAAFP
Family and Sports Medicine Physician, Musculoskeletal Faculty, Naval Hospital
Jacksonville Family Medicine Residency, Assistant Professor of Family Medicine,
Uniformed Services University of the Health Sciences, Jacksonville, Florida

SILVIA BLAUSTEIN, MD
Assistant Professor of Pediatrics, Icahn School of Medicine at Mount Sinai, New York,
New York

CARINA M. BROWN, MD
Assistant Professor, Department of Family Medicine, The University of North Carolina at Chapel Hill, Cone Health Family Medicine Residency, Greensboro, North Carolina

CATHERINE F. CASEY, MD
Department of Family Medicine, University of Virginia, Charlottesville, Virginia

HEATHER CASSELLA, MS
Visiting Professor, Counseling Education, School Psychology and Human Services, University of Nevada - Las Vegas, Las Vegas, Nevada

JENNIFER J. CHANG, MD, AAHIVS
Associate Physician, Department of Infectious Diseases, Kaiser Permanente at Los Angeles Medical Center, Los Angeles, California

ANASTASIA COSSETTE, BA
Global Health Corps Fellow, Covenant House New Jersey, Newark, New Jersey

LESLEY COTTRELL, PhD
Professor, Department of Pediatrics, Director of Center for Excellence in Disabilities, West Virginia University, Morgantown, West Virginia

COURTNEY CUNDIFF, MD
Assistant Professor, Department of Emergency Medicine, West Virginia University, Morgantown, West Virginia

DANIELLE M. DAVIDOV, PhD
Assistant Professor, Department of Social and Behavioral Sciences, West Virginia University, Morgantown, West Virginia

STEPHANIE D'COSTA, PhD, LP
Assistant Professor of School Psychology, Department of Education and Leadership, California State University - Monterey Bay, Monterey Bay, California

ANGELA DIAZ, MD, PhD, MPH
Jean C. and James W. Crystal Professor, Departments of Pediatrics and Environmental Medicine and Public Health, Icahn School of Medicine at Mount Sinai, Director, Mount Sinai Adolescent Health Center (MSAHC), New York, New York

DANIELLE G. DOOLEY, MD, MPhil
Medical Director, Community Affairs and Population Health, Child Health Advocacy Institute, Children's National Health System, Washington, DC

JULIA EINBOND, JD
Director of Strategy and Learning, Covenant House New Jersey, Newark, New Jersey

SWATI V. ELCHURI, MD
Pediatric Endocrinology, Pediatric Diagnostic Center, Ventura, California

GRETCHEN K. GAROFOLI, PharmD, BCACP
Clinical Associate Professor, Department of Clinical Pharmacy, West Virginia University School of Pharmacy, Morgantown, West Virginia

MARK GAROFOLI, PharmD, MBA, BCGP, CPE
Clinical Assistant Professor, Director of Experiential Learning, West Virginia University School of Pharmacy, Clinical Pain Management Pharmacist, WVU Medicine Center for Integrative Pain Management, Morgantown, West Virginia

FERN R. HAUCK, MD, MS
Spencer P. Bass, MD Twenty-First Century Professor of Family Medicine, Professor of Public Health Sciences, Department of Family Medicine, University of Virginia, Charlottesville, Virginia

B. TATE HINKLE, MD, MPH
Total Healthcare at Russell Medical Center, Alexander City, Alabama; Clinical Assistant Professor, Department of Family Medicine, UAB Huntsville Regional Medical Campus, Huntsville, Alabama

ROANNA KESSLER, MD, FAAP
Medical Director, Johns Hopkins University Student Health and Wellness Center, Homewood Student Affairs, Baltimore, Maryland

KACIE M. KIDD, MD
Adolescent Medicine Fellow, Center for Adolescent and Young Adult Health, UPMC Children's Hospital of Pittsburgh, University of Pittsburgh School of Medicine, Pittsburgh, Pennsylvania

PATRICE M. LEVERETT, PhD, NCSP
Assistant Professor of School Psychology, Counseling Education, School Psychology and Human Services, University of Nevada - Las Vegas, Las Vegas, Nevada

MEREDITH LINGER, MSN, RN
SANE Coordinator, Department of Emergency Medicine, WVU Medicine J.W.Ruby Memorial Hospital, Morgantown, West Virginia

JENNIFER J. MOMEN, MD, MPH
Assistant Professor, Division of Physician Assistant Studies, Department of Human Performance and Applied Exercise Science, West Virginia University School of Medicine, Morgantown, West Virginia

AMY MOYERS, MD
Assistant Professor, Department of Family Medicine, WVU Medicine, Morgantown, West Virginia

ALEX MROSZCZYK-McDONALD, MD, CAQSM
Family and Sports Medicine Physician, Kaiser Permanente Department of Family Medicine, Fontana, California

PAMELA J. MURRAY, MD, MHP
Department of Pediatrics, West Virginia University, Morgantown, West Virginia

STEVE NORTH, MD, MPH
Medical Director, Health-e-Schools, Center for Rural Health Innovation, Spruce Pine, North Carolina

DEBRA J. PAULSON, MD, FACEP, FAAEM
Professor, Department of Emergency Medicine, West Virginia University, Morgantown, West Virginia

NADIA T. SAIF, MD
Resident Physician, Department of Family Medicine, University of Virginia, Charlottesville, Virginia

ROSALYN SCRIVEN, JD
Equal Justice Works Crime Victims Justice Corps Fellow, Covenant House New Jersey, Newark, New Jersey

PAUL SEALES, MD, MS
Family Medicine Physician, Staff Physician, Fleet Surgical Team 4, Norfolk, Virginia

MANAN SHAH, MD
Service Chief, Child and Adolescent Day Hospital, Division of Child and Adolescent Psychiatry, Sheppard Pratt Health System, Towson, Maryland

BENJAMIN SILVERBERG, MD, MSc, FAAFP
Assistant Professor, Departments of Emergency Medicine and Family Medicine, WVU Medicine; Medical Director, Division of Physician Assistant Studies, Department of Human Performance, West Virginia University School of Medicine, Morgantown, West Virginia, USA

LALITHA SWAMINATHAN, MBBS
Assistant Professor, Department of Family Medicine, University of Virginia, Charlottesville, Virginia

CAITLIN THORNBURGH, MSW, LSW
Clinical Social Worker, Center for Adolescent and Young Adult Health, UPMC Children's Hospital of Pittsburgh, Pittsburgh, Pennsylvania

SUZY MASCARO WALTER, PhD, APRN
Assistant Professor, West Virginia University School of Nursing, Morgantown, West Virginia

Contents

Disorders of Pubertal Onset   189

Swati V. Elchuri and Jennifer J. Momen

Evaluation of the child with abnormal pubertal development can be challenging for the primary care provider. Understanding the factors associated with timing of pubertal onset and the normal sequence of pubertal changes is useful in evaluation of children with puberty disorders. A thorough workup includes assessment of growth rate, Tanner staging, and rate of pubertal progression, in addition to an extensive history and physical examination to identify signs and symptoms of disorders associated with abnormal pubertal timing. Initial diagnostic studies will most often include a bone age, levels of gonadotropins, and levels of estradiol (for girls) or testosterone (for boys).

Adolescent Vaccines: Current Recommendations and Techniques to Improve Vaccination Rates   217

Megan Adelman, Ashleigh L. Barrickman, and Gretchen K. Garofoli

With multiple vaccines for adolescents recommended, it is imperative providers remain up to date with the current recommendations. With misinformation of vaccine safety and effectiveness in the mainstream media and social media, adolescents are a vulnerable population that needs to be reviewed and educated. Adolescents are typically only just starting to take ownership of their health care. Consequently, they may represent a more vulnerable population in need of education. This article reviews the current guidelines, recommended vaccinations and schedules, and methods to improve compliance rates.

School-Based Health Care   231

Steve North and Danielle G. Dooley

School-based health care encompasses a variety of health care professionals and practice models, including school nursing, school-based health centers, and school-based mental health programs. Services can be delivered in person or via telehealth. School-based health care is an important mechanism for removing barriers to health care services and for reaching adolescent patients. This article illustrates the various models of school-based health care, the particular benefit of school-based health care for adolescents, and opportunities and challenges in maintaining and sustaining a school-based health program.

Headache is a common episodic and chronic pain syndrome in adolescents. Evaluation of headaches in primary care requires a comprehensive assessment including lifestyle behaviors and physical examination, as well as an understanding of when to pursue appropriate testing. Primary headache disorders seen in adolescents include migraine and tension-type headache. Pharmacologic management for primary headache includes both acute and prophylactic treatment strategies.

Musculoskeletal care of the adolescent patient involves unique knowledge of their rapidly changing physical and psychological health. In this article, the importance of preventing early sports specialization is elucidated, and an encouragement of the safety and necessity of resistance training in adolescents is undertaken. It also explores two common conditions, one affecting the immature skeleton (apophysitis), and one affecting the improperly developed muscular system (patellofemoral syndrome), both of which are diagnosed clinically, and require little advanced imaging. Finally, a brief overview of relative energy deficiency in sport is given.

Transgender and gender diverse youth (TGDY) experience modifiable health disparities and difficulty accessing the physical and mental health care systems. Providers and staff should understand the unique needs of this population and provide affirming spaces where these resilient young people can thrive. In addition to addressing social, setting, and system level barriers to access, providers should consider offering comprehensive gender care because this reduces barriers to medical services and can improve health outcomes. This article educates providers about TGDY, reviews the role of mental health care, and provides an overview of medical interventions for gender affirmation.

This article describes the current scope of immigration to the United States, defines the different categories of immigrants, and describes the Centers for Disease Control and Prevention–mandated overseas and postarrival medical assessment of adolescent refugees. Guidelines for primary care physicians who care for refugee youth are provided, including diagnosis and treatment of common medical and mental health conditions. Special considerations in caring for this vulnerable population include acknowledging prior traumas, acculturation and challenges to education such as bullying, and adjustment to a new health care system that emphasizes preventive care in addition to curative medical care.

and economic factors. Strategies for screening and prevention of HIV infection, including universal screening, behavioral counseling, and preexposure prophylaxis, are reviewed, and the initial treatment approach to a diagnosis of HIV in adolescents is outlined.

Development of SOGIE (sexual orientation and gender identity and expression) is not unique to minority populations, as all adolescents grapple with their sexuality and identity. Health care providers straddle the unique positions of authority figure and advocate and can help these young people establish behaviors that will allow them to flourish as adults. This article discusses the appropriate language to use while conducting a sexual history, summarizes the epidemiologic data on sexually transmitted infections, and reviews the screening and reporting guidelines set forth by the United States Preventive Services Task Force and the Centers for Disease Control and Prevention.

Adolescent substance abuse is America's #1 public health problem as per the National Center on Addiction and Substance Abuse. People are most likely to begin abusing drugs during adolescence, and the longer adolescents defer experimentation, the less likely they are to develop long-term drug abuse problems. The CRAFFT and DAST questionnaires are brief, reliable tools for adolescent substance abuse screening. Health care professionals can help continue low adolescent substance utilization rate by having open conversations with adolescents regarding all substances and medications, including illicit substances.

PRIMARY CARE:
CLINICS IN OFFICE PRACTICE

SERIES OF RELATED INTEREST

Medical Clinics (http://www.medical.theclinics.com)
Physician Assistant Clinics (http://www.physicianassistant.theclinics.com)

THE CLINICS ARE AVAILABLE ONLINE!
Access your subscription at:
www.theclinics.com

Foreword

Culture Shock and Changing Times

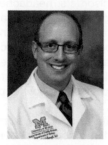

Joel J. Heidelbaugh, MD, FAAFP, FACG
Consulting Editor

I remember the culture shock of entering high school in 1984 like it was yesterday. Being an only child, and not having much exposure to children older than I was, I didn't have much of a reference point for what "becoming a teenager" really meant. Transitioning from a small private school in Connecticut to a larger public school in upstate New York opened my eyes very quickly. The first week of school I saw a classmate get his locker searched: The school officials found marijuana, and that's pretty much the last we ever saw of that guy. I think back then they might have given him a life sentence. I remember learning in health class about sexually transmitted infections (STIs) and condoms (and abstinence); how cigarettes, drugs, and too much alcohol were bad for you; and about something called human immunodeficiency virus (HIV) that nobody really knew much about. I didn't learn about human trafficking, sexual assault, human papilloma virus, or what it means to be transgender. At the time, those things just didn't garner significant attention on a national and global level, much less my high school health class.

As the parent of two teenagers, I am experiencing adolescence all over again, albeit vicariously, but the challenges and issues seem much greater than those my wife and I experienced. We have family discussions centered on various issues, deciphering and debunking myths, while striving to raise the bar on basic parenting skills. Yet, the world seems to be a very different place than it was 36 years ago, with a lot more opportunity for adolescents to get exposure to seemingly "adult" issues at an earlier age before they may be adequately prepared to process their meaning and ramifications.

While the "typical" adolescent visit in my practice seems to center on sports physicals and completion of the requisite forms, inquiries by young women about birth control and STI testing, mental health issues, and the occasional injury, we find it a formidable challenge to cover the ground we need to cover discussing the many other pertinent aspects of preventive adolescent health that also need to be addressed. The advent of school-based health clinics for adolescents has provided many of these

Prim Care Clin Office Pract 47 (2020) xiii–xiv
https://doi.org/10.1016/j.pop.2020.03.001
0095-4543/20/© 2020 Published by Elsevier Inc.

resources at a convenience, with the opportunity for continuity of care, yet somewhat parallel to primary care practices.

The scope of this issue of *Primary Care: Clinics in Office Practice* is quite different from comparative issues in that Dr Benjamin Silverberg and his colleagues have addressed many very timely and socially relevant topics. Guideline-based reviews on diagnosis and treatment of STIs, HIV, substance abuse disorders, headaches, and musculoskeletal issues provide a solid foundation for providers caring for adolescents in daily practice. Impressively, detailed articles on human trafficking, crisis counseling, and sexual assault provide cogent information and resources to assist adolescents in a timely and caring fashion. As vaccination becomes more and more "questioned" and refused by patients and their families, another article herein provides an outstanding blueprint on how to best address the need for interval vaccines and how to provide appropriate education that can improve vaccination rates.

I am indebted to Dr Silverberg and his expert authors for rising to the formidable challenge of creating a unique compendium of articles on timely topics in adolescent health. I hope that our readers will learn as much as I have, and become better health care providers, mentors, and parents.

Joel J. Heidelbaugh, MD, FAAFP, FACG
Departments of Family Medicine and Urology
University of Michigan Medical School
Ann Arbor, MI 48103, USA

Ypsilanti Health Center
200 Arnet Street, Suite 200
Ypsilanti, MI 48198, USA

E-mail address:
jheidel@umich.edu

Preface

Too Much Go, Not Enough Slow: Navigating the Challenges of Adolescence

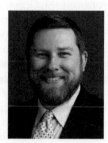

Benjamin Silverberg, MD, MSc, FAAFP
Editor

According to the German-American psychologist Erik Erikson,[1] individuals are wrestling with their sense of identity during adolescence. This includes both vocation (purpose) and sexuality (reproduction): Who am I, and what can I be? Teenagers invent and reinvent themselves. They try to stand out, and they try to fit in. They may anguish over their body image as they develop secondary sex characteristics. They may experiment with drugs or engage in other risky behaviors. They compare their family's values to those of their peers and mentors. Ascribing to particular ideals shapes and guides their behavior, though pressure to assume a certain identity can lead to rebellion, poor self-image, and unhappiness. Adolescents frequently challenge authority figures, potentially impeding effective communication with their medical provider, for example. Individuals with a strong sense of self are thought to feel more independent and in control; conversely, those who are uncertain of their beliefs feel insecure about their place in society. This so-called "role confusion" or identity crisis may lead to further experimentation. Nonetheless, successful navigation of this, the fifth stage of psychosocial development, yields the virtue of fidelity, the Shakespearian trait of being true to oneself and one's principles.

Adolescence roughly corresponds to the second decade of life, though recently-expanded definitions suggest it extends as late as age 25.[2] Chronological age, however, does not necessarily indicate an individual's emotional (or physical) maturity. There is indeed some truth to the idea that girls mature faster than boys. For instance, compared with adolescent girls, adolescent boys are less engaged in primary care, resulting in higher levels of unmet health care needs (eg, immunizations, risk prevention) and greater mortality.[3] It has been said that adolescents are like a car with a functioning gas pedal but weak brakes: The drive is there but the restraint is not. In this installment of *Primary Care: Clinics in Office Practice*, the authors–a constellation of

Prim Care Clin Office Pract 47 (2020) xv–xvi
https://doi.org/10.1016/j.pop.2020.03.002
0095-4543/20/© 2020 Published by Elsevier Inc.

academics, clinicians, nurses, pharmacists, lawyers, counselors, and social workers–explore risk, privacy, health care disparities, intersectionality, and other medical concerns particularly relevant for adolescents.

An appropriate starting point for this issue, Elchuri and Momen detail the causes, evaluation, and treatment of precocious and delayed puberty. Next, Adelman, Barrickman, and Garofoli review adolescent vaccines and suggest ways to improve their utilization. In the first of two case-based articles, North and Dooley describe the provision of physical and mental health care services in primary and secondary schools. Thereafter, Walter, Banvard-Fox, and Cundiff offer a survey of primary headaches and their treatment. Bernstein, Seales, and Mroszczyk-McDonald then comment on several issues in adolescent sports medicine, including apophysitis, patellofemoral pain syndrome, and relative energy deficiency in sport. Transgender and gender-diverse youth are the focus of the contribution by Kidd and her colleagues, as the reader is introduced to gender-affirming clinical environments and medical interventions. Brown and her colleagues follow with an excellent analysis of the issues refugees and immigrants confront upon arriving in the United States. Human trafficking, which does not necessarily include movement across international borders, is the subject of the case-based article by Einbond and her colleagues. In response to an unfortunate sign of the times, Leverett and her colleagues discuss crisis counseling for those impacted by school shootings and suicide, and Banvard-Fox and her colleagues provide a guide for compassionate evaluation of the victim of sexual assault. Risk, screening, and treatment of human immunodeficiency virus are covered by Chang and Ashcraft, and, subsequently, Kessler and her colleagues address other sexually transmitted infections. Finally, Garofoli concludes the conversation on risk with his composition on adolescent substance abuse.

It is my hope that these articles serve as both reference and inspiration as together we help our next generation of leaders navigate the winding–and at times, bumpy-road ahead of them.

This issue is dedicated to my mother, Joann Silverberg, PhD, who was my first (and continues to be my best) teacher.

Benjamin Silverberg, MD, MSc, FAAFP
Departments of Emergency Medicine, Family Medicine, and
Human Performance
West Virginia University School of Medicine

WVU Student Health
390 Birch Street
Morgantown, WV 26506, USA

E-mail address:
benjamin.silverberg@hsc.wvu.edu

REFERENCES

1. Erikson EH. Identity: youth and crisis. New York: WW Norton; 1968.
2. Sawyer SM, Azzopardi PS, Wickremarathne D, et al. The age of adolescence. Lancet Child Adolesc Health 2018;2(3):223–8.
3. McGarry ML. Male adolescent health: addressing a critical need (chapter 5). In: Quallich SA, Lajiness M, Mitchell K, editors. Manual of men's health: primary care guidelines for APRNs and PAs. New York: Springer; 2019. p. 45–55.

Disorders of Pubertal Onset

Swati V. Elchuri, MD[a], Jennifer J. Momen, MD, MPH[b],*

KEYWORDS

- Central precocious puberty • Peripheral precocious puberty • Precocious puberty
- Premature adrenarche • Premature thelarche • Delayed puberty • Hypogonadism

KEY POINTS

- Differentiating normal from abnormal pubertal development can be challenging for the primary care provider; however, the distinction is important because of the potential for long-term medical and psychosocial complications.
- Precocious puberty may result from early activation of the hypothalamic-pituitary-gonadal (HPG) axis (central precocious puberty) or exposure to sex steroids independent of HPG axis activation (peripheral precocious puberty).
- A significant proportion of children with central precocious puberty have no underlying abnormality, but it is important to exclude disorders of the central nervous system.
- Delayed puberty may result from functional failure of the gonads or impaired function at the level of the hypothalamus or pituitary gland.
- Although a basic workup is helpful in identifying a possible cause of early or delayed puberty, referral to a pediatric endocrinologist is often indicated for management.

INTRODUCTION

The primary care provider (PCP) plays a vital role in the recognition of abnormal pubertal development in children. Effective management of children with disorders of puberty requires an understanding of the physiology of pubertal development, the timing and sequence of normal pubertal development, and the underlying pathophysiology of disorders associated with abnormal pubertal timing.

Initial evaluation of a child with abnormal pubertal timing may be conducted by the PCP and includes a thorough history, physical examination (including careful assessment of growth and pubertal stage), and initial diagnostic studies. A specific diagnosis may be possible following initial evaluation, but referral to a pediatric endocrinologist is often necessary for more specific diagnostic testing and overall management.

[a] Pediatric Diagnostic Center, 300 Hillmont Avenue, Building 340, Suite 302, Ventura, CA 93003, USA; [b] Division of Physician Assistant Studies, Department of Human Performance and Applied Exercise Science, West Virginia University School of Medicine, 1 Medical Center Drive, PO Box 9226, Morgantown, WV 26506-9226, USA
* Corresponding author.
E-mail address: jjmomen@hsc.wvu.edu

Prim Care Clin Office Pract 47 (2020) 189–216
https://doi.org/10.1016/j.pop.2020.02.001
0095-4543/20/© 2020 Elsevier Inc. All rights reserved.

primarycare.theclinics.com

Close coordination between the PCP and pediatric endocrinologist is essential in follow-up of children with disorders of pubertal timing. The PCP can facilitate periodic and regular follow-up to monitor growth velocity, progression of pubertal changes, and adverse effects of treatment. In addition, PCPs with a long-term relationship with the child and family will be well suited to provide psychosocial support.

PRECOCIOUS PUBERTY

Onset of pubertal development is initiated by reactivation of the previously suppressed hypothalamic-pituitary-gonadal (HPG) axis, an event influenced by both genetic and environmental factors.[1-8] Reactivation of the HPG axis involves a shift in the balance of excitatory and inhibitory stimulation of gonadotropin-releasing hormone (GnRH) neurons in the hypothalamus, resulting in activation of the hypothalamic GnRH pulse generator.[9-12] Activation of the hypothalamic pulse generator leads to an increase in the amplitude and frequency of GnRH secretion and a subsequent increase in the pulsatile release of luteinizing hormone (LH) and follicle-stimulating hormone (FSH) from the pituitary, which initially occurs at night during sleep. These gonadotropins are responsible for enlargement of the ovaries in girls and enlargement of the testes in boys and the increased production of estradiol and testosterone, respectively.[8,12] Onset of puberty is recognized clinically by the appearance of secondary sexual characteristics: breast development in girls and testicular enlargement in boys. Descriptions of the standardized stages of regular pubertal development are provided in **Tables 1** and **2**.

Classification of Disorders of Premature Pubertal Onset

The most widely accepted definition of precocious puberty is the onset of breast development in girls less than 8 years old and the onset of testicular enlargement in boys less than 9 years old.[12-14] **Fig. 1** categorizes central, peripheral, and variant causes.

Central precocious puberty (CPP) results from activation of the HPG axis before the normal age of pubertal onset[1,16] and is further categorized based on its cause: insult

Table 1
Sexual maturity rating (Tanner stages) in girls

Stage	Breast Development	Pubic Hair Development
1	Preadolescent; elevation of papilla only	Preadolescent, no pubic hair
2	Breast bud; elevation of breast and papilla as a small mound; enlargement of areola	Hair is sparse long, downy, straight (or only slightly curled); mainly along labia
3	Further enlargement of breast and areola; no separation of their contours	Hair darker, more course, and more curled; extends sparsely over the junction of the pubes
4	Areola and papilla form a secondary mound above the level of the breast	Adult type hair; covers less area than in most adults; no spread to medial thighs
5	Mature adult stage; projection of papilla only	Adult quantity, type, and distribution (inverse triangle); spread to medial thighs

Data from Marshall WA, Tanner JM. Variations in pattern of pubertal changes in girls. Arch Dis Child. 1969;44:291-303.

Stage	Genital Development	Pubic Hair Development
	Table 2 **Sexual maturity rating (Tanner stages) in boys**	
1	Preadolescent; testes, scrotum, and penis childhood size	Preadolescent, no pubic hair
2	Enlargement of testes and scrotum with reddening and change in texture of scrotal skin	Hair is sparse long, downy, straight (or only slightly curled); mainly at base of penis
3	Growth of penis has begun; continued growth of testes and scrotum	Hair darker, more course and more curled; spreads sparsely over the junction of the pubes
4	Penis further enlarged with development of glans; continued growth of testes and scrotum; darkening of scrotal skin	Adult type hair; covers less area than in most adults; no spread to medial thighs
5	Adult size and shape of testes, scrotum, and penis	Adult quantity, type, and distribution (inverse triangle); spread to medial thighs

Data from Marshall WA, Tanner JM. Variations in the pattern of pubertal changes in boys. Arch Dis Child. 1970;45:13-23.

to, or disorder of, the central nervous system (CNS); or idiopathic, in which no underlying disorder can be identified.[16–18]

Peripheral precocity results from gonadal secretion of testosterone or estrogen independent of activation of the HPG axis or exposure to sex steroids from a nongonadal endogenous or exogenous source.[1,16,17]

Variants of precocious puberty, which are listed in **Table 3**, include premature thelarche (Isolated breast development in girls before the normal age of puberty) and premature pubarche (development of pubic hair in either sex before the normal age of puberty).[1,8,14,16]

Factors Associated with Timing of Pubertal Onset

Both genetic and environmental factors influence timing of pubertal onset.[1–13] Mutations involving 4 distinct genes are known to cause CPP (**Box 1**).[18,19,20] Early pubertal

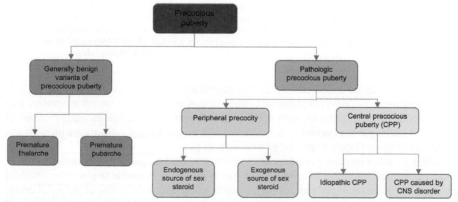

Fig. 1. Classification of precocious puberty. (*Data from* Refs.[8,14,15])

Table 3
Variants of precocious puberty

	Premature Thelarche	Premature Pubarche (Premature Adrenarche)[a]
Clinical features	• Isolated breast development before normal age of puberty[1,8,16] • May be unilateral or bilateral[1]; may regress or persist[1] • Enlargement may wax and wane over time[14] • Complete regression more common with onset before 2 y of age[16] • Normal growth rate and bone age[1,8,16] • Not accompanied by other signs of pubertal development[1,8,16] • Most common between infancy and 3 y of age[16] • Progression to CPP seen in small number of patients[14,16]	• Development of pubic hair in boys or girls before the normal age of puberty[1,8,16] • Increase in hair growth over time is typical[16] • Growth rate and skeletal maturation may be slightly advanced[16]; most will not have an obvious growth spurt[8] • Not accompanied by other signs of puberty[14,16] • Axillary hair, body odor, and/or acne may be present[1,16] • Most cases caused by premature adrenal maturation (premature adrenarche) with increased levels of dehydroepiandrosterone (DHEA) and dehydroepiandrosterone sulfate (DHEAS)[8,14,16]
Primary care evaluation	• History of exposure to exogenous estrogens, lavender oil, or tea tree oil[1] • Bone age[16] • Physical examination and assessment of growth rate every 3–6 mo[16]	• Physical examination for signs of virilization (presence may indicate late-onset CAH or virilizing (androgen-secreting) tumor • Growth rate[16] • Bone age[16]
Indications for endocrine referral	• Increased breast enlargement over a 4- to 6-mo period[14] • Increase in growth rate[14]	• Significant virilization[16] • Increase in growth rate[16] • Advanced bone age[16]

Specialist considerations (differential diagnosis)	• Feminizing disorders[8]
	  ○ Luteinized follicular cyst
	  ○ Aromatase excess syndrome
	• May be initial sign of CPP[14,16]
		• Virilizing tumor[16]
		• Late-onset CAH[16]; corticotropin (ACTH) stimulation testing can help distinguish[1]

[a] Although associated with a normal onset of puberty and normal adult height, premature adrenarche is no longer considered a "benign" variant of pubertal development.[16] Some girls with premature pubarche due to premature adrenarche will develop PCOS in adolescence,[1,16] and premature adrenarche is now thought of as representing 1 point on the spectrum of metabolic syndrome.[16]

development may be a component of a recognized chromosomal syndrome (eg, Williams syndrome).[21] Timing of pubertal onset in boys and girls can be influenced by pubertal timing of both parents, with children tending to experience an earlier onset of puberty if either parent had early pubertal development as well.[6] Given the inverse association between body mass index and age at pubertal onset in girls,[1–3,13,14,17] it is not clear to what degree the association with parental pubertal timing indicates genetic control of initiation of puberty versus shared food behaviors and/or lifestyle choices.[7] Studies have demonstrated an association between timing of pubertal onset and/or age at menarche and socioeconomic factors, stressful family experiences, and

> **Box 1**
> **Genetic causes of central precocious puberty**
>
> Monogenic causes:
> - KISS1 (kisspeptin) gain-of-function mutations
> - KISS1R (kisspeptin receptor) gain-of-function mutations
> - MKRN3 (makorin ring finger protein 3) loss-of-function mutations
> - DLK1 (Delta-like homolog 1) loss-of-function mutations
>
> Chromosomal disorders that may include CPP as a manifestation:
> - Williams syndrome
> - Prader-Willi syndrome
> - Russel-Silver syndrome
> - Temple syndrome
>
> *Data from* Refs.[18,19,20]

adverse childhood experiences.[4,5,21] Earlier onset of puberty has also been associated with low birth weight and following international adoption.[22] Childhood exposure to endocrine disrupting chemicals including organochlorine compounds (eg, polychlorinated biphenyls, DDT, dioxin) may be associated with an earlier onset of puberty, but the evidence is inconclusive.[5,13,18,22,23]

Central Precocious Puberty

CPP (gonadotropin-dependent) results from activation of the HPG axis before the normal age of pubertal onset.[1,16] Because the underlying physiology of CPP is identical to that of normal puberty, pubertal changes in children with CPP will always be isosexual (ie, appropriate for the sex of the child).[16] Girls often present to the PCP with breast development; boys may not present for evaluation until genital and pubic hair development are noted, because testicular enlargement may initially go undetected.[16] The rate of progression of pubertal changes, as well as growth rate and skeletal maturation for age, is typically increased.[16,17,19] Indeed, premature fusion of the growth plates with potential for compromised adult height[8,13] is one of the main indications for treatment.[14,19,24]

CPP may be idiopathic or caused by a wide range of CNS disorders (**Box 2**).[16–18,19] Girls with CPP are much more likely than boys to have the idiopathic form.[16,24,25] Specifically, only about 10% of girls with CPP have underlying CNS pathologic condition,[16,18,25] whereas 70% to 90% of boys with CPP have a CNS lesion.[18,22]

Diagnosis of CPP is based on demonstration of activation of the HPG axis.[16,18,19] Affected children often have an elevated (pubertal) baseline level of LH of greater than 0.3 mIU/mL and a pubertal LH level (>5 mIU/mL) in response to stimulation with a GnRH agonist.[8,17,25] Regardless of the underlying cause, bone age is typically more than 2 standard deviations (SD) above normal for age.[13] Following confirmation of the diagnosis, MRI of the brain is indicated to rule out a structural CNS abnormality.[8,14,16]

A central goal in the treatment of precocious puberty itself is to extend the period of skeletal growth and preserve adult height potential.[19,24,27] Another important goal is to minimize the psychological impact experienced by early maturing children.[8,17,28] Treatment of any underlying CNS abnormality is indicated in addition to treatment aimed at slowing the rate of pubertal progression; in most cases, this will require specialty consultation.

The cornerstone of treatment of CPP is the use of GnRH agonists, which slows the progression of puberty by overriding pulsatile release of endogenous GnRH via delivery of a constant serum level of GnRH activity.[25] GnRH agonists are available in a

---

Box 2
Disorders associated with central precocious puberty

- Tumor of hypothalamic pituitary region
  - Hamartoma
  - Glioma
  - Astrocytoma
  - Germinoma
  - Ependymoma
  - Pinealoma
  - Craniopharyngioma

- Hydrocephalus

- Suprasellar arachnoid cyst

- Septooptic dysplasia

- Chiari malformations

- Myelomeningocele

- CNS infection

- Intracranial bleeding

- Cranial irradiation

- Traumatic brain injury

- Cerebral palsy

- Neurofibromatosis type 1, Sturge-Weber syndrome, tuberous sclerosis

- CNS granulomatous disease

Data from Refs.[18,19,21,26]

---

variety of forms, including depot intramuscular (IM) injections given monthly or every 3 months (leuprolide) or every 6 months (triptorelin), and a subcutaneous implant marketed for annual use (histrelin).[24] Despite differences in route and dosing, all available GnRH agonists are effective,[29] and the choice of agent is largely dependent on patient and physician preference. They are generally well tolerated[24]: systemic adverse effects include headaches and hot flashes, neither of which usually results in discontinuation of treatment.[29] Patients with local adverse events (eg, pain, erythema, inflammatory reaction) may require a change in formulation.[29] Sterile abscess formation has been reported with the use of IM injection.[24]

Monitoring during treatment with GnRH agonists should include assessment of Tanner stage and growth velocity every 3 to 6 months.[29] Bone age should also be obtained periodically.[29] Effective treatment is suggested by a decrease in both growth velocity and rate of bone age advancement.[29]

Gain in height following treatment is most pronounced in girls with onset of puberty less than 6 years of age.[25,29] The decision to initiate treatment in girls with onset of puberty greater than 6 years old should be individualized.[29] Insufficient data exist to relate age at pubertal onset to treatment outcome (height gain) for boys; treatment should be considered for all boys with onset of CPP less than 9 years of age.[29] Conclusive data do not exist to demonstrate that treatment of CPP lessens the psychosocial impact of the condition.[29]

The decision to stop treatment should be individualized, and height potential, chronologic age, and psychosocial factors should be taken into consideration.[24,25,29]

Peripheral Precocity

Pubertal changes in children with peripheral precocity result from exposure to sex steroids in the absence of activation of the HPG axis. As a group, the disorders are characterized by suppressed LH and FSH levels in the setting of elevated levels of testosterone or estradiol.[13] Accurate diagnosis is critical, because it is always associated with underlying pathologic condition or exogenous steroid exposure.[8] Causes and features of peripheral precocity in boys and girls are listed in **Table 4**.

Treatment of peripheral precocity is directed at the underlying disorder. Steroid replacement is indicated in congenital adrenal hyperplasia (CAH). Management of gonadal or adrenal tumors may consist of surgical management, chemotherapy, or radiation therapy (or some combination thereof) and will likely require coordination with multiple specialists. Exposure to endogenous steroids is treated by elimination of the source. Aromatase inhibitors and selective estrogen-receptor modulators have been used to counteract the action of estrogens in children with McCune-Albright syndrome.[22] Treatment of boys with familial male limited precocious puberty has included ketoconazole, spironolactone, and testolactone (an aromatase inhibitor).[17]

Evaluation of the Child with Precocious Puberty

Overall goals of evaluation are to answer the following questions[12,13]:

- Is the pubertal development occurring outside the range of normal?
- Are the rate of progression of pubertal development and growth rate abnormally rapid?
- Are the pubertal changes a result of activation of the HPG axis?
- Whether or not there is activation of the HPG axis, does an organic disorder exist that requires specific treatment?

PCPs should obtain a thorough personal and family history with a focus on identifying risk factors for premature pubertal onset, the rate of progression of pubertal changes, and symptoms suggestive of an underlying disorder requiring specific evaluation and treatment (**Box 3**). Physical examination should include a determination of Tanner stage and an examination for signs of an underlying disorder associated with early pubertal development. For example, children with progressive CPP will often advance from 1 pubertal stage to the next within 3 to 6 months.[22] Determination of growth rate is an important component of the evaluation and will guide further studies.

Initial diagnostic studies should include bone age, FSH, LH, and either testosterone or estradiol.[14] FSH and LH levels should ideally be obtained in the morning and should ideally be measured using an ultrasensitive assay with detection limits adapted to pediatric values.[19,22] Children with precocious puberty (in contrast to those with premature thelarche or premature pubarche) will typically have an advanced bone age (>2 SD greater than normal for age) and growth acceleration, with a growth rate of more than about 6 cm per year.[13,22] Children with CPP are likely to have a high (pubertal) baseline level of LH. If the LH is not clearly elevated, a GnRH stimulation test is necessary to confirm the diagnosis[14,22] and will be done following referral to a pediatric endocrinologist.

MRI of the brain should be obtained for all children with progressive CPP following diagnosis and is especially important in children with signs or symptoms of a CNS lesion.[13,22]

Testing for a genetic mutation may be done in children with CPP who have a normal brain MRI starting with the most common mutation, MKRN3.[21]

Table 4
Cause and features of disorders associated with peripheral precocity

	Sex	Hormonal Imbalance	Associated Features	Other Comments
Genetic mutations				
CAH: • 21-hydroxylase deficiency • 3β-hydroxysteroid dehydrogenase deficiency • 11-hydroxylase deficiency	♀, ♂	Defective steroidogenesis → ↓ cortisol production and ↑ ACTH secretion, with shunting of steroid precursors into the intact androgen pathway(s) → ↑ adrenal androgen production	Signs of virilization (eg, axillary and pubic hair, body odor, clitoromegaly or penile enlargement); ↑ growth rate and advanced bone age; in boys, testicular volume remains prepubertal	Most common cause of abnormal postnatal virilization in children; except in rare cases, boys will not have increases in testicular volume; diagnosis should be considered in children with isolated development of pubic hair
McCune-Albright syndrome	♀ > ♂	Unregulated sex steroid production from gonads and generalized, autonomous hyperfunction of endocrine glands (ie, pituitary, thyroid, parathyroid)	Irregular café-au-lait spots, polyostotic fibrous dysplasia, gigantism, hyperprolactinemia, hyperthyroidism, hyperparathyroidism; affected boys may have asymmetric testicular enlargement	More common in girls; sexual precocity rare in affected boys; clinical presentation highly variable, but affected girls may progress to central (GnRH-dependent) puberty
Familial male-limited precocious puberty (testotoxicosis)	♂	Activating mutation of LH receptor gene → serum testosterone in adult male range	Testicular enlargement and signs of virilization; premature fusion of the growth plates	Typically presents by age 4; autosomal dominant inheritance and sporadic mutations
Neoplasia				
Adrenal tumors	♀, ♂	↑ Serum adrenal androgen[a]	Signs of virilization	Adenocortical adenomas and carcinomas are a very rare causes of precocious puberty and most are malignant
Ovarian tumors	♀	↑ Serum estrogen[b]	Signs of feminization; palpable abdominal mass, distension, and ascites	May present in infancy, but average age is 10 y old; granulosa cell tumors are most frequent ovarian tumor causing precocious puberty

			Signs of virilization	
Testicular tumors	♂	↑ Serum testosterone		Leydig cell tumors are often benign in children and are the most common gonadal stromal tumor causing precocious puberty in boys
Nongonadal germ cell tumors (eg, chorionic gonadotropin-secreting tumors)	♀ < ♂	Ectopic β-hCG mimics action of LH on testicular Leydig cells (↑ serum testosterone)	↑ Tumor markers (α-fetoprotein, β-hCG, pregnancy-specific β1-glycoprotein)	More common in boys; tumor may arise in numerous locations, including liver, lungs, and mediastinum
Other causes				
Transiently functioning ovarian cysts (feminizing benign follicular cyst)	♀	↑ Ovarian estradiol secretion	Waxing and waning breast development	May represent transient activation of HPG axis, an unusual form of McCune-Albright syndrome, or unidentified mutation of FSH receptor
Aromatase excess syndrome	♀, ♂	↑ Conversion of androgens to estrogen	Premature breast development in girls and gynecomastia in boys	
Van Wyk-Grumbach syndrome	♀, ♂	Severe, untreated hypothyroidism	↓ Growth rate and delayed bone age	Due to partial structural homology between thyrotropin (TSH) and the gonadotropins LH and FSH

[a] Rarely associated with estrogen production and signs of feminization (eg, gynecomastia in boys).
[b] Uncommonly associated with androgen production and signs of virilization.
Data from Refs. [1,8,12,13,16,17,22,23,26]

Box 3
Evaluation of the child with precocious puberty

Family history
- Age at pubertal onset for both parents and siblings
- Mother's age at menarche
- Parental height

Personal history
- Pubertal changes
  - Age at first sign of puberty
  - Rate of progression of pubertal changes
  - Presence of vaginal bleeding and timing of bleeding in relation to breast development
- Exposure to exogenous sex steroids
  - Oral contraceptives
  - Transdermal estrogen creams
  - Testosterone gels
- Exposure to aromatic oils
  - Lavender
  - Tea tree
- Neurologic insult
  - CNS trauma
  - Meningitis
  - Hypoxic-ischemic injury
  - Histiocytosis
  - Neurofibromatosis
- Review of systems
  - Presence of body odor, acne, and/or axillary hair
  - Vaginal bleeding or discharge
  - Symptoms associated with CNS disorder (eg, headache, cognitive changes, visual impairment, visual field deficit, seizures, increased head circumference, polyuria, polydipsia)
  - Abdominal pain
  - Signs/symptoms of hypothyroidism
  - Bone pain (due to polyostotic fibrous dysplasia in McCune-Albright syndrome)

Physical examination
- Assessment of growth velocity and body mass index
- Determination of sexual maturity stage (Tanner stage)
  - Breast and pubic hair development in girls
  - Genital and pubic hair development in boys (include estimation of testicular volume)
- Signs of an underlying disorder
  - Hyperpigmented skin lesions
  - Nystagmus
  - Signs of virilization (eg, increased muscle mass, voice change, facial hair, clitoromegaly)
  - Abdominal or pelvic mass
  - Testicular asymmetry or palpable mass

Diagnostic studies
- Bone age
- Serum estradiol (girls)
- Serum testosterone (boys)
- LH and FSH
- Additional studies as indicated (often done in referral setting)
  - FSH and LH following stimulation with a GnRH agonist
  - Brain MRI (in all confirmed cases of central precocious puberty)
  - Pelvic ultrasound to evaluate for uterine or ovarian enlargement or ovarian cysts/tumors
  - Testicular ultrasound to evaluate for testicular pathologic condition
  - TSH and free thyroxine in suspected severe, untreated hypothyroidism (especially in the setting of slow growth velocity)
  - Adrenal cortisol precursors in isolated precocious pubarche or suspected adrenal disorder (eg, CAH)
  - Abdominal ultrasound and/or CT scan to evaluate for adrenal tumor

Data from Refs.[14,16,22]

Children with premature puberty and a declining growth rate require evaluation for hypothyroidism (TSH and free T4).[13,14,17]

Additional diagnostic testing is indicated when peripheral precocity is suspected (ie, suppressed LH and FSH levels in the setting of elevated levels of testosterone or estradiol). Ultrasound of the ovaries or testes should be performed to rule out a gonadal tumor.[22] Girls with pubic hair development in the absence of breast development and boys with prepubertal testicular volume should be evaluated for an adrenal disorder (eg, CAH) by checking serum levels of DHEAS and 17-hydroxyprogesterone.[13,22] In rare cases, an abdominal ultrasound or computed tomography (CT) scan may be necessary to rule out an adrenal tumor.

Complications of Precocious Puberty and Indications for Referral

Children with early pubertal onset may experience long-term medical and psychological complications.[7,8,21] The most prevalent complication of CPP is diminished adult height[18] resulting from rapid bone maturation and premature fusion of the epiphyseal growth plates.[8,19] Children with premature puberty may experience emotional difficulties related to the discordance between physical development and emotional maturity[16,18] and/or an awareness of being different from peers.[8] Girls undergoing menarche at an earlier age appear to be at increased risk for disorders associated with longer periods of estrogen exposure, such as breast cancer and endometrial cancer.[5,7,18]

Referral to a pediatric endocrinologist is indicated for the following:

- All children with confirmed central or peripheral precocious puberty
- Girls with pubertal changes younger than 6 years of age
- Girls with progressive breast development younger than 8 years of age, especially when growth rate is increased[14]
- Boys with pubertal changes (eg, penile or testicular enlargement) younger than 9 years of age[14]
- Children with precocious puberty and neurologic symptoms or a disorder known to be associated with precocious puberty
- Children with rapid progression through pubertal stages

Whenever referral is indicated, periodic follow-up by the PCP every 4 to 6 months to evaluate growth and progression of pubertal changes is an important component of management.[14]

Children with premature thelarche or premature pubarche may be managed by the PCP provided that appropriate diagnostic studies have been performed and close follow-up is assured to evaluate growth rate and progression of pubertal changes.[14]

Take-Away Points

- The PCP plays a critical role in the recognition of abnormal pubertal development, initial evaluation, and identification of the need for pediatric endocrine referral.
- Children with premature thelarche or premature adrenarche require close clinical follow-up to rule out early presentation of a pathologic condition.
- Key elements in the evaluation of precocious puberty include rate of growth, bone age, and the rate of progression of pubertal changes.
- GnRH agonists are the only medication class currently available for the treatment of CPP.
- Further studies of the underlying molecular basis of the initiation of puberty will likely lead to new treatments for children with precocious puberty.[19]

- Following referral, the PCP and endocrinologist should continue to work in concert to monitor the progress of pubertal development and response to treatment while providing education and psychosocial support to the patient and family.

DELAYED PUBERTY

Delayed puberty is defined as the absence of secondary sexual characteristics by an age at which 95% of the children of that sex and culture have experienced initiation of puberty. In the United States, delayed puberty is the absence of breast development in girls by age 13 years, and the absence of testicular development by age 14 years in boys. Ethnicity also contributes to variation in pubertal timing.[30] Children usually complete puberty within 4 years of the start of pubertal development. Puberty can be considered stalled if not complete within this 4-year period.

It is the fine balance of communication between the hypothalamus, pituitary, and gonads that ensures appropriate pubertal development and progression. The most common cause of a delay in initiation is inadequate production of GnRH from the hypothalamus. Causes of this can include underlying chronic illness, disorders involving the HPG axis, malnutrition, and constitutional delay of growth and puberty (CDGP). Delayed puberty affects more than 2% of the adolescent population and can have adverse effects, including compromised bone and psychosocial health, and short stature.[31] A retrospective study of 232 subjects (158 boys, 74 girls) found CDGP to be the most common cause of delayed puberty (53% of subjects, 63% of boys and 30% of girls), and those with spontaneous but delayed development compromising a smaller percentage of the cohort with functional hypogonadotropic hypogonadism affecting 19% of subjects. Permanent hypogonadotropic hypogonadism was reported in 12% of subjects, and permanent hypergonadotropic hypogonadism was reported in 13% of subjects.[32] Causes of hypogonadism are listed in **Box 4**.

Hypergonadotropic Hypogonadism

Because of functional failure at the level of the gonads, the hormonal profile is characterized by elevated LH and FSH levels with low sex steroids (estrogen or testosterone).

Turner syndrome

Turner syndrome affects 1:2000 to 1:2500 live births and is the most common sex chromosome abnormality in girls. It is characterized by complete or partial absence of one X chromosome. A little less than half of all live births have X monosomy (45,X), and roughly half have a mosaic karyotype (eg, 45, X/46, XX, 45,X/47, XXX, or 45,X with other anomalous X chromosomes, such as isochromosome Xq, ring chromosome X, or partial deletions on X). A smaller percentage has Y chromosomal material resulting in a variable phenotype and an increased risk of gonadoblastoma.[33–37] Features include short stature, webbed neck, low posterior hairline, retrognathia, high arched palate, and cardiac anomalies, such as coarctation of the aorta or bicuspid aortic valve. Girls may present during adolescence with absence of pubertal development and short stature with a declining height velocity. Primary ovarian failure is a classic feature. Pubic or axillary hair may still be present because of the production of adrenal androgens. Most patients are born with streak ovaries of mainly fibrous tissue. In most girls, ovarian deterioration is complete before birth, but in some this can occur in or after adolescence. Therefore, although most girls with Turner syndrome do not undergo spontaneous puberty, because of the variable timing of ovarian functional impairment, a small percentage of girls may experience spontaneous puberty with pubertal failure or even achieve menarche and experience early menopause.[38,39] Diagnosis is made by karyotype from peripheral blood cells.

Box 4
Causes of hypogonadism

Hypergonadotropic hypogonadism
Congenital (female)
- Turner syndrome
- Swyer syndrome
- Mixed gonadal dysgenesis
- Galactosemia

Congenital (male)
- Klinefelter syndrome
- Congenital anorchia
- Noonan syndrome[a]

Acquired
- Autoimmune polyglandular syndrome
- Infectious causes (eg, mumps)
- Chemotherapy (eg, alkylating agents)
- Radiation exposure
- Toxins
- Trauma

Hypogonadotropic hypogonadism
Genetic
- Prader-Willi syndrome
- Bardet-Biedl syndrome
- CHARGE syndrome

Functional/acquired
- Functional hypothalamic amenorrhea
- Gonadotropin-releasing hormone deficiency (eg, Kallman syndrome)
- Tumors (eg, prolactinoma, craniopharyngioma)
- Panhypopituitarism

[a] Noonan syndrome can be seen in both sexes. Boys more commonly present with hypergonadotropic hypogonadism, whereas girls usually present with delayed puberty or without evidence of hypogonadism.

Growth hormone therapy and estrogen therapy should be considered and are prescribed and managed typically by a pediatric endocrinologist.

Klinefelter syndrome
Klinefelter syndrome affects 1:500 to 1:1000 live births and is due to X chromosome polysomy with X disomy being the most common, 47,XXY. It is the most common sex chromosome disorder in boys. Most cases are sporadic. Diagnosis before puberty is rare, with a mean age of diagnosis in the mid-30s.[40] Features include small testes, gynecomastia, learning difficulties, hypergonadotropic hypogonadism, and infertility. The timing of puberty in affected boys is comparable to nonaffected peers with normal levels of LH, FSH, and testosterone in early puberty. However, gonadotropin levels eventually increase with a decrease in testosterone to a low or low-normal range.

Peripheral blood karyotype can confirm the diagnosis, although a low degree of mosaicism can be missed. If clinical suspicion is high, gonadal mosaicism may be detected with testicular biopsy. Testosterone therapy should be initiated at the beginning of puberty with the onset of increase in gonadotropin levels. Lifelong treatment with testosterone is required and may benefit muscle mass and strength, sexual activity, bone health, and areas of cognition.[41] Adolescents in the early stages of puberty may have sperm in ejaculate, but sperm analysis and cryopreservation should be considered given future risk of infertility. Testicular sperm extraction and intracytoplasmic sperm injection have been shown to be successful methods in combating infertility in adult men with Klinefelter syndrome and azoospermia.[42]

Noonan syndrome

Noonan syndrome affects 1:100 to 1:2500 live births and is typically an autosomal dominant condition,[43] with one-half of cases caused by gain-of-function mutation in the PTPN11 gene. Disease expression is variable, and other disorders (eg, Turner syndrome) may have similar physical features.[43,44] Characteristics of Noonan syndrome include triangular-shaped face with down-slanting eyes, ptosis, low-set ears, webbed neck, right-sided congenital heart disease, short stature, and coagulopathy.[39,43,44] Cryptorchidism or small testes can be seen in men. Although some boys may experience spontaneous puberty, they may have slow pubertal progression. Laboratory evaluation may show an elevated FSH, normal LH, and low-normal testosterone. Girls may present with delayed or normal puberty.[39]

Anorchia

Congenital anorchia is the absence of testes with normal external male genitalia. The exact cause is unknown, but familial cases do exist. It is important to distinguish anorchia from cryptorchidism. Imaging studies can be helpful in differentiating and in identifying gonadal tissue; however, inability to detect intraabdominal or intrainguinal testes does not exclude the presence of testicular tissue because they can be difficult to visualize. Biochemical markers can therefore be helpful. Anti-Müllerian hormone levels are undetectable in bilateral anorchia. In addition, low testosterone in response to human-chorionic gonadotropin (hCG) stimulation with increased levels of FSH and low inhibin B are characteristic of absent testicular tissue.[45,46] High suspicion of congenital anorchia warrants laparoscopy, and blind stump endings of testicular arteries are diagnostic. Remaining testicular tissue is removed to reduce concerns for malignancy. Testosterone therapy is required for pubertal induction and continued lifelong for maintenance of sexual health.

Hypogonadotropic Hypogonadism

Impaired function at the level of the hypothalamus or pituitary gland results in low LH and FSH levels with resultant low sex steroids. Functional causes include chronic illnesses, malnutrition, excessive exercise, or constitutional delay of growth of puberty. In these cases, puberty can occur spontaneously but at a much slower pace. Genetic causes are listed in **Table 5**.

Normoestrogenic menstrual irregularity can arise from a variety of causes related to ovarian or adrenal dysfunction.

Hypothyroidism

Primary or central hypothyroidism can delay puberty. However, severe juvenile primary hypothyroidism can be associated with isosexual precocious puberty (eg, Van Wyk-Grumbach syndrome, in which there is also a delayed bone age). Menstrual disorders can range from shortened cycles to cessation of menses. In some cases, prolactin levels may also be elevated in the setting of hypothyroidism, further exacerbating menstrual disturbances.

Functional hypothalamic amenorrhea

Functional hypothalamic amenorrhea (FHA) is a state of chronic anovulation owing to stressors (eg, significant weight loss, intense physical activity, or eating disorders) that decrease the GnRH drive, thereby resulting in insufficient gonadotropin production from the pituitary and subsequent low estrogen production. Ovulatory function can

Table 5			
Genetic syndromes associated with hypogonadotropic hypogonadism			
	Mutation/Defect	Frequency	Characteristic Features
Prader-Willi syndrome[a]	Absence of paternally imprinted genes at 15q11.2-q13 (paternal deletion, maternal uniparental disomy, or imprinting defect)	1:10,000–25,000 live births	Infantile hypotonia, small hands and feet, hypothalamic obesity, short stature, insatiable appetite, obesity, and hypothalamic hypogonadism
Bardet-Biedl syndrome	Genetic heterogeneity, autosomal recessive	1:140,000–160,000 live births	Developmental delay, obesity, retinal degeneration, renal anomalies, and polydactyly
CHARGE syndrome	Mutations in CHD7 gene	1:12,000 live births	Coloboma, heart disease, choanal atresia, growth retardation, genital anomalies, and ear abnormalities (+/- deafness)

[a] A small percentage may undergo spontaneous puberty and achieve menarche but will likely develop irregular menses. The need for hormonal therapy should be determined on an individual basis and bone mineral density monitored starting in the early teenage years.
Data from Refs.[39,47,48]

be restored with amelioration of the instigating factors. The diagnosis should be considered when menstrual cycle interval is greater than 45 days and/or when amenorrhea lasts $\geq$3 months.[49] FHA is a diagnosis of exclusion following thorough evaluation for an organic cause. In suspected cases, obtaining a detailed history is critical related to extent of exercise, perfectionist tendencies, weight disturbances, sleep patterns, fracture history, and substance abuse, in addition to personal and family history of eating disorders or menstrual irregularity. Six or more months of amenorrhea and/or malnutrition can increase risk of impaired bone health, and baseline bone mineral density measurement by dual-energy x-ray absorptiometry is recommended. Achieving an appropriate energy balance by improving nutrition and caloric intake and by decreasing exercise is the key to treating FHA. Psychological therapies may also be considered to aid in encouraging behavioral changes. Oral contraceptive pills are not preferred for reestablishing menses or optimizing bone health, because they may mask the onset of spontaneous menses. Following behavioral modifications, should menses not spontaneously resume, a short course of transdermal estradiol therapy with cyclical oral progestin in adolescents can be considered. With concerns for bone health, calcium 1500 mg/d with vitamin D 400 IU/d should be prescribed.[49]

GnRH deficiency
GnRH is released from the arcuate nucleus in the hypothalamus and binds to receptors on gonadotrophs in the anterior pituitary gland, stimulating secretion and synthesis of LH and FSH, which then have target effects on the gonads. GnRH neurons are the only CNS neurons originating peripherally and during embryonic development migrate with olfactory neurons from the olfactory placode to the forebrain.[50] Disruption of this migratory process can result in idiopathic hypogonadotropic hypogonadism (IHH) or Kallman syndrome. GnRH deficiency is characteristic of both diagnoses

with impairment of the olfactory sense seen in the latter. The degree of gonadotropin deficiency can vary in both IHH and Kallman syndrome, ranging from failure to enter puberty to adult onset of hypogonadotropic hypogonadism following normal spontaneous pubertal development and even reversal of hypogonadism. Kallman syndrome presents with anosmia and low gonadotropins. Although stature is normal, pubertal growth spurt is stunted. Boys may have cryptorchidism or micropenis, or normal male external genitalia, and girls will have no breast development. Anosmia can be confirmed with a smell test. Hormonal therapy with estrogen or testosterone should be considered on an individual basis for pubertal induction or for maintenance therapy.[38]

Pituitary tumors

Tumors originating from the pituitary can negatively impact function. Prolactinomas are the most common pituitary tumor to cause menstrual irregularity.[51] Microadenomas are less than 1 cm, and larger tumors are macroadenomas. Symptoms include cessation of menses, menstrual irregularity, and/or galactorrhea. A diagnosis is made by an elevated prolactin level and evidence of an adenoma on pituitary MRI. Hyperprolactinemia secondary to medications such as tricyclic antidepressants, metoclopramide, prostaglandins, cimetidine, phenothiazines, methyldopa, or benzodiazepines can cause levels less than 150 ng/dL. Use of these medications should be excluded as a cause of elevated prolactin levels before initiating pharmacologic therapy.[52] Switching to a different drug within the same class not known to elevate prolactin levels may help in identifying an iatrogenic cause of hyperprolactinemia if prolactin levels normalize within levels 72 hours following the switch.[52] Presentations of a microadenoma or idiopathic hyperprolactinemia with normal estrogen or testosterone levels may require minimal intervention and can be followed with serial measurements of prolactin. Of those who are symptomatic, most will require a dopamine agonist to decrease tumor size and normalize prolactin levels. Cabergoline is preferred over bromocriptine, because it is better tolerated with fewer side effects. Dosing ranges from 0.25 to 0.5 mg with once or twice weekly dosing. With tumor shrinkage and improvement in prolactin levels, cabergoline can be gradually weaned off. Treatment failure with a dopamine agonist warrants surgical attention, with a consideration for a transsphenoidal approach. Radiation therapy is a consideration in cases when medical and surgical therapy fail for treatment of a macroadenoma.[52,53]

Craniopharyngiomas are the most common tumor in childhood to originate in the pituitary and usually present between 5 and 14 years of age with headaches, vision concerns, and poor linear growth. Forty percent of patients can experience gonadotropin deficiency. Treatment involves surgery with radiotherapy as an adjunct. Pituitary compromise following surgery is not uncommon, and should gonadotropin insufficiency be a concern, hormone therapy should be prescribed.[51]

Anabolic steroids

Abuse of anabolic androgenic steroids (AAS) by adolescents should be considered, especially in boys. Supraphysiologic amounts can increase hematocrit and blood viscosity, in addition to elevating liver enzymes. Estradiol levels may increase, which can lead to gynecomastia, impaired pubertal development, and premature epiphyseal fusion, resulting in compromised final adult height. Elevated levels of testosterone can feed back to the pituitary and suppress gonadotropin release, thereby impairing pubertal development and negatively impacting sperm health and count. AAS use can induce a psychological dependence, and cessation may not always completely reverse negative physiologic effects. Treatment involves comprehensive care with mental health providers and endocrinology.[39,54,55]

Illicit drugs
Chronic alcohol abuse in boys can lower LH, FSH, and subsequently testosterone levels, causing delayed puberty.[56]

Constitutional delay of growth and puberty
CDGP, a pronounced delay of pubertal onset and development in an otherwise healthy child, is seen in both girls and boys, although it is diagnosed more commonly in boys, likely because of referral bias. It is the most common cause of delayed puberty and is not due to an underlying pathologic condition but instead represents a normal variant in which pubertal onset is at a later age compared with peers, and pubertal tempo may be slower as well. In up to 50% of cases, there is a family history, oftentimes with 1 or more parent having had a similar pattern of growth and development. Birth weight and length are normal, but weight gain and height velocity can decrease as early as 6 months, with growth eventually resuming a normal rate, however, at lower percentiles than expected given familial genetic expectations. Around the anticipated time of puberty, the height can further shift from the expected curve because of pubertal delay. Children will have a delayed bone age and prepubertal gonadotropins. Ultimately, sexual maturation will complete normally, and a normal adult height will be achieved.

It may be difficult to distinguish hypogonadotropic hypogonadism from CDGP. There is no definitive test to effectively distinguish CDGP from hypogonadotropic hypogonadism, and close monitoring of pubertal progression is the recommended method. If by a chronologic age of 18 years, bone age of 13 years in girls and 15 years in boys, there is no pubertal development in the absence of exogenous steroid administration, and prepubertal gonadotropins and sex steroids with an age-appropriate DHEAS, hypogonadotropic hypogonadism is the likely diagnosis.[57]

In those children who are struggling psychosocially, a short course of testosterone can be considered, with referral to a pediatric endocrinologist for management.

Polycystic Ovary Syndrome
Girls within 2 years of menarche can display a menstrual pattern different from most adult patterns, with 50% of those within the second year having a menstrual cycle that is 21 to 45 days in length, with low progesterone levels.[58,59] The average adult cycle is 28 days in length, with a range of 24 to 35 days. Time to regulatory cycles is related to age of menarche. For girls who experience menarche at age less than 12 years, 50% will have ovulatory cycles by 1 year, in contrast to those between 12 to 13 years and 13 and 15 years of age, whereby 50% are ovulatory by 3 years and 4.5 years, respectively. More than 50% of girls who achieve menarche by 15 years of age remain oligomenorrheic by age 18 years.[60,61] Irregular menses are normal within the first year after menarche but thereafter irregular cycle length is defined as follows[62,63]:

- Greater than 1 to less than 3 year after menarche: less than 21 to greater than 45 days
- Greater than 3 years after menarche to perimenopause: less than 21 or greater than 35 days or less than 8 cycles per year
- Greater than 1 year after menarche: greater than 90 days for any cycle
- Primary amenorrhea by age 15 years or greater than 3 years after onset of breast development

Polycystic ovary syndrome (PCOS) is the most common endocrine disorder affecting women of reproductive age. The cause of PCOS is unknown but thought to be due to a complex interaction of various factors including heritable traits and environmental influences. In adults, PCOS classically presents with chronic anovulation, polycystic ovarian morphology, hirsutism, and infertility.[64] Three international consensus statements describing diagnostic criteria for PCOS have been developed, and they present somewhat different, but overlapping, definitions. The National Institutes of Health conference criteria (1990) include irregular menses or loss of menstruation with biochemical or clinical evidence of hyperandrogenism (such as hirsutism or acne).[65] The Rotterdam Consensus Workshop (2003) is broader and includes 2 out of 3 criteria, including anovulation or oligomenorrhea, biochemical or clinical evidence of hyperandrogenism, and polycystic ovarian morphology.[66] The Androgen Excess-PCOS Society (2006) suggested hyperandrogenemia (clinical and/or biochemical) and ovarian dysfunction (irregular menses or absent menarche and/or polycystic ovaries).[67]

The ultrasonographic finding of polycystic ovaries as a diagnostic criterion remains controversial because cystic morphology may not always be present concordantly with other features of PCOS and can also be detected in women who otherwise display no other features of PCOS. Follicle counts should also not be used as a diagnostic criterion. However, an enlarged ovarian volume could be considered as greater than 12 cm^3 (by formula for prolate ellipsoid).[68] Although obesity, hyperinsulinemia, and insulin resistance are associated features of PCOS, they are also not diagnostic criteria for PCOS. Diagnosis in adolescents remains a challenge because the classic adult features could be considered normal physiology in this age group.[68]

Hyperandrogenism is a consistent criterion for diagnosis. (Other causes of adolescent hyperandrogenism are listed in **Box 5**). Clinical hyperandrogenemia includes persistent and severe acne, seborrhea, and moderate to severe hirsutism, which must be distinguished from hypertrichosis (a generalized distribution of vellus hair in a nonsexual pattern). An example of a standardized scale to assess gradation of sexual hair growth is the Ferriman-Gallwey score, which has limitations because of its subjective nature and differences between racial/ethnic groups. A score ≥8 in African American or white reproductive age women in the United States indicates hirsutism.[69] Biochemical hyperandrogenemia can be detected by persistent elevation (>2 SD above the mean for the specific assay) of serum total and/or free testosterone levels using appropriate assays, such as liquid chromatography-tandem mass spectrometry. Androstenedione and DHEAS could be considered should total and/or free testosterone not be elevated. Caution should be exercised in interpreting laboratory tests relative to ongoing hormonal therapy. Assessment of biochemical hyperandrogenism should be conducted when having been off hormonal contraception for ≥3 months.[63]

Adoption of healthy lifestyle changes related to diet and exercise are a mainstay of treatment. Pharmacotherapy is available with a combined hormone pill (ie, oral contraceptive) with estrogen and progesterone being first-line therapy. Use of this medication can regulate menstrual cycles, decrease risk of endometrial hyperplasia or cancer, and may also improve acne and hirsutism. Recommended formulations have an average estrogen component of ~30 μg/d of estradiol and an average progesterone component with antiandrogenic properties.[38] Adjunct therapies include metformin, which has suggested insulin-sensitizing and antiandrogenic properties,[70] and spironolactone, an antiandrogen that works by binding to and blocking the androgen receptor, and can help with hirsutism. Other methods of hair removal include waxing, threading, shaving, topical depilatory creams, and laser hair removal.

Box 5
Causes of adolescent hyperandrogenism

Functional gonadal hyperandrogenism
- Primary (dysregulation) functional ovarian hyperandrogenism
- Secondary polycystic ovary syndrome
  - Poorly controlled classic congenital adrenal hyperplasia
  - Ovarian steroidogenic blocks
  - Syndromes of severe insulin resistance
  - Portohepatic shunting
  - Epilepsy or valproic acid therapy
- Adrenal rests
- Ovotesticular disorder of sexual differentiation
- Chorionic gonadotropin related

Functional adrenal hyperandrogenism
- Primary (dysregulational) functional adrenal hyperandrogenism
- Congenital adrenal hyperplasia
- Prolactin or growth hormone excess
- Dexamethasone-resistant functional adrenal hyperandrogenism
  - Cushing syndrome
  - Cortisol resistance
  - Apparent cortisone reductase deficiency

Peripheral androgen overproduction
- Obesity
- Idiopathic hyperandrogenism

Tumoral hyperandrogenism

Androgenic drugs

From Rosenfield RL, Cooke DW, Radovick S. Puberty and its disorders in the female. In: Sperling MA, editor. Pediatric endocrinology. 3rd edition. Philadelphia: Saunders Elsevier 2008. p. 586; with permission.

Approach to a Patient with Delayed Puberty

Most patients with a temporary or functional delay in puberty who eventually experience spontaneous puberty will progress naturally and achieve their growth potential. Those with an organic cause of delayed puberty, however, will require early intervention to ensure appropriate development of secondary sexual characteristics and optimization of linear growth. A detailed history should be obtained to assess for chronic medical conditions, therapeutic exposures, or family history that all could contribute to impaired pubertal development (**Box 6**).

Box 6
Pertinent history for absent or delayed puberty

- Chronic medical conditions

- Abnormal eating patterns

- Therapeutic exposures (eg, glucocorticoid use, chemotherapy, and/or radiation exposure)

- Competitive athletics

- History of anosmia or hyposmia

- Family history of delayed puberty
  - Constitutional delay of growth and puberty

Height and weight measurements should be verified and assessed longitudinally. Poor weight gain or rapid weight loss can be a sign of malnutrition. Poor height velocity can suggest underlying pathologic condition. Features suggestive of a syndromic diagnosis should be noted and body proportions assessed; for instance, Klinefelter syndrome can present with an increased arm span (arm span >5 cm of the height) and eunuchoid body habitus,[71] and Turner syndrome, as another example, may present with short stature, low posterior hairline, widened carrying angle, and webbed neck. A thorough CNS examination can help evaluate for possible intracranial pathologic condition. A lack of the sense of smell could indicate Kallman syndrome, associated with hypoplastic olfactory nerves and hypogonadotropic hypogonadism. Examination should focus on Tanner staging for pubic hair in both sexes and breast development in girls and testicular development in boys. Absence of breast or testicular development with evidence of adrenarche can signal gonadal dysgenesis or gonadotropin deficiency.

Initial laboratory evaluation should include assessment of gonadotropins (LH and FSH), ideally obtained early in the morning and performed using an ultrasensitive pediatric assay. Caution should be exercised when interpreting levels in children under 12 years of age because the HPG axis can be quiescent. Sex steroids (estradiol or total testosterone) should be obtained only when pubertal changes are appreciated on examination, because they are otherwise low. Daytime levels of sex steroids indicative of pubertal onset are estradiol level of 9 pg/mL and plasma testosterone level of 45 ng/dL, in girls and boys, respectively.[39] Additional laboratory tests include DHEAS as an assessment of adrenarche, comprehensive metabolic panel and urinalysis (to assess hepatic and renal function), complete blood count (to evaluate bone marrow function and assess for possible anemia), erythrocyte sedimentation rate (to identify an inflammatory state), celiac screen, free thyroxine and thyroid stimulating hormone (to assess for potential thyroid dysfunction), and prolactin (to assess for hyperprolactinemia). Bone age, estimated with a standardized x-ray of the left hand and wrist and most commonly interpreted using the method of Greulich and Pyle, is helpful in comparing skeletal age to chronologic age and in helping predict adult height relative to midparental height.[72,73] Findings on examination suggestive of Turner syndrome or Klinefelter syndrome warrant a chromosomal analysis. A brain MRI is to be considered should there be a suspicion of a neurologic cause (**Figs. 2** and **3**).

Management of Delayed Puberty

Routine monitoring is recommended in suspected temporary delay of puberty, such as constitutional delay of puberty; however, a short course of hormonal therapy can be considered in those with psychosocial concerns owing to delayed development. Identification of treatable underlying causes of delayed puberty (eg, chronic illness, malnutrition, or excessive exercise) should be appropriately addressed. Treatment with exogenous sex steroids in those with gonadotropin deficiency should be conducted in a gradual manner so as to mimic normal physiology. Those with permanent gonadotropin deficiency will require lifelong therapy.

Various estrogen therapies for women are available, including transdermal or oral preparations (**Table 6**). Although either formulation can be used in pubertal induction and maintenance therapy (**Box 7**), transdermal estrogens have a higher bioavailability, have better mimic normal physiology, and avoid first-pass through the liver in comparison to oral estrogens.[74] Low doses are initiated and gradually increased over 6-month intervals over a 2-year period. Breast development should

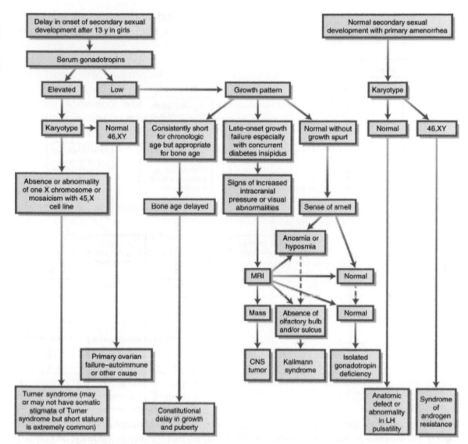

Fig. 2. Flow chart for delayed puberty in girls. (*From* Styne DM. Physiology and disorders of puberty. In: Melmed S, Auchus RJ, Goldfine AB, et al, editors. Williams textbook of endocrinology.14th edition. Philadelphia: Elsevier; 2020. p. 1023–1164; with permission.)

be assessed every 6 months. Once appropriate estrogenization is achieved or breakthrough uterine bleeding is appreciated on estrogen therapy, cyclical progesterone therapy is added for menstruation, with withdrawal bleeding usually occurring in the subsequent 3 to 10 days (see **Table 6**). Unopposed estrogen therapy in these first 1 to 2 years does not increase risk for endometrial malignancy. Suggested protocols for feminization and maintenance of estrogen therapy for girls with Turner syndrome are available.[75–77] Adult dosing options include a weekly estrogen patch with oral progesterone or a combined hormone pill of estrogen and progesterone.

Boys also require a gradual dose increase of testosterone over a 2- to 3-year period with adult dosing of testosterone of 200 to 300 mg every 2 to 4 weeks (**Box 8**). Once virilization is appropriately induced and final adult height is reached using IM injections of testosterone, other formulations, such as gels or patches, can be used for maintenance therapy. Clinical development and testosterone levels should be monitored accordingly. When starting IM testosterone therapy, trough serum testosterone levels with IM injections should be obtained 1 day before the second injection. Baseline liver function tests and hematocrit should be obtained as well as 3 months following

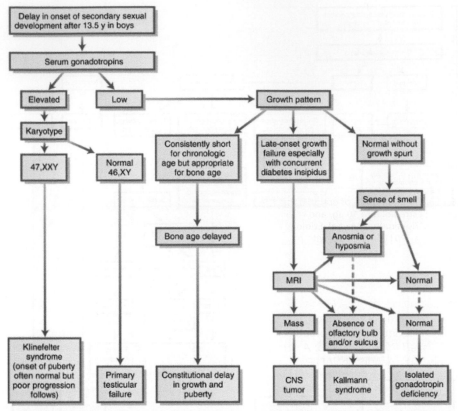

Fig. 3. Flow chart for delayed puberty in boys. (*From* Styne DM. Physiology and disorders of puberty. In: Melmed S, Auchus RJ, Goldfine AB, et al, editors. Williams textbook of endocrinology.14th edition. Philadelphia: Elsevier; 2020. p. 1023–1164; with permission.)

initiation of therapy and every 6 months thereafter, with annual measurement of lipids.[39] Topical in comparison to IM formulations of testosterone better mimic normal physiology. Caution should be exercised when using topical androgen preparations because virilization in female partners has been described.

Take-Away Points

There are multiple causes for delayed puberty with CDGP being most common. Although a basic workup for evaluation is helpful in identifying a possible cause, referral to a pediatric endocrinologist may be indicated for management. Referral should be considered when[38]

- No signs of puberty in girls older than 13 years of age
- No signs of puberty in boys older than 14 years of age
- Greater than 4 years between first signs of puberty and menarche in girls, or between onset and completion of puberty in boys
- Boys with CDGP and psychosocial compromise who may benefit from testosterone therapy
- A diagnosis of an underlying genetic condition that is associated with hypogonadism

Table 6
Estrogen formulations

Type of Estrogen	Trade name	Available Strengths (Doses)
Oral estradiol	Estrace	0.5, 1, 2 mg
	Gynodiol	0.5, 1, 2 mg
Oral esterified estrogen	Menest	0.3, 0.625, 1.25, 2.5 mg
	Ogen	Equivalent to 0.625 mg and above
	Ortho-Est	Equivalent to 0.625 mg and above
Oral conjugated equine estrogen	Premarin	0.3, 0.45, 0.625, 0.9, 1.25 mg
Estradiol patches	Vivelle	0.025, 0.0375, 0.05, 0.075, 0.1 mg/d
	Menostar	0.014 mg/d
Estradiol gel	Divigel	0.5 mg estradiol per 5 g gel

Equivalent adult doses of oral therapy are micronized estradiol 2 mg, esterified estrogen 1.25 mg, ethinyl estradiol 8 to 10 μg, and conjugated estrogens 1.25mg.
From Viswanathan V, et al. Etiology and treatment of hypogonadism in adolescents. Pediatr Clin North Am. 2011;58(5):1192; with permission.

Resources for Families

Precocious Puberty: A Guide for Families–Pediatric Endocrinology Fact Sheet (American Academy of Pediatrics and Pediatric Endocrine Society). https://www.aap.org/en-us/Documents/soen_precocious_puberty.pdf.

Delayed Puberty in Girls: A Guide for Families–Pediatric Endocrinology Fact Sheet (American Academic of Pediatrics and Pediatric Endocrine Society). https://pediatrics.wustl.edu/portals/endodiabetes/PDFs/DelayedPubertyGirls.pdf.

Delayed Puberty in Boys: A Guide for Families–Pediatric Endocrinology Fact Sheet (American Academic of Pediatrics and Pediatric Endocrine Society). https://pediatrics.wustl.edu/portals/endodiabetes/PDFs/DelayedPubertyBoys.pdf.

Box 7
Female pubertal induction and maintenance

Conjugated equine estrogens
- 0.3 mg daily for first 6 months
- 0.625 mg daily for the second 6 months
- Followed by 0.6 to 1.2 mg starting in the second year

Ethinyl estradiol
- 0.02 mg daily for first 6 months
- 0.1 mg daily for the second 6 months
- 0.2 mg thereafter

Transdermal estradiol
- Advance slowly over 2 years to a daily dose of 0.025 to 0.1 mg per day
- At the end of 2 years or when breakthrough bleeding occurs, add cyclical progesterone

Medroxyprogesterone (Provera)
- 10 mg on days 20 to 30 at the cycle

Micronized progesterone (Prometrium)
- 200 mg on days 20 to 30 at the cycle

Data from Kappy MS, Allen DB, Geffner ME. Pediatric practice endocrinology, 2nd edition. New York: McGraw Hill Education. 2014. p. 116–39.

Box 8
Testosterone therapy for pubertal induction and maintenance therapy

Constitutional delay of growth and puberty:
- Testosterone (cypionate or enanthate) 40 to 50 mg/m^2 IM every 4 weeks for 6 months

Pubertal initiation:
- Testosterone (cypionate or enanthate) 50 mg IM every 4 weeks for 6 months, followed by 100 mg IM every 4 weeks; gradual increase in dosing by 50 mg as indicated and increase in frequency until adult dosing achieved

Adult dosing:
- Testosterone (cypionate or enanthate) 200 to 300 mg IM every 2 to 4 weeks (most common dosing 20 0 mg IM every 2 weeks)
- Androderm 5 to 7.5 mg/d, apply nightly to clean, dry area on intact skin of back, abdomen, upper arm, or thigh
- Androgel 5 to 10 g apply once daily (preferably morning) to dry area on intact skin of shoulder, upper arm, or abdomen

Data from Kappy MS, Allen DB, Geffner ME. Pediatric practice endocrinology, 2nd edition. New York: McGraw Hill Education; 2014. p. 116–39; and Sarafoglou, K. Pediatric endocrinology and inborn errors of metabolism. New York: McGraw-Hill Companies; 2009. p. 557-600.

ACKNOWLEDGMENTS

The authors thank Grace Shearer for her assistance in preparing this article.

DISCLOSURE

The authors have nothing to disclose.

REFERENCES

1. Escobar O, Viswanathan P, Witchel SF. Pediatric endocrinology. In: Zitelli BJ, McIntire SC, Nowalk AJ, editors. Atlas of pediatric physical diagnosis. 7th edition. Philadelphia: Elsevier; 2018. p. 341–77.

2. Bygdell M, Kindblom JM, Celind J, et al. Childhood BMI is inversely associated with pubertal timing in normal-weight but not overweight boys. Am J Clin Nutr 2018;108:1259–63.

3. Rosenfeld RL, Lipton RB, Drum ML. Thelarche, pubarche, and menarche attainment in children with normal and elevated body mass index. Pediatrics 2009; 123(84):84–8.

4. Sun Y, Mensah FK, Azzopardi P, et al. Childhood social disadvantage and pubertal timing: a national birth cohort from Australia. Pediatrics 2017;139(6):1–10.

5. Yermachenko A, Dvornyk V. Nongenetic determinants of age at menarche: a systematic review. Biomed Res Int 2014;2014:1–14.

6. Wohlfarhrt-Vege C, Mouritsen A, Hagen CP, et al. Pubertal onset in boys and girls is influenced by pubertal timing of both parents. J Clin Endocrinol Metab 2016; 101(7):2667–74.

7. Witchel SF. Disorder of puberty: take a good history. J Clin Endocrinol Metab 2016;101(7):2643–6.

8. Rosenfield RL, Cooke DW, Radovick S. Puberty and its disorders in the female. In: Sperling MA, editor. Pediatric endocrinology. 4th edition. Philidelphia: Saunders; 2014. p. 569–663.

9. Chulani VL, Gordon LP. Adolescent growth and development. Prim Care 2014; 41(3):465–87.
10. Bordini B, Rosenfield RL. Normal pubertal development: part I: the endocrine basis of puberty. Pediatr Rev 2011;32(6):223–9.
11. Lomniczi A, Wright H, Ojeda SR. Epigenetic regulation of female puberty. Front Neuroendocrinol 2015;36:90–107.
12. Wolfgram PM. Disorders of puberty. In: Kliegman RM, Lye PS, Bordini BJ, et al, editors. Nelson pediatric symptom-based diagnosis. Philadelphia: Elsevier; 2018. p. 774–90.
13. Palmert MR, Dunkel L, Witchel SF. Puberty and its disorders in the male. In: Sperling MA, editor. Pediatric endocrinology. 4th edition. Philadelphia: Saunders; 2014. p. 697–733.
14. Kaplowitz P, Bloch C. Evaluation and referral of children with signs of early puberty. Pediatrics 2016;137(1):1–6.
15. Klein DA, Emerick JE, Sylvester JE, et al. Disorders of puberty: an approach to diagnosis and management. Am Fam Physician 2017;96(9):590–9. Available at: https://www.aafp.org/afp/2017/1101/p590.html.
16. Haddad NG, Eugster EA. Precocious puberty. In: Jameson JL, De Groot LJ, de Kretser DM, et al, editors. Endocrinology adult and pediatric. 7th edition. Philadelphia: Elsevier; 2016. p. 2130–41.
17. Styne DM, Grumbach MM. Physiology and disorders of puberty. In: Shlomo M, Polonsky KS, Larsen PR, et al, editors. Williams textbook of endocrinology. Philadelphia: Elsevier; 2016. p. 1074–218.
18. Soriano-Guillen L, Argente J. Central precocious puberty, functional and tumor-related. Best Pract Res Clin Endocrinol Metab 2019;1–21. https://doi.org/10.1016/j.beem.2019.01.003.
19. Aguirre RS, Eugster EA. Central precocious puberty: from genetics to treatment. Best Pract Res Clin Endocrinol Metab 2018;32:343–54.
20. Valadares LP, Meireles CG, De Toledo IP, et al. MKRN3 mutations in central precocious puberty: a systematic review and meta-analysis. J Endocr Soc 2019;3(5): 979–95.
21. Latronico AC, Brito VN, Carel JC. Causes, diagnosis, and treatment of central precocious puberty. Lancet 2016;4:265–74.
22. Carel JC, Leger J. Precocious puberty. N Engl J Med 2008;358(22):2366–77.
23. Alotaibi MF. Physiology of puberty in boys and girls and pathological disorders affecting its onset. J Adolesc 2019;71:63–71.
24. Eugster EA. Treatment of central precocious puberty. J Endocr Soc 2019;3(5): 965–72.
25. Fuqua JS. Treatment and outcomes of precocious puberty: an update. J Clin Endocrinol Metab 2013;98(6):2198–207.
26. Bramswig J, Dubbers A. Disorders of pubertal development. Dtsch Arztebl Int 2009;106(17):295–304.
27. Liu S, Liu Q, Cheng X, et al. Effects and safety of combination therapy with gonadotropin-releasing hormone analogue and growth hormone in girls with idiopathic central precocious puberty: a meta-analysis. J Endocrinol Invest 2016;39: 1167–78.
28. Wales JKH. Disordered pubertal development. Arch Dis Child Educ Pract Ed 2012;97:9–16.
29. Carel JC, Eugster EA, Rogol A, et al. Consensus statement on the use of gonadotropin-releasing hormone analogs in children. Pediatrics 2009;123(4): e752–62.

30. Crowly WF Jr, Pitteloud N. Approach to the patient with delayed puberty. Post TW, ed. UpToDate. Waltham (MA): UpToDate Inc. Available at: https://www.uptodate.com. Accessed June 20, 2019.
31. Howard SR, Dunkel L. The genetic basis of delayed puberty. Neuroendocrinology 2018;106:283–91.
32. Sedlmeyer IL, Palmert MR. Delayed puberty: analysis of a large case series from an academic center. J Clin Endocrinol Metab 2002;87:1613–20.
33. Wolff DJ, Van Dyke DL, Powell CM, et al. Laboratory guideline for Turner syndrome. Genet Med 2010;12(1):52–5.
34. Furguson-Smith MA. Karyotype-phenotype correlations in gonadal dysgenesis and their bearing on the pathogenesis of malformations. J Med Genet 1965; 2:142.
35. Simpson JL. Gonadal dysgenesis and abnormalities of the human sex chromosomes: current status of phenotypic-karyotypic correlations. Birth Defects Orig Artic Ser 1975;11:23.
36. Jacobs P, Dalton P, James R, et al. Turner syndrome: a cytogenetic and molecular study. Ann Hum Genet 1997;61:471.
37. Backeljauw P. Clinical manifestations and diagnosis of Turner syndrome. Post TW, ed. UpToDate. Waltham (MA): UpToDate Inc. Available at: https://www.uptodate.com. Accessed June 20, 2019.
38. Kappy MS, Allen DB, Geffner ME. Pediatric practice endocrinology. 2nd edition. New York: McGraw Hill Education; 2014. p. 116–39.
39. Sarafoglou K. Pediatric endocrinology and inborn errors of metabolism. New York: McGraw-Hill Companies; 2009. p. 557–600, 592–93, 560–70.
40. Growth KA, Skakkebaek A, Host C, et al. Clinical review: Klinefelter syndrome–a clinical update. J Clin Endocrinol Metab 2013;98(1):20–30.
41. Cherrier MM, Asthana S, Plymate S, et al. Testosterone supplementation improves spatial and verbal memory in healthy older men. Neurology 2001;57:80–8.
42. Schiff JD, Palermo GD, Veeck LL, et al. Success of testicular sperm injection in men with Klinefelter syndrome. J Clin Endocrinol Metab 2005;90:6263–7.
43. Sarkozy A, Conti E, Seripa D, et al. Correlation between PTPN11 gene mutations and congenital heart defects in Noonan and LEOPARD syndromes. J Med Genet 2003;40(9):704–8.
44. Bhambhani V, Muenke M. Noonan syndrome. Am Fam Physician 2014;89(1): 37–43.
45. Thorup J, Petersen BL, Kvist K, et al. Bilateral vanished testes diagnosed with a single blood sample showing very high gonadotropins (follicle-stimulating hormone and luteinizing hormone) and very low inhibin B. Scand J Urol Nephrol 2011;45(6):425–31.
46. Niedzielski JK, Oszukowska E, Slowikowska-Hilczer J. Undescended testis–current trends and guidelines: a review of the literature. Arch Med Sci 2016; 12(3):667–77.
47. Burman P, Ritzen EM, Lindgren AC. Endocrine dysfunction in PWS: a review with special reference to GH. Endocr Rev 2001;22(6):787–99.
48. Khan SA, Muhuammad N, Khan MA, et al. Genetics of human Bardet-Bieldl syndrome, an update. Clin Genet 2016;90(1):3–15.
49. Gordon CM, Ackerman KE, Berga SL. Functional hypothalamic amenorrhea: an Endocrine Society clinical practice guideline. J Clin Endocrinol Metab 2017; 102-(5):1413–39.
50. Rugarli E. Kallman syndrome and the link between olfactory and reproductive development. Am J Hum Genet 1999;65(4):943–8.

51. Lafferty AR, Chrousos GP. Pituitary tumors in children and adolescents. J Clin Endocrinol Metab 1999;84(12):4317–23.
52. Molitch ME, Drummond J, Korbonits M. Prolactinoma management. Endotext. Sept. 20, 2018.
53. Snyder P. Management of hyperprolactinemia. Post TW, ed. UpToDate. Waltham (MA): UpToDate Inc. Available at: https://www.uptodate.com. Accessed June 20, 2019.
54. Tanner SM, Miller DW, Alongi C. Anabolic steroid use by adolescents: prevalence, motives, and knowledge of risks. Clin J Sport Med 1995;5:108–15.
55. Malone DA Jr, Dimeff RJ. The use of fluoxetine in depression associated with anabolic steroid withdrawal, a case series. J Clin Psychiatry 1992;53:130–2.
56. Diamond F Jr, Ringenberg L, MacDonald D, et al. Effects of drug abuse upon pituitary-testicular function in adolescent males. J Adolesc Health Care 1986;7: 28–33.
57. Stanhope R, Preece MA. Management of constitutional delay of growth and puberty. Arch Dis Child 1988;63:1104–10.
58. Sperling MA. Pediatric endocrinology. 3rd edition. Saunders Elsevier; 2008. p. 586–93.
59. Lemarchand-Beraud T, Zufferey MM, Reymond M, et al. Maturation of the hypothalamo-pituitary-ovarian axis in adolescent girls. J Clin Endocrinol Metab 1982;54(2):241–6.
60. Apter D, Vihko R. Serum pregnenolone, progesterone and 17-hydroxyprogesterone, testosterone and 5-alpha dihydrotestosterone during female puberty. J Clin Endocrinol Metab 1977;45(5):1039–48.
61. Apter D, Vihko R. Early menarche, a risk factor for breast cancer, indicates early onset of ovulatory cycles. J Clin Endocrinol Metab 1983;57(1):82–6.
62. van Hooff MH, Voorhorst FJ, Kaptein MB, et al. Predictive value of menstrual cycle pattern, body mass index, hormone levels and polycystic ovaries at age 15 years for oligo-amenorrhea at age 18 years. Hum Reprod 2004;19(2):383–92.
63. Teede HJ, Misso ML, Costello MF, et al. Recommendations from the international evidence-based guideline for the assessment and management of polycystic ovary syndrome. Hum Reprod 2018;33(9):1602–18.
64. Stein IF, Leventhal ML. Amenorrhea associated with bilateral polycystic ovaries. Am J Obstet Gynecol 1935;29:181–91.
65. Zawadzki J, Dunaif A. Diagnostic criteria for polycystic ovary syndrome: towards a rational approach. In: Dunaif A, Givens JR, Haseltine FP, et al, editors. Polycystic ovary syndrome, vol. 4. Boston: Blackwell Scientific Publications; 1992. p. 377–84.
66. Rotterdam ESHRE/ASRM-Sponsored PCOS Consensus Workshop Group. Revised 2003 consensus on diagnostic criteria and longterm health risks related to polycystic ovary syndrome. Fertil Steril 2004;81:19–25.
67. Azziz R, Carmina E, Dewailly D, et al. The Androgen Excess and PCOS Society criteria for the polycystic ovary syndrome: the complete task force report. Fertil Steril 2009;91:456–88.
68. Witchel S, Oberfield A, Rosenfeld R, et al. Polycystic ovary syndrome during adolescence. Horm Res Paediatr 2015;83:376–89.
69. Escobar-Morreale HF, Carmina E, Dewailly D, et al. Epidemiology, diagnosis and management of hirsutism: a consensus statement by the Androgen Excess and Polycystic Ovary Syndrome Society. Hum Reprod Update 2012;18(2):146–70.
70. Geller DH, Pacaud D, Gordon CM, et al. Drug therapeutics committee of the Pediatric Endocrine Society. State of the art review: emerging therapies: the use of

insulin sensitizers in the treatment of adolescents with polycystic ovary syndrome (PCOS). Int J Pediatr Endocrinol 2011;2011:9.

71. Bojesan A, Gravholt CH. Klinefelter syndrome in clinical practice. Nat Clin Pract Urol 2007;4(4):192–204.

72. Bayley N, Pinneau SR. Tables for predicting adult height from skeletal age: revised for use with the Greulich-Pyle hand standards. J Pediatr 1952;40(4): 423–41.

73. Melmed S, Williams RH. Williams textbook of endocrinology. 12th edition. Philadelphia: Elsevier/Saunders; 2011. Chapter 25, Puberty: ontogeny, neuroendocrinology, physiology and disorders.

74. Kenigsberg L, Balachandar S, Prasad K, et al. Exogenous pubertal induction by oral versus transdermal estrogen therapy. J Pediatr Adolesc Gynecol 2013; 26(2):71–9.

75. Davenport ML. Approach to the patient with Turner syndrome. J Clin Endocrinol Metab 2010;95(4):1487–95.

76. Shankar RK, Backeljauw PF. Current practice in management of Turner syndrome. Ther Adv Endocrinol Metab 2018;9(1):33–40.

77. Gravholt CH, Andersen NH, Conway GS, et al. Clinical practice guidelines for the care of girls and women with Turner syndrome: proceedings from the 2016 Cincinnati International Turner Syndrome Meeting. Eur J Endocrinol 2017;177(3): G1–70.

Adolescent Vaccines
Current Recommendations and Techniques to Improve Vaccination Rates

Megan Adelman, PharmD, BCPS, BCGP*,
Ashleigh L. Barrickman, PharmD, BCACP,
Gretchen K. Garofoli, PharmD, BCACP

KEYWORDS

- Adolescent • Vaccination • Meningococcal vaccines • Influenza vaccines
- Papillomavirus vaccines

KEY POINTS

- Every clinical encounter should be used as an opportunity to immunize; providers should be screening for adherence to recommended vaccine schedules.
- Important adolescent vaccines include influenza, meningococcal, and human papillomavirus.
- Providers can improve adherence to recommended schedules through appropriate education and counseling and collaboration with other health care team members.

IMPORTANCE OF VACCINES

Vaccines are a hot topic in society and a key way to prevent life-threatening diseases. Smallpox, a disease that once infected many people, has now been eradicated as a result of vaccination efforts.[1] We usually start our lives with some protection against disease due to passive immunity from our mothers, but vaccinations later build active immunity. Starting shortly after birth, most children receive vaccines to protect them throughout their lifetime. During adolescence, booster doses of some childhood vaccines are recommended, in addition to new vaccines. Vaccinating children and adolescents provides protection not only to them but also to those around them ("herd immunity").[2] The 2019 measles outbreak highlights the importance of childhood vaccination. All health care providers should be aware of the recommendations for vaccinations to ensure that all patients are fully protected.

Department of Clinical Pharmacy, West Virginia University School of Pharmacy, PO Box 9520, Morgantown, WV 26506 USA
* Corresponding author.
E-mail address: melavsky@neomed.edu

Prim Care Clin Office Pract 47 (2020) 217–229
https://doi.org/10.1016/j.pop.2020.02.002
0095-4543/20/Published by Elsevier Inc.

primarycare.theclinics.com

SCHEDULES

In February of each year, the Centers for Disease Control and Prevention (CDC) releases updated immunization schedules. These include the pediatric schedule, which covers the recommended vaccinations from birth through 18 years, and the adult schedule for those 19 years and older. Both the pediatric and adult schedules cover the recommended immunizations by age groups, as well as the recommended immunizations by medical conditions and other indications. There is also a catch-up schedule available as part of the birth–18 schedule, which provides information on the shortest allowable timeframes between vaccinations to get a patient caught up with the recommended vaccinations if not given during the recommended timeframe. These schedules are reviewed and updated annually by the Advisory Committee on Immunization Practices (ACIP). In 2019, the schedules were reformatted for readability, and now include information on using the schedules, a list of vaccinations with trade names, and important contact information. It is recommended that all providers have the most up-to-date immunization schedules available to make appropriate recommendations for their patients (available at www.cdc.gov/vaccines/schedules/).[3]

Meningococcal Disease

Meningococcal infections are rare but can lead to diseases with high mortality rates, such as meningitis and septicemia. Caused by *Neisseria meningitidis*, meningococcal infections are common in patients aged 15 to 24 years. Virulence of the bacteria is variable over time, and is based on the expression of different polysaccharides. There are at least 12 types of bacteria (serogroups) with serogroups A, B, C, W, and Y causing most cases of meningococcal disease.[4] Although the incidence of the disease has decreased since its peak in the 1990s, between 800 and 1200 cases are still reported annually in the United States alone.[5] There are currently 2 available categories of meningococcal vaccines in the United States: meningococcal conjugate vaccines (MenACWY) and serogroup B meningococcal vaccines (MenB).

Serogroup ACWY

The meningococcal conjugate vaccine (MenACWY) was first recommended for adolescents in 2005. The ACIP and the CDC recommend administration of MenACWY as a 2-dose series, with the initial dose given at 11 to 12 years and the booster at 16 years. If an individual has missed the recommended timing, 1 dose can be given between 13 and 15 years, with the second given at 16 to 18 years, with a minimum of 8 weeks between the 2 doses. Adolescents who receive a first dose after their 16th birthday require only 1 dose and do not require a booster unless they are at increased risk for meningococcal disease (ie, those living in close quarters, such as college dormitories or military barracks). According to the CDC, the vaccine is not routinely recommended for those aged 19 to 21 years but may be administered up to age 21 as catch-up vaccination for those who have not received a dose after their 16th birthday.

Booster doses are necessary because antibody levels decline 3 to 5 years after a single dose.[6] Vaccine effectiveness studies suggest that many adolescents are not protected 5 years after vaccination, leaving a gap in protection during a potentially critical age.[7] Based on these findings, a column for 16-year-old patients was added to the CDC pediatric vaccine schedule in 2017 to highlight the importance of a visit at this age to administer the MenACWY booster and any other necessary vaccinations.[8]

Two inactive, conjugated versions of the MenACWY vaccine are currently approved by the Food and Drug Administration (FDA) (**Table 1**): Menactra and Menveo. Vaccine effectiveness is between 85% and 100% in adolescents.[9] Overall, the 2 vaccines are interchangeable, and 1 can be substituted for another at the time of the booster.[10] The vaccines are administered intramuscularly, and the most common adverse events include injection site pain, swelling or redness, malaise, and headache.[10]

The US Department of Health and Human Services' "Healthy People 2020" established a target of ≥80% coverage for adolescents aged 13 to 15 years with ≥1 MenACWY doses.[11] Unfortunately, opportunities for adolescent vaccinations are often missed; one study published in 2013 reviewed findings from health records for adolescents aged 11 to 18 years who visited a pediatric clinic in Seattle, Washington. Missed vaccination opportunities were defined as visits in which a patient was eligible for vaccination but did not receive ≥1 recommended vaccine. During the study period, 1628 adolescents made 9180 visits; opportunities to vaccinate with MenACWY were missed in 57% of preventive care visits, 86% of vaccine-only visits, and 96% of non–preventive care visits. Overall, 82% of visits were missed vaccination opportunities for the first dose of MenACWY.[12] Data from the 2017 National Immunization Survey-Teen (NIS-Teen) showed that 85.1% of adolescents aged 13 to 17 years had been vaccinated with at least 1 dose of MenACWY, which continues to increase from the initial survey collection in 2006.[9,13] Although not reported in the 2017 reports, rates of successful administration of the booster dose were lower at approximately 40%.[9]

Serogroup B

The ACIP updated its meningococcal B (MenB) vaccine recommendations in adolescents in 2015 following accelerated FDA approvals of the vaccines in 2014 and 2015, precipitated by 2 university outbreaks.[14] The ACIP and the CDC recommend administration of the MenB vaccine as a multidose series with the initial dose given to high-risk individuals aged 16 to 23 years (preferably 16–18). The ACIP encourages individual clinical decision-making regarding vaccination against serogroup B meningococcus but has not issued a firm recommendation for routine vaccination given the low prevalence of disease as well as a significant decline in protective antibodies at 12 months following vaccination (category B recommendation).[15] Two vaccines are available (see **Table 1**): Bexsero and Trumenba. Both are 2-dose vaccines, with the booster dose given at 1 or 6 months after the initial dose, respectively, based on the vaccine administered (Bexsero or Trumenba). A third dose of Trumenba is warranted if the second dose is administered less than 6 months following the first; this

---

Table 1
Commercially available meningococcal vaccines[3,10,17]

Trade Name[a]	Type of Vaccine	Approved Ages	Interval Between Doses	Serogroups Included
Menactra	Conjugate	9 mo–55 y	Minimal 8 wk apart	A, C, W, Y
Menveo	Conjugate	9 mo–55 y	Minimal 8 wk apart	A, C, W, Y
Trumenba	Protein	10–25 y	2 doses: 6 mo between 1st and 2nd dose 3 doses: 1–2 mo between 1st and 2nd, 6 mo between 1st and 3rd	B
Bexsero	Protein	10–25 y	Minimum 4 wk apart	B

[a] Menomune was discontinued in 2017 and is no longer commercially available.[67]

third dose should be administered more than 4 months after the second dose. The reason for this is that Trumenba was initially approved as a 3-dose series and then was later updated and approved for only 2 doses if given at recommended intervals.[7]

Effectiveness of the MenB vaccines is 57% to 98% based on serum antibody levels.[15,16] In contrast to MenACWY, the 2 MenB vaccines are not interchangeable, and the same vaccine must be used for completion of the series.[17] If a patient receives 1 dose of Bexsero and 1 dose of Trumenba, the provider should choose 1 brand to complete the recommended schedule. Both vaccines are administered intramuscularly, and the most common adverse events include injection site pain, swelling or redness, fatigue, myalgia, and headache.[17]

There are no current published data on vaccine administration rates for MenB, as it is a category B recommendation. The National Meningitis Association indicates only that "many teens have not received the meningococcal serogroup B vaccine since it was just permissively recommended by CDC in 2015."[18] Studies indicate that antibody levels start to wane 1 year after completion of the MenB series, but the CDC does not currently recommend booster doses after series completion. Recommendations may incorporate this information when deciding on boosters in the future.[17] Both MenACWY and MenB vaccines can be given at the same provider visit or at any time before or after one another.[10]

Influenza

Influenza is an acute respiratory illness that is often characterized by fever, cough, sore throat, congestion, muscle aches, chills, and fatigue, although not all patients will experience all symptoms, including fever.[19,20]

The seasonal influenza vaccine is developed annually and is designed to stimulate production of antibodies to the most common influenza strains predicted during the upcoming flu season. This is determined by using surveillance information from the World Health Organization and different strains may be recommended for the northern hemisphere compared with the southern hemisphere.[21,22] Antibodies take approximately 2 weeks to develop after the administration of the vaccine, so patients should be educated to get influenza vaccines before the start of flu season to ensure adequate protection.[20]

Influenza vaccines can contain 3 or 4 strains of influenza virus. Trivalent influenza vaccines offer protection against 2 A strains and 1 B strain. Quadrivalent influenza vaccines protect against 2 A strains and 2 B strains.[20]

Multiple influenza vaccines are currently available in the United States, as shown in **Table 2**. The CDC recommends that all patients ≥6 months of age receive an annual influenza vaccine and suggests the use of any licensed, age-appropriate vaccine. Multiple studies have demonstrated that most influenza-related deaths in pediatric patients are in unvaccinated children and adolescents.[23,24] Shang and colleagues[25] found that between 2010 to 2015, influenza was reported to have led to the deaths of 675 children: only 31% of patients older than 6 months had been vaccinated, and 50% of the patients had no preexisting medical conditions.

In 2018, the CDC included the live attenuated influenza vaccine (LAIV) as an option for patients for the 2018 to 2019 flu season, but no preference was provided regarding the use of an inactivated influenza vaccine or the live actuated influenza vaccine.[20] In the previous 2 flu seasons, the LAIV was not listed as an appropriate option for patients, as studies indicated a lack of effectiveness against one particular strain of influenza (H1N1) among patients aged 2 to 17 years. Incorporation of a new vaccine component that showed effectiveness against H1N1 stimulated the recommendation to include LAIV as a possible option for the 2018 to 2019 season.[26-28] The American

Table 2
Commercially available influenza vaccines[3,20,22]

Trade Name	Type of Vaccine	Vaccine Category	Site of Administration	Approved Ages	Notes
Fluzone	IIV4	Inactivated	IM	6 mo and older	
Fluvirin	IIV3	Inactivated	IM	4 y and older	
Fluarix	IIV4	Inactivated	IM	6 mo and older	
FluLaval	IIV4	Inactivated	IM	6 mo and older	
Afluria	IIV3 or IIV4	Inactivated	IM	6 mo and older	
Fluzone High-Dose	IIV3	Inactivated	IM	65 y and older	
Flucelvax	ccIIV4	Inactivated	IM	4 y and older	Cell-cultured
Flublok	RIV3 or RIV4	Inactivated	IM	18 y and older	Recombinant
Fluad	IIV3	Inactivated	IM	65 y and older	Adjuvant to enhance immune response
FluMist	LAIV4	Live attenuated	Intranasal	2 y to 49 y	

Abbreviations: ccIIV4, cell-cultured quadrivalent inactivated influenza vaccine; IIV3, trivalent inactivated influenza vaccine; IIV4, quadrivalent inactivated influenza vaccine; IM, intramuscular; LAIV4, quadrivalent live attenuated influenza vaccine; RIV3, recombinant trivalent influenza vaccine; RIV4, recombinant quadrivalent influenza vaccine.

Academy of Pediatrics (AAP) preferred the use of the inactivated influenza vaccine over LAIV for the 2018 to 2019 flu season and recommended the use of LAIV only for patients who would not otherwise get vaccinated.[29]

The inactivated influenza vaccines are administered intramuscularly, and adverse effects include soreness, redness, or swelling at the injection site; headache; fever; nausea; and muscle aches.[20] The LAIV is administered intranasally, and adverse effects include rhinorrhea, wheezing, headache, muscle aches, and fever.[26]

The AAP reported that as of mid-November 2018, only 46% of pediatric patients had been vaccinated with the influenza vaccine that season. This is an improvement from the 2017 to 2018 season (38.8%) but is still suboptimal.[30,31] Vaccination rates were highest among children 6 months to 4 years (57%), whereas teenagers had the lowest vaccination rates (35%).[30]

There are many misconceptions about the influenza vaccine that likely contribute to suboptimal vaccination rates. Common misconceptions include the fear of getting the flu from the vaccine and skepticism about the vaccine's effectiveness. It is important to address these misconceptions and educate patients that the influenza vaccine does not cause the flu, as the vaccine is inactivated, or in the case of the LAIV, the virus is attenuated and not potent enough to cause an active influenza infection in immunocompetent patients. Patients may not feel well after receiving a vaccine, and it is important for clinicians to not dismiss their concerns, but to address them by explaining that flu-like symptoms can be a normal part of building immunity.

Human Papillomavirus

Human papillomavirus (HPV) infection is the most common sexually transmitted disease in the United States. It is estimated that approximately 80 million Americans are currently infected by HPV, with 14 million new cases annually, 50% of which will occur in those 15 to 24 years old.[32–34] Most sexually active adults will acquire the virus at some time in their life, as HPV can be transmitted through vaginal, anal, and oral sex.[32,33] HPV can cause genital warts, as well as cervical, vaginal, and vulvar cancers in female individuals, penile cancers in male individuals, and anal and oropharyngeal cancers in both sexes.[32,33] Approximately 32,000 people are diagnosed with cancers caused by HPV infections each year in the United States, and because cervical cancer is the only HPV-cancer that physicians routinely screen for, prevention of HPV infection with a vaccine is vital.[33]

"Healthy People 2020" set a national goal for HPV vaccination coverage at 80% for adolescents between 13 and 15 years of age.[32] There is only 1 vaccine currently available for prevention of HPV, Gardasil (HPV 9-valent vaccine, recombinant), which protects against 9 strains of HPV. This includes HPV 16 and HPV 18, which account for 70% of HPV-associated cancers.[35,36] The CDC and the ACIP currently recommend that all male and female adolescents receive HPV9 between the ages of 11 and 12, but adolescents can be vaccinated anytime between 9 and 26 years of age. The appropriate age for administration should be *before* sexual activity, so the patient is protected before being exposed to HPV. Studies have indicated that HPV infection typically occurs within a few years of becoming sexually active, with 1 study showing a probability of infection rate of 38.9% 2 years after the first sexual intercourse.[35] If adolescents are not vaccinated before first having intercourse, it is recommended to administer the HPV9 series to protect from any strains of HPV that the adolescent has not previously been exposed to.[33] The HPV9 vaccine series can be given as either a 2-dose series or a 3-dose series, depending on the age at which the vaccination series is initiated. Based on immunogenicity evidence, adolescents between the ages of 9 and 14 years can receive a 2-dose series, with the second dose being given 6 to 12 months after the first dose. The antibody response of the 2-dose series in this age group has been shown to be as good as or better than the antibody response after a 3-dose series in older adolescents.[37]

Adolescents who initiate the HPV9 vaccine series after their 15th birthday should receive a 3-dose series, with the second and third doses being given at 1 and 6 months after the first dose, respectively.[36] Any immunocompromised adolescent should receive the 3-dose series as well, regardless of their age at initiation.[36] According to the current ACIP recommendations, adolescents who completed the HPV vaccine series with a previous version of the HPV vaccine (HPV2 or HPV4) are considered adequately vaccinated and do not need to repeat the series with HPV9.[36]

In October 2018, the FDA expanded the approval for the HPV9 vaccine for ages 27 to 45 years in an attempt to further decrease the prevalence of HPV-related diseases and cancers.[38] However, the CDC and ACIP have not yet developed recommendations on routine vaccinations in that age group for the HPV9 vaccine.

The HPV9 vaccine is administered intramuscularly, and the most common side effects include pain, redness or swelling at the injection site, dizziness, nausea and headache. Fainting can also occur on administration and is more common in adolescents receiving the vaccine.

Studies have shown an improvement in HPV-associated clinical outcomes in the United States since the recommendation of the vaccine in 2006.[33,34] From 2006 to 2014, HPV infections responsible for most HPV-associated cancers and genital warts decreased by 61% and 71% in young women and adolescent girls, respectively.[33] Claims from US health plans indicate the presence of anogenital warts declined from 2.9 per 1000 person-years in 2006 to 1.8 in 2010 in adolescent girls and young women aged 15 to 19 years.[34] Cervical cancer precursor lesions are more challenging to monitor as it is not recommended for female individuals to get cervical cancer screenings until the age of 21, or routine HPV screenings until the age of 30, so data with associated cancers may not be evident for decades.[34,39]

Despite having a vaccine that is both safe and highly effective at reducing HPV infections and HPV-associated cancers, vaccination rates remain suboptimal.[9,36] In 2017, only 65.5% of adolescents had received ≥1 dose of the HPV vaccine, and only 48.6% had completed the HPV series. Interestingly, coverage with ≥1 dose of the HPV vaccine (73.3%) or completion of the HPV vaccine series (53.7%) was higher in adolescents living below the federal poverty level when compared with those living at or above the poverty level (62.8% and 46.7%, respectively).[9]

There are many barriers that have been identified to possibly explain the suboptimal vaccination rates of the HPV vaccine. Some evidence indicates that vaccine rates could be improved by involving adolescents in the decision to be vaccinated.[40] Another study concluded that reducing parents' uncertainties toward the HPV vaccine increased the likelihood of the adolescent receiving the HPV vaccine.[41] The fact that HPV is spread through sexual contact creates an additional challenge to vaccination, as there is associated social, philosophic, and religious stigma among some parents and guardians.[32] Other studies of caregiver attitudes indicate that in addition to concerns about vaccine safety and efficacy, there is an unwillingness to vaccinate adolescents who parents do not presume are sexually active yet.[42] These individuals presume that HPV vaccination may encourage adolescents to engage in sexual activity, so it is imperative to educate caregivers that no evidence has been found to establish correlation between the receipt of the HPV vaccine and an increase in risky sexual behaviors.[32,43]

VACCINE RECOMMENDATIONS FOR SPECIAL POPULATIONS

The CDC recommends specific vaccines before, during, and after pregnancy. The 2 main vaccines that are recommended during every pregnancy include the influenza vaccine and the tetanus, diphtheria, and acellular pertussis (TdaP) vaccine. Pregnant patients should receive only the inactivated influenza vaccine, as live vaccines are contraindicated during pregnancy, and it is safe to get the influenza vaccine at any time during the pregnancy. The TdaP vaccine, which primarily protects the infant from pertussis (whooping cough) in the early months of life, should be administered during each pregnancy, ideally between 28 and 32 weeks' gestation.[44] Most other vaccines should be deferred until after delivery.

OUTBREAK UPDATES

With the growing epidemic of measles (total count for 2019: 839 in 23 states), all adolescents should be screened for adherence to childhood vaccination recommendations.[45] The CDC currently recommends individuals who do not have evidence of immunity should receive at least 1 dose of the MMR vaccine. Acceptable evidence of immunity includes written documentation, laboratory evidence of immunity (titers), or laboratory confirmation of measles infection. The CDC states health care providers should not accept verbal reports of vaccination without written documentation as presumptive evidence of immunity.

IMPLEMENTING PRACTICE CHANGES TO IMPROVE VACCINE ADHERENCE

It is important to educate the public about the safety and importance of vaccinations.[46,47] Parental beliefs also play a vital role in vaccination rates among adolescent patients. One study showed that children of vaccinated adults were 2.77 times more likely to receive a vaccination than children of unvaccinated parents.[48]

Improvement in vaccination rates should be a primary concern when serving the adolescent population and should be a key component during appointments. Studies have shown a clinician's strong recommendation is a powerful and persuasive method to build confidence and acceptance among young patients and parents.[49,50] Every encounter, including sports and camp physicals and routine visits for chronic illnesses, should be considered a potential vaccine visit. Minimize necessary follow-up nursing visits by administering multiple vaccine doses during a single visit, as feasible.[51,52]

Within one's practice, reminders can be used to notify staff and providers when vaccines are due. Information and flags can be added to a clinic's electronic medical record to enable practices to quickly determine a patient's vaccine status. Vaccine screening checklists, available through the Immunization Action Coalition, can help identify adolescents with contraindications and precautions.[53] Offices should have policies and procedures in place to enable minors who present for care without a guardian to receive a vaccination. Policies vary by state but can include obtaining written informed consent from parents in advance, getting verbal informed consent telephonically at the time of visit, using email as consent, or having processes that allow minors to provide their own informed consent.[54]

Recommendations and monitoring for vaccinations should be a team approach. Based on state laws, partnering with local community pharmacies may also improve vaccination rates.[55] For example, pharmacists in West Virginia are able to administer influenza and HPV vaccines to adolescents between 11 and 18 years of age with a prescription and parental consent. Because this age group typically visits their physician only annually, this provides an optimal opportunity for collaboration so patients could receive the first dose of the HPV vaccine at the annual wellness visit, and the remaining dose(s) can be administered at the pharmacy, which could be more convenient for the patients.

ADDRESSING VACCINE HESITANCY

Vaccine hesitancy refers to the delay in a vaccination or vaccination series or refusal of vaccines despite availability.[56] Despite the known benefit of vaccinations in preventing 2 to 3 million deaths per year, vaccine hesitancy has been identified by the World Health Organization as one of the top 10 threats to global health in 2019.[57] Hesitancy can be influenced by multiple factors, including cultural, psychosocial, political, and spiritual beliefs.[58] There are multiple known causes of vaccine hesitancy, although one of the most documented reasons is the antivaccine movement, which started in the 1980s and gained in popularity in 1998 following the retracted article published in The Lancet by Andrew Wakefield and colleagues.[59,60]

Previous studies demonstrate that a recommendation from the provider is the strongest indicator for a patient to receive a vaccine, if initially hesitant.[61,62] Simple statements such as "I strongly recommend your child receive these vaccines today" can positively impact vaccination rates.[61] Taking a proactive approach (eg, "your child is indicated for these vaccines today") versus a more passive one (eg, "which vaccines would you like us to administer") can increase compliance to recommended vaccine schedules. Having multiple discussions that highlight the importance of vaccines also has been shown to increase vaccination rates, and these continual discussions are an important concept for all providers. Other studies have demonstrated minimal benefit with patient alerts, written education, and messages, although these results have not been consistently demonstrated across the literature.[61,63,64] For patients and parents seeking further education and information, providers can refer them to resources provided by the Immunization Action Coalition andCDC.[65,66] Vaccine hesitancy is a relatively new focus for research, and further evaluation is necessary to provide insight on beneficial interventions to reduce hesitancy.

SUMMARY

This article summarizes selected vaccination recommendations in the adolescent population and strategies to aid with increasing compliance rates. Vaccination education for providers and patients is critical to ensure the population remains fully protected. Additional strategies to improve vaccination compliance are warranted. Providers should review recommendations annually to ensure consistency with practice guidelines.

DISCLOSURE

The authors have nothing to disclose.

REFERENCES

1. World Health Organization. Smallpox. WHO - emergencies preparedness, response. 2019. Available at: https://www.who.int/csr/disease/smallpox/en/. Accessed April 2, 2019.
2. US Department of Health and Human Services - National Vaccine Program. Vaccines protect your community 2017. Available at: https://www.vaccines.gov/basics/work/protection. Accessed May 6, 2019.
3. CDC. Immunization Schedules. 2019. Available at: www.cdc.gov/vaccines/schedules/index.html. Accessed May 6, 2019.
4. Schmitz JE, Stratton CW. Neisseria meningitidis. Mol Med Microbiol Second Ed 2015;3(3):1729–50. Available at: https://www.sciencedirect.com/book/9780123971692/molecular-medical-microbiology.
5. Centers for Disease Control and Prevention. Epidemiology and prevention of vaccine-preventable diseases. Washington, DC: Pink B; 2015. p. 231–46.
6. Cohn AC, MacNeil JR, Clark TA, et al. Prevention and control of meningococcal disease: recommendations of the Advisory Committee on Immunization Practices (ACIP). MMWR Recomm Rep 2013;62(RR-2):1–28. Available at: http://www.ncbi.nlm.nih.gov/pubmed/23515099.
7. Cohn AC, MacNeil JR, Harrison LH, et al. Effectiveness and duration of protection of one dose of a meningococcal conjugate vaccine. Pediatrics 2017;139(2): e20162193.
8. Robinson C, Romero J, Kempe A, et al. Advisory Committee on Immunization Practices Recommended Immunization Schedule for Children and Adolescents Aged 18 Years or Younger — United States, 2017 Advisory Committee on Immunization Practices Recommended Immunization Schedule for Children and Adolescents. MMWR Morb Mortal Wkly Rep 2017;66(5):134–5.
9. Walker TY, Elam-Evans LD, Yankey D, et al. Morbidity and mortality weekly report national, regional, state, and selected local area vaccination coverage among adolescents aged 13-17 years-United States, 2017. MMWR Morb Mortal Wkly Rep 2018;67(33):874–82. Available at: https://www.cdc.gov/mmwr/cme/conted_info.html#weekly.

10. Immunization Action Coalition. Ask the Experts - Meningococcal ACWY. CDC. 2019. Available at: http://www.immunize.org/askexperts/experts_meningococcal_acwy.asp. Accessed February 20, 2019.

11. Office of Disease Prevention and Healthy Promotion. Healthy people 2020 - immunization and infectious diseases. Healthy people 2020 2019. Available at: www.healthypeople.gov/2020/topics-objectives/topic/immunization-and-infectious-diseases/objectives. Accessed February 20, 2019.

12. Wong C, Taylor J, Wright J, et al. Missed opportunities for adolescent vaccination, 2006-2011. J Adolesc Health 2013;53(4):492–7.

13. Centers for Disease Control and Prevention (CDC). National immunization survey - teen (NIS-Teen). National Immunization Surveys (NIS). 2019. Available at: https://www.cdc.gov/vaccines/imz-managers/nis/datasets-teen.html. Accessed March 28, 2019.

14. Centers for Disease Control and Prevention (CDC). Department of Health and Human Services Centers for Disease Control and Prevention Advisory Committee on Immunization Practices Record of the Proceedings. 2015. Available at: https://www.cdc.gov/vaccines/acip/meetings/downloads/min-archive/min-2006-10-508.pdf. Accessed March 28, 2019.

15. Patton M, Stephens D, Moore K, et al. Updated recommendations for use of MENB-FHBP serogroup B meningococcal vaccine - Advisory Committee on Immunization Practices, 2016. MMWR Morb Mortal Wkly Rep 2017;66(19):509–13.

16. Lacy I. A broadly effective meningitis B vaccine has been proved effective in a Danish study. Clin Neurol News 2017. Available at: https://www.mdedge.com/clinicalneurologynews/article/154387/vaccines/broadly-effective-meningitis-b-vaccine-has-been-proved. Accessed March 28, 2019.

17. Immunization Action Coalition. Ask the Experts - Meningococcal B. CDC2. 2019. Available at: http://www.immunize.org/askexperts/experts_meningococcal_b.asp. Accessed February 20, 2019.

18. National Meningitis Association. Statistics and disease facts 2019. Available at: www.healthypeople.gov/2020/topics-objectives/topic/immunization-and-infectious-diseases/objectives. Accessed February 20, 2019.

19. Taubenberger JK, Morens DM. The pathology of influenza virus infections. Annu Rev Pathol 2007. https://doi.org/10.1146/annurev.pathol.3.121806.154316.071015171337001.

20. Centers for Disease Control. Key facts about flu vaccine 2004. Available at: https://www.cdc.gov/flu/protect/keyfacts.htm. Accessed March 18, 2019.

21. Centers for Disease Control. Influenza - how influenza vaccines are made 2018. Available at: https://www.cdc.gov/flu/protect/vaccine/how-fluvaccine-made.htm. Accessed April 2, 2019.

22. World Health Organization. Influenza - vaccine viruses. Influenza - vaccine viruses. 2018. Available at: https://www.who.int/influenza/vaccines/virus/recommendations/2019_south/en/. Accessed April 2, 2019.

23. Flannery B, Reynolds SB, Blanton L, et al. Influenza vaccine effectiveness against pediatric deaths: 2010–2014. Pediatrics 2017;139(5):e20164244.

24. Brammer L, Shang M, Olsen S, et al. Influenza-associated pediatric deaths in the United States, 2010–2015. Online J Public Health Inform 2017;9(1):2010–6.

25. Shang M, Blanton L, Olsen S, Fry A, Brammer L. Influenza-Associated Pediatric Deaths in the United States, 2010–2016, Abstract. Presented at: The Epidemic Intelligence Service Conference, April 2017; Atlanta, GA. Available at: https://www.cdc.gov/eis/downloads/eis-conf.

26. Centers for Disease Control. Live attenuated influenza vaccine (LAIV) [the nasal spray flu vaccine]. National Center for Immunization and Respiratory Diseases (NCIRD). 2018. Available at: https://www.cdc.gov/flu/about/qa/nasalspray.htm. Accessed April 2, 2019.

27. Walter EB, Sokolow LZ, Grohskopf LA, et al. Update: ACIP recommendations for the use of quadrivalent live attenuated influenza vaccine (LAIV4) — United States, 2018–19 influenza season. MMWR Morb Mortal Wkly Rep 2018;67(22): 643–5.

28. McLean H, Caspart H, Griffin M, et al. Association of prior vaccination with influenza vaccine effectiveness in children receiving live attenuated or inactivated vaccine. JAMA Netw Open 2018;1(6):e183742.

29. AAP Committee on Infectious Diseases. Recommendations for prevention and control of influenza in children, 2013-2014. Pediatrics 2014;132(4):2018–9.

30. Jenco M. CDC: flu vaccination rates improved, still too low. Am Acad Pediatr News J 2018. Available at: https://www.aappublications.org/news/2018/12/14/fluvaccine121418.

31. National early-season flu vaccination coverage, US, November 2017. Centers for Disease Control - FluVax View. 2017. Available at: https://www.cdc.gov/flu/fluvaxview/nifs-estimates-nov2017.htm. Accessed April 2, 2019.

32. Fava JP, Colleran J, Bignasci F, et al. Adolescent human papillomavirus vaccination in the United States: opportunities for integrating pharmacies into the immunization neighborhood. Hum Vaccin Immunother 2017;13(8):1844–55.

33. Center for Disease Control and Prevention. HPV vaccine information for clinicians. Atlanta, GA: Cent Dis Control Prev; 2015. p. 1–4. Available at: http://www.cdc.gov/std/HPV/STDFact-HPV-vaccine-hcp.htm.

34. Markowitz LE, Gee J, Chesson H, et al. Ten years of human papillomavirus vaccination in the United States. Acad Pediatr 2018;18(2):S3–10.

35. Markowitz LE, Dunne EF, Saraiya M, et al. Human papillomavirus vaccination: recommendations of the Advisory Committee on Immunization Practices (ACIP). MMWR Recomm Rep 2014;63(RR-05):1–30. Available at: http://www.ncbi.nlm.nih.gov/pubmed/25167164.

36. Meites E, Kempe A, Markowitz L. Use of a 2-dose schedule for human papillomavirus vaccination - update from the advisory Committee on Immunization Practices. MMWR Morb Mortal Wkly Rep 2016;65(49):1405–8.

37. Centers for Disease Control. Clinician FAQ: CDC recommendations for HPV vaccine 2-dose schedules. 2016. Available at: https://www.cdc.gov/hpv/downloads/hcvg15-ptt-hpv-2dose.pdf. Accessed April 2, 2019.

38. Food and Drug Administration. FDA approves expanded use of Gardasil 9 to include individuals 27 through 45 years old. 2018. Available at: https://www.fda.gov/newsevents/newsroom/pressannouncements/ucm622715.htm. Accessed April 2, 2019.

39. American Cancer Society. Guidelines for the prevention and early detection of cervical cancer. 2018. Available at: https://www.cancer.org/cancer/cervical-cancer/prevention-and-early-detection/cervical-cancer-screening-guidelines.html. Accessed April 2, 2019.

40. Forster AS, Mahendran KA, Davies C, et al. Development and validation of measures to evaluate adolescents' knowledge about human papillomavirus (HPV), involvement in HPV vaccine decision-making, self-efficacy to receive the vaccine and fear and anxiety. Public Health 2017;147:77–83.

41. VanWormer JJ, Bendixsen CG, Vickers ER, et al. Association between parent attitudes and receipt of human papillomavirus vaccine in adolescents. BMC Public Health 2017;17(1):1–7.

42. Vielot NA, Butler AM, Brookhart MA, et al. Patterns of use of human papillomavirus and other adolescent vaccines in the United States. J Adolesc Health 2017;61(3):281–7.

43. Dreweke J. Promiscuity propaganda: access to information and services does not lead to increases in sexual activity. Guttmacher Inst 2019;22:29–36. Available at: https://www.guttmacher.org/sites/default/files/article_files/gpr2202919.pdf.

44. Swamy GK, Heine RP. Vaccinations for pregnant women. Obstet Gynecol 2015; 125(1):212–26.

45. Centers for Disease Control and Prevention. Measles cases and outbreaks. 2019. Available at: https://www.cdc.gov/measles/cases-outbreaks.html. Accessed April 2, 2019.

46. Rogers CJ, Bahr KO, Benjamin SM. Attitudes and barriers associated with seasonal influenza vaccination uptake among public health students; a cross-sectional study. BMC Public Health 2018;18(1):1–8.

47. Doherty M, Schmidt-Ott R, Santos JI, et al. Vaccination of special populations: protecting the vulnerable. Vaccine 2016;34(52):6681–90.

48. Robison SG, Osborn AW. The concordance of parent and child immunization. Pediatrics 2017;139(5):e20162883.

49. Centers for Disease Control and Prevention. In: Hamborsky J, Kroger A, Wolfe S, editors. Immunization strategies for healthcare practices and providers. 13th edition. Washington, DC: Public Health Foundation; 2015.

50. Centers for Disease Control and Prevention (CDC). Influenza vaccination coverage among pregnant women. MMWR Morb Mortal Wkly Rep 2014;63(37): 816–21.

51. Centers for Disease Control and Prevention (CDC). General best practices recommendations for immunization 2018. Available at: https://www.cdc.gov/vaccines/hcp/acip-recs/general-recs/index.html. Accessed February 19, 2019.

52. National Vaccine Advisory Committee. Standards for child and adolescent immunization practices. Pediatrics 2003;112(4):958–63.

53. Stone MJ, Stone DU. Screening checklist for contraindications to vaccines for children and teens. 2016;4060:16-7.Available at: https://www.immunize.org/catg.d/p4060.pdf

54. English A, Ford C, Kahn J. Adolescent consent for vaccination: a position paper of the Society for Adolescent Health and Medicine. Am J Prev Med 2009;36(3): 278–9.

55. Islam JY, Gruber JF, Lockhart A, et al. Opportunities and challenges of adolescent and adult vaccination administration within pharmacies in the United States. Biomed Inform Insights 2017;9. 117822261769253.

56. World Health Organization. Improving vaccination demand and addressing hesitancy 2019. Available at: https://www.who.int/immunization/programmes_systems/vaccine_hesitancy/en/. Accessed November 1, 2019.

57. World Health Organization. Ten threats to global health in 2019. 2019. Available at: https://www.who.int/emergencies/ten-threats-to-global-health-in-2019. Accessed November 1, 2019.

58. Dubé E, Laberge C, Guay M, et al. Vaccine hesitancy: an overview. Hum Vaccin Immunother 2013;9(8):1763–73.

59. Wakefield A, Murch S, Anthony A, et al. Ileal-lymphoid-nodular hyperplasia, non-specific colitis, and pervasive developmental disorder in children. Lancet 1998; 351:637–41.
60. Rosenberg J. Unpacking the root causes and consequences of vaccine hesitancy. Am J Manag Care 2019. Available at: https://www.ajmc.com/focus-of-the-week/unpacking-the-root-causes-and-consequences-of-vaccine-hesitancy. Accessed November 1, 2019.
61. Shen S, Dubey V. Addressing vaccine hesitancy: clinical guidance for primary care physicians working with parents. Can Fam Physician 2019;65:175–81.
62. Nyhan B, Reifler J, Richey S, et al. Effective messages in vaccine promotion: a randomized trial. Pediatrics 2014;133(4). https://doi.org/10.1542/peds.2013-2365.
63. Loehr J, Savoy M. Strategies for addressing and overcoming vaccine hesitancy. Am Fam Physician 2016;94(2):94–6. Available at: https://www.aafp.org/afp/2016/0715/p94.pdf.
64. Williams SE, Rothman RL, Offit PA, et al. A Randomized trial to increase acceptance of childhood vaccines by vaccine-hesitant parents: a pilot study. Acad Pediatr 2019;13(5):475–80.
65. Need Help Responding to Vaccine-Hesitant Parents? Immunization Action Coalition. Available at: https://www.immunize.org/catg.d/p2070.pdf. Accessed November 1, 2019.
66. Centers for Disease Control and Prevention. Provider resources for vaccine conversations with parents 2015. Available at: https://www.cdc.gov/vaccines/hcp/conversations/index.html. Accessed November 1, 2019.
67. Centers for Disease Control and Prevention. Clinical update - menomune (meningococcal polysaccharide vaccine) discontinuation. Atlanta, GA: CDC - Travelers' Health; 2017. Available at: https://wwwnc.cdc.gov/travel/news-announcements/menomune-discontinuation.

School-Based Health Care

Steve North, MD, MPH[a],*, Danielle G. Dooley, MD, MPhil[b]

KEYWORDS

- School-based health care • Adolescent • Mental health • Telehealth
- School nursing

KEY POINTS

- In response to changing medical and societal needs, school-based health care has evolved over time.
- School-based health care is an important mechanism for reaching underserved populations, particularly adolescents, and demonstrates positive health outcomes for youth.
- Challenges include workforce development, integration of technology, financing and sustainability, and alignment of health and education objectives.

INTRODUCTION

The connection between educational performance and health outcomes is clear and bidirectional. In the United States, graduating from high school increases one's lifespan by at least 7 years compared with students who do not graduate.[1] Students who can see better, hear better, and breathe better all have higher academic achievement.[2] Aside from sleeping, attending school is the most common activity for children in the United States. Addressing their health care needs at school is essential for their long-term success in life.

Accessing confidential and culturally sensitive health care is a major challenge for adolescents.[3] They often use multiple sources of care, such as urgent care clinics, mobile vans, emergency rooms, and primary care offices, resulting in fragmentation.[4] Adolescents living in underresourced communities have high rates of physical and behavioral health needs and have less access to regular well-child checks.[5] School nursing, school-based health centers (SBHCs), school-based mental health (SBMH) services, and telehealth, independently and collaboratively, impact academic outcomes, chronic absenteeism, and health outcomes.

HISTORY

School health emerged in the mid-nineteenth century, with the release of the Shattuck report.[6] Lemuel Shattuck chaired the Sanitary Commission of Massachusetts and recognized schools as a vehicle for health education. An outbreak of smallpox in

[a] Health-e-Schools, Center for Rural Health Innovation, 120 Oak Street, Spruce Pine, NC 28777, USA; [b] Children's National Hospital, Goldberg Center for Community Pediatric Health and Child Health Advocacy Institute, 111 Michigan Ave NW, Washington, DC 20010, USA
* Corresponding author.
E-mail address: steve.north@crhi.org

Prim Care Clin Office Pract 47 (2020) 231–240
https://doi.org/10.1016/j.pop.2020.02.003
0095-4543/20/© 2020 Elsevier Inc. All rights reserved.

New York City in the 1860s led to the inspection of children in schools by the Board of Health, and medical inspection programs spread to Boston, Chicago, and Philadelphia to assess for communicable diseases in schools.

The first school nurse, Lina Rogers, worked in New York City in 1902 and demonstrated that nurse oversight could reduce school absenteeism and communicable disease among students.[2] The school nurse model spread rapidly, and by 1911, 102 cities across the country had school nurses. With the passage of the Education for All Handicapped Children Act in 1975, school nurses became advocates for special needs children in the school setting.[1,2] School nursing continues to evolve, from an initial focus on communicable disease to a broader portfolio including care coordination, health education, and population health.

The first SBHCs began in the 1960s, and there are now more than 2500.[4] With the growth of SBHCs, the breadth of services available has expanded from an initial focus on family planning and support for pregnant and parenting teens to a more holistic model of comprehensive primary care services, including mental and oral health services.[4,7] Funding for SBHCs initially came from the American Academy of Pediatrics (AAP) Community Access to Child Health grants and federal Title X Family Planning Program funds.[2] Other funders such as the Robert Wood Johnson Foundation, and local and state governments began funding the SBHC model, and the federal government joined in 1995.[2,4]

GUIDING PRINCIPLE:
WHOLE SCHOOL, WHOLE COMMUNITY, WHOLE CHILD MODEL

In 2014, the Centers for Disease Control and Prevention (CDC) and the Association for Supervision and Curriculum Development launched a new model to promote integration and coordination of the education and health sectors: the Whole School, Whole Community, Whole Child (WSCC) model.[3] This model advocates that children should be healthy, safe, engaged, supported, and challenged.[5] Previously, the health sector had relied on the Coordinated School Health (CSH) approach,[8] also developed by the CDC, to incorporate health promotion and practices into the school setting (**Table 1**). A constraint of the CSH approach was that it was viewed primarily as a health sector effort. The WSCC Model expands the number of components and strengthens the role of the community in supporting the growth of children.[9] Children frequently receive services focused on improving their overall success from multiple agencies who struggle with coordinating care. The WSCC model can serve as a guide to improving this challenging and convoluted task by focusing on the school and community as a continuum of interrelated programs and influences impacting the child.

TYPES OF SCHOOL HEALTH SERVICES

Health professionals working in schools include school and public health nurses; social workers; psychologists; doctors; dentists and dental hygienists; speech pathologists; physical and occupational therapists; athletic trainers; and others. The provision of health care services in the school setting requires an understanding of the intersection of FERPA (Family Educational Rights and Privacy Act) and HIPAA (Health Insurance Portability and Accountability Act) to ensure confidentiality.[10] Care is provided in schools through multiple delivery models, 4 of which are detailed here.

School Nursing

According to the National Association of School Nursing (NASN), there are more than 95,000 full-time equivalent school nurses spread throughout elementary, middle, and high schools in the United States.[11] NASN defines school nursing as "a specialized

Table 1	
Comparison of the Centers for Disease Control and Prevention Whole School, Whole Community, Whole Child model (2016) to the Centers for Disease Control and Prevention Coordinated School Health model (1987)	
WSCC Model	**CSH Model**
Physical education and physical activity	School physical education
Nutrition environment and services	School food service
Health education	School health education
Physical environment	School health environment
Health services	School health services
Counseling, psychological, and social services	School counseling
Employee wellness	School site health promotion programs for faculty and staff
Community involvement	Integrated school and community health promotion efforts
Social and emotional school climate	
Family engagement	

practice of nursing that advances the well-being, academic success, and lifelong achievement and health of students.[12]" School nurses render individual care and health education to students and serve as advocates and care coordinators, connecting students and families to broader resources and championing policies and programs that promote health in the school setting. Most school nurses in the United States are funded through education budgets; other funding sources include health departments and local, state, and federal organizations and agencies. Both the AAP and the NASN recommend that all students have daily access to a full-time nurse; however, approximately 25% of schools do not have a school nurse, and 27% only have a school nurse part-time.[13] School nurses are a mainstay of school health and play a vital role in bridging the health and education sectors.

School-Based Health Centers

The 2016 to 2017 National School-Based Health Care Census identified 2584 SBHCs across the United States, which represents a doubling since the late 1990s.[4] In addition, the census identified that 13% of public schools and 10% of public school students have access to an SBHC. SBHCs provide a range of services, such as primary care, behavioral health, oral health, health education, nutrition, ophthalmic care, and care coordination.[14] Although most SBHCs offer pregnancy testing and contraceptive counseling, more than 60% are unable to dispense contraception because of limitations imposed by their jurisdiction or sponsoring partner.[13] Related to adolescent health care, 81% of SBHCs are located in schools serving students in sixth grade and above. Research has shown that adolescents feel comfortable accessing health care services in the school-based setting and prefer the convenience of SBHCs.[15] The census identified 4 models of care delivery (**Table 2**),[16] with the most common being traditional SBHCs. Access to SBHC services requires parental consent, although many jurisdictions permit adolescents to self-consent for confidential services, including sexual and reproductive health, substance abuse, and mental health.[17,18] Funding for SBHCs comes from a variety of sources, including hospitals and academic medical centers, patient care revenue, public and private grants, school

Table 2	
School-based health care delivery models	
Delivery Model	**Definition**
Traditional SBHC	A SBHC that is physically located on campus
School-linked SBHC	A SBHC that is located on a fixed site near campus
Mobile SBHCs	A mobile unit located on or near campus
Telehealth exclusive SBHC	A fixed site on campus where students can see a remote provider

Adapted from Love, H., Soleimanpour, S., Panchal, N., Schlitt, J., Behr, C., Even, M. 2016-17 National School-Based Health Care Census Report. School-Based Health Alliance. Washington, D.C.

districts, and the most common source, federally qualified health centers (FQHCs).[13] SBHCs operated by FQHCs have access to a variety of state and federal funding streams that are not open to other SBHCs. The potential for increased funding has led to more than 50% of SBHCs being operated by FQHCs.[1] The range of services varies between SBHCs depending on resources available.[4] The School-Based Health Alliance has defined 7 core competencies for SBHCs (**Table 3**) to "achieve excellence in delivering health care in a school setting."[19]

School-Based Mental Health Services

Schools are an important setting in which children receive mental health care, because 1 in 5 children in the United States has a mental health condition,[20] and children spend a significant amount of time in school.[14,20] SBMH services have a multitiered system of supports[21]:

- Tier 1: Universal school-wide prevention to promote healthy social and emotional understanding and skills
- Tier 2: Targeted interventions for students exhibiting risky behaviors
- Tier 3: Indicated interventions for individual students that exhibit serious mental health issues

Table 3	
School-based health alliance core competencies	
Theme	**Summary**
Access	The SBHC assures students' access to health care and support services to help them thrive
Student-focus	The SBHC team and services are organized explicitly around relevant health issues that affect student well-being and academic success
School integration	The SBHC, although governed and administered separately from the school, integrates into the education and environment to support the school's mission of student success
Accountability	The SBHC routinely evaluates its performance against accepted standards of quality to achieve optimal outcomes for students
School wellness	The SBHC promotes a culture of health across the entire school community
Systems coordination	The SBHC coordinates across relevant systems of care that share in the wellbeing of its patients
Sustainability	The SBHC uses sound management practices to ensure a sustainable business

From School-Based Health Alliance. Core competencies. Available at: https://www.sbh4all.org/resources/core-competencies/; with permission.

Implementation of specific tiers varies by school needs and community resources with staffing driven by these decisions. Community partnerships frequently play a role in staffing and implementing SBMH services. Funding includes federal programs, such as Medicaid or the Individuals with Disabilities Education Act, state and local funding streams, and private foundation grants. Consent procedures differ across the country; generally, for preventive mental health programs that are integrated into the curriculum, active parental consent is not obtained. However, when providing direct treatment to a student, schools may obtain active consent from a parent or guardian.[22]

Telehealth

Telehealth has evolved into an important mechanism for delivery of all forms of health care in schools and addresses challenges, such as staffing shortages and transportation times to the nearest health care provider. By removing barriers to access and expediting the connection to care for a student, telehealth is patient- and family-centered. Telehealth requires a trained presenter or facilitator to be onsite at the school and manage the technology. The medical skills of the presenter directly impact the ability of the distant provider to diagnose specific illnesses; for example, an athletic trainer is highly qualified to examine the ligaments of an injured knee but is not trained to palpate lymph nodes in the evaluation of a sore throat. Telehealth services can range from health education to diagnosis and treatment of medical conditions, and research has shown that students, parents, and school staff report a high degree of satisfaction with telehealth services in schools.[23]

Each of these service delivery frameworks reflects principles of the WSCC model and strives to coordinate and align services in order to optimize health and academic outcomes for children and adolescents.

CASE STUDIES
Service Delivery Framework: Telehealth

Program name: Health-e-Schools (www.healtheschools.com)
Overview: Health-e-Schools (HeS) improves access to health care for students in more than 80 elementary, middle, and high schools in 6 rural counties in North Carolina (as of June 2019) through telemedicine. The technology is based on high-definition videoconferencing using specially equipped stethoscopes and cameras, so that a centrally located health care provider can examine students at multiple schools without traveling. The program was started to enhance access to care in rural areas and was modeled after traditional SBHCs. Family Nurse Practitioners work remotely, are employed by HeS, and see patients in collaboration with the school nurse, who serves as the presenter. Services are provided at no cost to the school, other than in-kind contributions, such as physical space to conduct the visit in a manner that respects patient privacy, school nurse time for training and presenting patients via telehealth, and Information Technology support.

Patient population: Students, faculty, and staff at the schools are eligible to use HeS. Minors must have written permission from their parent/guardian before services are provided. HeS accepts Medicaid and other insurances, and uninsured students and adults are billed on a sliding fee scale. No patient is turned away based on inability to pay.

Partnerships: Critical partnerships include the school district, school staff and leadership, primary care providers, and community health leadership. HeS connects with community health coalitions and leaders, in order to learn more about the health needs in that particular community. In addition, HeS proactively shares information about what they do and how the service works with primary care providers in the community. The data collected by HeS demonstrate that they reach populations that would not otherwise have access to a primary care provider.

Funding and sustainability: HeS blends multiple state, private, and foundation funding sources with clinical revenue to provide services and is viewed as a safety net provider. Claims and patient copays cover approximately 15% of program operations. The leaders of the program serve as paid consultants in the area of school telehealth, which contributes to sustainability.

Impact and outcomes: In the 2018 to 2019 school year, HeS provided more than 1100 visits; 86% of patients returned to class or work after the visit, and 3% were cleared to return to school the next day. The most common conditions treated were upper respiratory infections, acute otitis media, sinusitis, strep throat, and skin rashes. HeS encounters problems with the equipment or facilitator in less than 1% of visits. HeS does not have a data-sharing agreement with schools, but does share with school nurses and administrators school and district level monthly volumes. Culturally, HeS is becoming incorporated into the school environment with principals and other school staff actively referring students and families.

Challenges and opportunities: A significant challenge is the hidden cost of telehealth. The volume of patients does not cover the set up and maintenance costs, including facilitating and marketing the program, administering the program, and providing wraparound services such as case management. Although HeS overcomes many obstacles associated with traditional office-based care, it still requires an office structure to do support tasks, such as billing. HeS offers care for all students in a school while continually refining and adapting the methodology to better serve students and families. The program can also enhance recruitment and retention of school nurses: access to telehealth services connects nurses with resources and colleagues decreasing professional isolation. HeS is committed to disseminating their information, experience, and expertise. There are no paywalls on their website, and they will share their work with other interested parties, creating opportunities for telehealth in the school setting to expand and serve more children and communities.

Service Delivery Framework: School-Based Mental Health

Program name: Mary's Center School-Based Mental Health Program (https://www.maryscenter.org/behavioral-health/children-and-teens/school-based-mental-health-program/)

Overview: Mary's Center is an FQHC in Washington, DC, serving 50,000 patients annually. Mary's Center recognized the large number of unmet mental health needs in Washington, DC schools, particularly among Latino students. School referrals to outside clinics did not work because students and families experienced many barriers, including transportation, work schedules, and language access, to attending clinic appointments. Mary's Center built on the DC Department of Behavioral Health school mental health program that located clinicians in schools. Collaborating with 19 DC public and public charter schools, the Mary's Center SBMH Program strives to increase student, family, and school communities' attainment of positive mental health and well-being. The SBMH Program operates in elementary, middle, and high schools, as well as an adult charter school, and supplements and enhances each school's wellness team by providing diagnostic assessments and behavioral health treatment to students. Licensed bilingual culturally competent therapists provide on-site diagnostic, therapeutic, and community referral services and connections to primary care services. The SBMH Program supports school staff through activities such as stress management and wellness practice workshops for teachers, monthly mental health newsletters for school staff to increase awareness of children's mental health, and consultation to teachers. Importantly, the SBMH Program also links children and families to primary care, dental care, and other social and legal services at Mary's Center and in the community.

Patient population: Any student in a school served by the SBMH Program is eligible to participate, and the Mary's Center clinician obtains consent from the parent and student. The SBMH Program accepts Medicaid and other forms of insurance; students are not billed for services.

Partnerships: Critical partnerships include school staff and leadership, school-based community programs, and SBHCs. The schools provide an in-kind donation of office space and contribute to the program's success through inclusion of SBMH Program staff in school activities. The connection to the FQHC, Mary's Center, enables students and schools to draw on the clinic's resources, including pediatricians, social services, and benefits enrollment coordinators. The SBMH Program also has a strong partnership with the DC government, with financial support from the DC Department of Behavioral Health enabling the SBMH Program to engage in school-wide practices, including teacher coaching and parent meetings.

Funding and sustainability: Data indicate that 96% of children in Washington, DC have health insurance.[24] The high rate of health insurance coverage in DC, and particularly Medicaid coverage, is important for the SBMH Program in terms of reimbursement for services, and the program is almost entirely funded through billables. The SBMH Program receives grants from Community Schools and the DC Department of Behavioral Health, along with private funders.

Impact and outcomes: In the 2018 to 2019 school year, 944 participants received individual, family, and group therapy, and 80 participants received community support services through 17,339 clinical encounters across 19 public and public charter school sites in DC. The average time from referral to intake was 3 weeks, and an average episode of care (intake to discharge) lasted approximately 5 months and included approximately 29 therapy sessions. The most common diagnoses were adjustment disorder, attention-deficit/hyperactivity disorder, posttraumatic stress disorder, depression, and anxiety. Surveys of school partners indicate 95% are satisfied overall with the SBMH Program and think it contributes to a culture of wellness in the school. Patient surveys reveal 95% feel better after participation and are satisfied overall with the program.

Challenges and opportunities: There are several challenges in the operation of the SBMH Program. First, collaboration is not funded, and for the program to be successful, the health and education systems need to come together. Schools and health partners need to team up in a way that is effective and impactful in order for the program to succeed, and this is challenging when academic and health outcomes are not aligned. Second, the SBMH Program constantly strives to balance prevention needs with acute intervention needs in the school setting, and students and families may require intensive case management support. Third, the SBMH Program recognizes that the work can be emotionally draining for staff, who may experience vicarious trauma and absorb a significant amount of stress. Thus, the program maintains a strong focus on supporting its workforce through high-quality supervision and clinician development, as well as team building and team appreciation opportunities. The SBMH Program offers the opportunity to meet students where they are, in school, and reduce barriers to accessing mental health services. In addition, it reduces the stigma of mental health services by integrating into the school setting. The success and strong foundations of the SBMH Program make it an important community resource and advocate, providing trainings beyond the school walls and serving as a leading voice for children's mental health in the District of Columbia and beyond.

Service Delivery Framework: School-Based Health Center

Program name: Bassett School-Based Health Centers (https://www.bassett.org/services/school-based-health-services)
Overview: Located in southern New York State, The Bassett Healthcare Network's School-Based Health Centers serve a predominately rural and underserved population and operate 20 SBHCs in 16 different school systems. The program is recognized as a Patient Centered Medical Home by the National Committee for Quality Assurance. Like most rural SBHCs, this program was developed to address barriers of distance and a lack of providers that result in poorer health outcomes for students compared with their suburban counterparts. Currently, all sites provide primary care, behavioral health care, and dental care. In 2016, the program received a Health Resources Services Administration Telehealth Network Program Grant to address asthma, obesity, behavioral health, diabetes, and oral health through partnerships with subspecialists outside of the health system.

Patient population More than 85% of students in each of the schools served by the SBHCs are enrolled.

Partnerships The mindset of the Bassett program has been to never solicit schools to open new SBHCs but to be highly responsive when they are asked to begin a discussion around the development of a new SBHC. This conversation and the development of a partnership can take many years; in 1 situation, it took 9 years to move from the initial conversation to the opening of an SBHC. In addition to the school districts, it is essential for the success of the SBHCs that other local partners be involved, including the local Health Department and a local collaborating physician to ensure that the SBHC is connected with the community. Historically, the program has engaged churches but is moving away from some of these relationships to ensure that students have access to reproductive health. Each SBHC partners with the district's School Health Advisory Council to coordinate efforts around population health and address issues unique to specific sites.

Funding and sustainability Bassett has developed a structure for launching new SBHCs that includes a clear division of expenses between the SBHC and the school district where the school takes responsibility for the physical plant, whereas the practice is responsible for staffing and all medical supplies. Before opening the SBHC, there must be 3 years of funding in place. Ongoing funding for the SBHCs is provided through a combination of clinical revenue, state support for SBHCs, state and federal grants, and private donors.

Impact and outcomes The Bassett program has done a significant amount of internal quality improvement work focused on health outcomes, return-to-class times, and school engagement. Their results reflect what is seen nationally in SBHCs: students who use the health centers have improved attendance and improved health outcomes. In 2006, they analyzed the impact of the SBHCs on emergency room use and found that, unlike prior studies in urban settings, the presence of a Bassett

SBHC increased emergency department use. There was an overall increase in emergency department use in the region during this time so additional contributing factors were difficult to identify.[25]

Opportunities and challenges Declining population in the region is resulting in new opportunities and challenges for the Bassett SBHCs. They are working to use SBHC staff to promote health literacy and health education in collaboration with schools as the volume of clinical services decreases. In addition, the SBHCs are exploring new models for engaging with physicians in new communities to expand the model, with administrative support provided by Bassett Health but medical care delivered by local providers. The expansion of services via telehealth has been successful in providing behavioral health care and nutrition services, but partnerships with outside specialists are limited because of scheduling challenges and an external telehealth program not taking a high priority in large health systems. The program is piloting how they can provide the state-mandated physician clearance for concussions via telemedicine in the schools.

FUTURE DIRECTIONS

School-based health care has experienced significant growth in the past 2 decades and remains a mainstay for providing access to health care for adolescent populations and improving academic outcomes. As school-based health care continues to evolve, several themes are critical. The first is workforce development, recruitment, and retention. A school-based health care workforce is on the front lines and may experience vicarious trauma and needs to be flexible and adaptable as modalities of care continue to change. The second is technology. With the expansion of telehealth models in particular, school-based health care has the potential to reach more schools, children, and communities. The integration of high-quality telehealth will require a commitment, at multiple levels, to invest in telehealth equipment and focused staff training. Finally, with SBHCs alone reaching more than 6 million children in the United States, the funding and sustainability models for school-based health care must be reexamined and reinforced, to ensure that this important lifeline for communities remains functioning and vibrant for decades to come.

DISCLOSURE

The authors have nothing to disclose.

REFERENCES

1. Allensworth D. Improving the health of youth through a coordinated school health programme. Promot Educ 1997;4(4):42–7.
2. Gustafson EM. History and overview of school-based health centers in the US. Nurs Clin North Am 2005;40(4):595–606.
3. ASCD Learning and Health. Available at: http://www.ascd.org/programs/learning-and-health.aspx. Accessed July 22, 2019.
4. Love HE, Schlitt J, Soleimanpour S, et al. Twenty years of school-based health care growth and expansion. Health Aff (Millwood) 2019;38(5):755–64.
5. Centers for Disease Control and Prevention, The Whole School, Whole Community, Whole Child model. Available at: https://www.cdc.gov/healthyyouth/wscc/pdf/wscc_fact_sheet_508c.pdf. Accessed June 25, 2019.
6. Shattuck L. Plan for the promotion of general and public health devised, prepared and recommended by the commissioners appointed under a resolve of the legislature of Massachusetts, relating to a sanitary survey of the state (part III, section

XXVI). Available at: https://biotech.law.lsu.edu/cphl/history/books/sr/. Accessed May 30, 2019.

7. Dryfoos JG. Full service schools: revolution or fad? J Res Adolesc 1995;5(2): 147–72.

8. A retrospective examination of the relationship between implementation quality of the coordinated school health program model and school-level academic indicators over time. J Sch Health 2009;79(3):144–6.

9. Chiang R, Meagher W, Slade S. How the Whole School, Whole Community, Whole Child model works: creating greater alignment, integration, and collaboration between health and education. J Sch Health 2015;85(11):775–84.

10. Kiel JM, Knoblauch LM. HIPAA and FERPA: competing or collaborating? J Allied Health 2010;39(4):e161–5.

11. National Association of School Nurses. School Nurses in the US. Available at: https://higherlogicdownload.s3.amazonaws.com/NASN/3870c72d-fff9-4ed7-833f-215de278d256/UploadedImages/PDFs/Advocacy/2017_School_Nurses_in_the_Nation_Infographic_.pdf. Accessed June 27, 2019.

12. National Association of School Nurses. The role of the 21st century school nurse. Available at: https://www.nasn.org/advocacy/professional-practice-documents/position-statements/ps-role. Accessed June 27, 2019.

13. Percentage of schools with full-time and part-time school nurses, by school type and selected school characteristics. Available at: https://nces.ed.gov/surveys/sass/tables/sass1112_20161115002_s12n.asp. Accessed July 7, 2019.

14. Barzel R, Holt K, eds. 2019. Promoting Oral Health in Schools: A Resource Guide (4th ed.). Washington, DC: National Maternal and Child Oral Health Resource Center.

15. Soleimanpour S, Geierstanger SP, Kaller S, et al. The role of school health centers in health care access and client outcomes. Am J Public Health 2010;100(9):1597–603.

16. Love H, Soleimanpour S, Panchal N, Schlitt J, Behr C, Even M. 2016-17 National School-Based Health Care Census Report. Washington, D.C.: School-Based Health Alliance; 2018.

17. Keeton V, Soleimanpour S, Brindis CD. School-based health centers in an era of health care reform: building on history. Curr Prob Pediatr Adolsec Health Care 2012;42(6):132–56.

18. An overview of consent to reproductive health services by young people 2019. Available at: https://www.guttmacher.org/state-policy/explore/overview-minors-consent-law. September 12, 2019.

19. School-based health alliance core competencies. 2019. Available at: www.sbh4all.org. Accessed June 27, 2019.

20. Mental health in schools. Available at: https://www.nami.org/Learn-More/Public-Policy/Mental-Health-in-Schools. Accessed June 25, 2019.

21. Freeman E, Stephan S. Providing school-based mental health services. Available at: https://safesupportivelearning.ed.gov/sites/default/files/05%20P2_Providing%20Scl-Based%20MH%20Svs%20FINAL.pdf [safesupportivelearning.ed.gov]. Accessed June 29, 2019.

22. Maag JW, Katsiyannis A. School-based mental health services: funding options and issues. J Disabil Policy Stud 2010;21(3):173–80.

23. Young T, Ireson C. Effectiveness of school-based telehealth care in urban and rural elementary schools. Pediatrics 2003;112(5):1088–94.

24. Children with health insurance: 0-17. Available at: http://www.dchealthmatters.org/indicators/index/view?indicatorId=200&localeId=130951. Accessed June 25, 2019.

25. Schwartz KE, Monie D, Scribani MB, et al. Opening school-based health centers in a rural setting: effects on emergency department use. J Sch Health 2016;86(4):242–9.

Evaluation and Treatment of Primary Headaches in Adolescents

Suzy Mascaro Walter, PhD, APRN[a],*, Christine Banvard-Fox, MD[b],
Courtney Cundiff, MD[c]

KEYWORDS

• Adolescent headache • Headache history • Lifestyle behaviors • Menstrual migraine

KEY POINTS

- Lifestyle behaviors play a significant role in adolescent headache; thus, evaluation of daily meals, sleep habits, caffeine use, and physical activity must be included in the overall assessment.
- Migraine is the most common form of primary adolescent headache that results in disability.
- Pharmacologic management of migraines includes both acute and prophylactic treatment.
- In addition to standard migraine therapy, menstrual migraines can be treated with triptans or nonsteroidal antiinflammatory drugs given before anticipated menstruation, and contraceptives.

INTRODUCTION

Adolescent headache is one of the most common referrals in pediatric neurology.[1] The estimated prevalence of headache in children and adolescents has been reported at 58.4%.[1] Gender differences in the pediatric population have been reported and, compared with boys, girls have a significantly higher rate of chronic migraine (CM), a significantly higher frequency of migraine with aura, and a significantly higher rate of onset after puberty.[2] Medical costs over a 1-year period for adolescents with headache were reported as significantly higher than for healthy adolescents ($4272 vs $1400).[3] In a recent study of 25 tertiary care hospitals in the United States, total pediatric

[a] West Virginia University School of Nursing, 64 Medical Center Drive, Morgantown, WV 26505, USA; [b] Department of Pediatrics, Division of Adolescent Medicine, WVU Medicine, West Virginia University, 6040 University Town Center Drive, Morgantown, WV 26501, USA; [c] Department of Emergency Medicine, WVU Medicine, West Virginia University, 1 Medical Center Drive, Morgantown, WV, 26505, USA
* Corresponding author.
E-mail address: swalters@hsc.wvu.edu

Prim Care Clin Office Pract 47 (2020) 241–256
https://doi.org/10.1016/j.pop.2020.02.004
0095-4543/20/© 2020 Elsevier Inc. All rights reserved.

emergency department visits for headache increased by 57.6% from 2003 to 2013 and admissions for pediatric headache increased by 300%.[4] Headache is a common cause of pain in adolescents[5,6] and, if improperly treated, is likely to persist into adulthood.[7] Given the high prevalence, social issues, and costs to society, it is important to obtain an understanding of the evaluation and treatment of this chronic pain syndrome.

APPROACH TO THE PEDIATRIC HEADACHE

The first step when evaluating an adolescent patient presenting with a headache is to obtain an adequate history to help differentiate primary from secondary headache and facilitate appropriate diagnostic studies (**Box 1**). Primary headaches are typically benign but recurrent problems in themselves, whereas secondary headaches are caused by some other underlying condition. Several illness-related factors are reported to be associated with recurrent headaches: idiopathic intracranial hypertension, classic Ehlers-Danlos syndrome, Chiari malformation type 1, medication overuse headache, intracranial neoplasm, intracranial hypotension, psychiatric disorders, sleep disorders, and obesity. Although most children presenting with headache have a primary headache disorder, rather than a serious neurologic disorder, secondary causes should always be considered in adolescent headache.[8]

Social history should include amount of physical activity, diet, and sleep habits. It has been well documented that lifestyle behaviors are associated with adolescent headache, and modification of these behaviors is reliant on the adolescent. Adolescents try to self-manage their headaches; however, they lack an understanding of how improving lifestyle behaviors results in better headache outcomes.[9] Thus, plans of care should include the adolescent in determining how to better self-manage lifestyle behaviors.[10]

Behaviors related to poor dietary and nutritional choices put adolescents at risk for recurrent headache. These behaviors include skipping meals, snacking between meals, and drinking soft drinks.[11–17] Caffeine has been reported as one of the most common triggers of headache,[18] and adolescents frequently consume caffeine in the form of coffee, tea, carbonated soft drinks, and energy drinks.[19,20] Caffeine withdrawal has been reported as the likely cause for triggering headache.[21] Because of the stimulatory effects of caffeine, adolescent caffeine use has also been attributed to adolescent sleep difficulties, which are, in turn, associated with headache.[22]

Mild dehydration is associated with headache, and a young person's hydration status effects not only health but also school performance.[23–25] In a nationally representative study of US children and hydration status, researchers found that more than half of all children, based on increased urine osmolality levels, were inadequately hydrated.[23] Adequate hydration of 4 to 6 235-mL (8-ounce) glasses of water a day has been recommended for adolescents with headache.[26]

The relationship between physical activity and headache has also been documented in the adult and adolescent populations.[27–29] Practice guidelines for children and adolescents with recurrent headache include physical activity as a part of non-pharmacologic management.[30,31] Exercise should be encouraged in those adolescents with chronic daily headache because they are more likely to miss school and become inactive.[31] These behaviors put the adolescents at increased risk for sleep disturbances, depression, and autonomic dysfunction.[31] Suggested amount of physical activity as a headache intervention varies from as little as 5 to 10 minutes a day to 30 minutes of aerobic activity 3 to 7 days per week.[30,31]

Both oversleeping and deviations in sleep schedule that reduce hours of sleep can cause headaches.[32] Headaches triggered by oversleeping typically occur in

---

Box 1
Headache history

- How many types of headache do you experience?

- When did you first experience a headache? Can you relate it to any event (head injury; infection; surgery; stress; or, for women, menses or pregnancy)?

- How often do you experience a headache?

- How long does your headache last? If you take a drug for your headache, how long will the headache last?

- In what part of your head to you feel the pain? Does the pain move around your head? Is the headache always on 1 side?

- During a headache, do you feel pain in your neck or shoulders?

- How would you rate the severity of your headaches on a scale of 1 (least) to 10 (most) severe?

- How would you describe the pain (throbbing, pulsating, tight headband, deep boring sensation, ache, viselike)?

- Do you have any warning that a headache will soon start? Do you see flashing lights or different colors? Do you have problems with your vision (loss of visual field, images look larger or smaller, blurred vision)? Before the headache, do you feel hungry, fatigued, loss of appetite, burst of energy, quick tempered?

- During a headache, do you have any associated symptoms (nausea, vomiting, dizziness, sensitivity to light or sound, facial flushing, nasal congestion, runny nose, tearing in either eye, eyelid droopy or swollen, ringing in the ears, blurred vision)?

- Can you identify any factor that precipitates your headache? Are you affected by certain foods; alcoholic beverages; skipping meals; skipping caffeine beverages; lack of sleep; changes in weather; certain drugs (nitrates, indomethacin); exercise; stress; or, for women, menses?

- How would you describe your sleep pattern? Do you experience difficulty falling asleep or staying asleep? Does the headache awaken you from a sound sleep? Do you awake and the headache has already started?

- Are you under stress at school? Have you missed work or school days because of the headaches?

- What are your medical and surgical histories? Have you ever been hospitalized for headaches?

- For women: what is your menstrual history? At what age did your periods start? Did you have headaches during your pregnancy? Are you on birth control pills or hormone supplements?

- What medications do you use for your headaches? Are you on any preventive medications for headaches? What medications have you tried previously for your headaches?

- Are you on medications for any other medical condition?

- Are you allergic to any medications? Do you have seasonal allergies? Do you have any food allergies?How many cups of coffee, tea, or caffeine-containing soda do you drink per day? Do you smoke?

- Do you drink alcoholic beverages on a daily basis? How often do you drink?

- Do you use any recreational drugs?

- Have you ever tried alternative therapies for your headaches (biofeedback, acupuncture, massage)?

- Are you using any herbal remedies for your headache?

From Messina E. Evaluation of the headache patient in the computer age. In: Diamond S, Cady RK, Diamond ML, et al, editors. Headache and migraine biology and management. New York: Academic Press; 2019. p. 22; with permission.

adolescents that sleep in later on weekends to make up for missed sleep hours during the week.[33] Studies have shown that sleep disruption occurring on 2 consecutive nights can precipitate migraine and tension-type headache.[34] The Academy of Sleep Medicine (ASM) recommends adolescents get 8 to 10 hours of sleep nightly.[35]

Sleep deprivation related to poor sleep hygiene is reversible through establishment of regular sleep/wake times, avoidance of technology before bedtime, and maintaining a positive sleep environment (eg, reduced noise). Studies have shown that, although adolescents are aware of sleep requirements, they have a poor understanding of the association of insufficient sleep on overall health.[36] Socially induced delayed sleep behaviors include peer pressure to stay awake, distractions from electronic devices, television, and gaming.[37] Thus, it is important to educate adolescents on the importance of adequate sleep as well as habits that may affect good sleep hygiene.

Performing a physical examination to differentiate between primary and secondary causes is also important.[38] Thorough neurologic examination may identify findings related to intracranial disorder. In 1 study, 94% of children with headaches secondary to brain tumors were found to have abnormal findings on ocular or neurologic examination at time of diagnosis, with 85% of these abnormalities occurring within 2 months of onset of headache.[38] The physical examination should include[38,39]:

- Vital signs (eg, hypertension)
- Full neurologic examination, including assessment of cranial nerves and motor, sensory, and cerebellar function
- Evaluation of pain in the facial and preauricular areas as well as the oral cavity (eg, temporomandibular disorder, oral caries)[40,41]
- Skin examination to rule out neurocutaneous stigmata (eg, neurofibromatosis)
- Ophthalmologic examination (eg, papilledema)
- Vascular examination to rule out bruits (eg, vascular malformation)
- Neck examination (eg, cervical spine abnormalities, musculoskeletal pain)
- Neck flexion and Brudzinski and Kernig signs (eg, meningismus)
- Müller maneuver (eg, sinus pressure)
- Assessment for signs of head trauma (eg, Battle sign, raccoon eyes)

The American Academy of Neurology (AAN) published practice parameters for evaluating children with headache recommending against routine laboratory studies, lumbar puncture, electroencephalogram (EEG), or neuroimaging in patients with no red flags on history and a normal neurologic examination.[42] Complete blood count or thyroid function studies may be ordered for suspicion of anemia or hypothyroidism/hyperthyroidism.[43] A lumbar puncture may be ordered if there are clinical concerns for:[43]

- Infection (eg, fever and stiff neck)
- Suspected increased intracranial pressure (eg, papilledema)
- Suspicion of a subarachnoid hemorrhage in the presence of normal computed tomography head (eg, first or worst headache)

An EEG should not be part of the work-up for the routine evaluation of headache, unless there are clinical concerns for seizure.[44]

The need to image adolescents presenting with headache depends on the history and physical examination. According to the AAN practice parameters, variables associated with the presence of space-occupying lesions are as follows[42]:

- Headache of less than 1 month's duration
- Absence of family history of migraine

- Abnormal neurologic findings on examination (eg, focal findings, signs of increased intracranial pressure, significant alteration of consciousness)
- Gait abnormalities
- Occurrence of seizures
- Change in type of headache

When appropriate, MRI is typically preferred because due to imaging detail and lack of radiation.

PRIMARY HEADACHES
Migraine Without Aura

Migraine is the most common form of primary headache that causes disability in childhood.[45] The impact of migraine in adolescents is considerable: 8% to 23% of teenagers experience migraines.[46] The morbidity associated with migraines is substantial and contributes to absenteeism and presenteeism (ie, physically at school but unable to function well) with poor scholastic achievement and reductions in extracurricular activity participation and social functions.[47–50] It is also associated with anxiety, school phobia, depression, poor self-esteem, sleep disorders, obesity, seizure disorders, eating disorders, and other mental and physical health conditions.[48–51]

Pediatric migraines have some recognized nuances that are different from the adult presentation, which include the duration, location, and associated symptoms. In adults, migraine headache is defined as an idiopathic recurring headache disorder manifesting in attacks lasting 4 to 72 hours, whereas adolescents tend to experience shorter headaches with attacks as short as 2 hours.[48] The location is more likely to be bilateral, often described as frontal or bitemporal, or the maxillary sinus area.[45,47,49] Gastrointestinal complaints such as nausea, vomiting, and abdominal pain are more prominent in children, as are vertigo[45] and dizziness.[48] Changes in vitals that accompany pain or dehydration may be accompanied by cutaneous allodynia as the only abnormal physical finding.[45,48] Cranial autonomic signs can be seen in migraines.[46,48] (**Box 2**).

Migraine with Aura

Approximately one-fourth of patients with migraines have migraine with aura.[45] Transient focal neurologic symptoms called auras most commonly (90%) are visual disturbances, such as scintillations, photopsia, or scotomas, and each symptom typically occurs for no longer than an hour.[52] Paresthesia or numbness, forms of sensory auras, are the next most common type.[45] Complex auras can include aphasia, weakness, confusion, or amnesia,[45] and a hallmark of an aura is the complete resolution as, or before, the headache begins. Individuals who experience auras may not consistently have auras with every migraine.

Auras are an important part of the history when caring for female adolescents who desire to be on contraception. Auras preclude the opportunity to use estrogen because of a 2- to 4-fold increased risk for ischemic stroke.[53] Therefore, according to the Centers for Disease Control and Prevention (CDC) Medical Eligibility Criteria and the World Health Organization (WHO), combined contraceptives (ie, estrogen with progestin) in the form of a pill, patch, or vaginal ring are considered an unacceptable health risk in persons with migraine with aura history.[54]

Other migraine syndromes seen in adolescents include 2 striking migraine with aura subtypes: the migraine with brainstem aura (previously called basilar migraine) and hemiplegic migraine.[45,51] The migraine with brainstem aura, seen more frequently in children and adolescents than in adults,[55] involves at least 2 of the following fully

---

Box 2
International classification of headache disorders, diagnostic criteria of migraines

Migraine without aura
A. At least 5 attacks fulfilling criteria B to D
B. Headache attacks lasting 4 to 72 hours (untreated or unsuccessfully treated)
C. Headache has at least 2 of the following characteristics:
   1. Unilateral location
   2. Pulsating quality
   3. Moderate or severe pain intensity
   4. Aggravation by or causing avoidance of routine physical activity (eg, walking or climbing stairs)
D. During headache at least 1 of the following:
   1. Nausea and/or vomiting
   2. Photophobia or phonophobia
E. Not better accounted for by another International Classification of Headache Disorder, Third Edition (ICHD-3) diagnosis

Migraine with aura
A. At least 2 attacks fulfilling criteria B and C
B. One or more of the following fully reversible aura symptoms:
   1. Visual
   2. Sensory
   3. Speech and/or language
   4. Motor
   5. Brainstem
   6. Retinal
C. At least 3 of the following 6 characteristics:
   1. At least 1 aura symptom spreads gradually over more than 5 minutes
   2. Two or more aura symptoms occur in succession
   3. Each aura symptom lasts 5 to 60 minutes
   4. At least 1 aura symptom is unilateral
   5. At least 1 aura symptom is positive
   6. The aura is accompanied, or followed within 60 minutes, by headache
D. Not better accounted for by another ICHD-3 diagnosis

From Headache Classification Committee of the International Headache Society (IHS). The international classification of headache disorders, 3rd edition. Cephalalgia 2018;38(1):19–20; with permission.

---

reversible symptoms: dysarthria, tinnitus, vertigo, ataxia, diplopia, hypacusis, or decreased level of consciousness.[51] The duration of the aura should follow that of a more typical aura.[48] The accompanying headache often is occipital.[52] Neuroimaging results are normal.[55] Hemiplegic migraine fulfills all of the necessary criteria of a migraine with aura, and, additionally, prolonged and fully reversible:

- Acute unilateral motor weakness, and
- Visual, sensory, or speech/language symptoms[45,48,51]

Hemiplegic migraine has autosomal-dominant inheritance with identifiable gene mutations but can also be sporadic. When there are no first-degree or second-degree relatives with the condition, testing should be performed.[51] Triptans are to be avoided in both subtypes.[45,48]

Acute confusional migraine of childhood, which is seen almost exclusively in late childhood to adolescence, is an abrupt alteration in mental status lasting minutes to hours.[55] Often accompanied by aphasia or impaired speech, the confusion state may be followed by headache and/or partial/complete amnesia of the episode.[52] The confusion episodes do not recur, but the development of migraine follows if the patient does not already have migraine.[55] The attack can be triggered by seemingly insignificant head trauma, and the initial episodes warrant a complete evaluation to rule out intoxications and other disorders.[52]

Chronic Migraine and Status Migrainosus

Chronic Migraine (CM),[52] a headache occurring on greater than or equal to 15 days/month for more than 3 months and that has the features of migraine headache on at least 8 days/month, is common in teenagers.[51] These adolescents typically have increasing frequencies of episodic migraines until they reach the frequency required for the diagnosis of CM.[52] Harsh symptoms that initially accompany the headache (eg, aura, emesis) diminish as the headaches become less severe and more frequent.[52] There may be exacerbations of severe head pain.[52]

Nearly 2% of adolescents meet the criteria for CM.[46] Based on a 2-year prospective study of patients 13 to 14 years old, risk factors for CM include obesity and a headache frequency of >7 days/month, lower household economic status, and female gender.[46,48] Careful attention to adequate (but not excessive) dosing of medication is necessary, because medication overuse contributes significantly to CM. Unlike adults, there is insufficient evidence that adolescent chronic migraineurs receiving regimented pericranial intramuscular injections of onabotulinumtoxinA experience a reduction in frequency of CM or headache days in general.[56]

Even with appropriately prescribed acute management, some debilitating migraines continue past 72 hours, and are considered status migrainosus.[51] Intravenous prochlorperazine, ketorolac, valproic acid, repetitive dosing of intravenous dihydroergotamine, and magnesium are some successfully used medications.[46,49,57] Opioids are to be avoided because their use is associated with increased chronicity of migraines and medication overuse headache.[49]

Menstrual Migraine

The precipitous physiologic decrease in estrogen levels a few days before menses lends itself to migraines in certain sensitive, ovulating adolescents.[58] A minority (10%) of women have migraine attacks associated with most of their periods.[51] Messenger RNA expression pattern studies reveal a genetic susceptibility for menstruation-related migraines.[46] To fulfill the criteria of menstruation-related migraines, migraines (with or without aura) occur during the time period of 2 days before menses up to the third day of menses in at least 2 of 3 monthly cycles.[51] Some women experience headaches at other times in the month; those with pure menstrual migraines do not.[51] Attacks during menstruation tend to be longer and more likely to be accompanied by severe nausea than when the migraineur is not on her menses.[51] Hormone fluctuations in those taking combined oral contraceptives (COCs) can also induce, or ameliorate, migraines.[58]

Menstrual migraine treatments include:

- Standard migraine therapy
- Strategic contraception[58]
- Triptans or nonsteroidal antiinflammatory drugs taken before the menstrual cycle[58]

Contraceptive options include:

- Low-estrogen monophasic COC (when no contraindication for estrogen exists), preferably the variety with 10 μg of ethinyl estradiol in the last week of the pill pack,[59] or with non–hormone-containing pills for 2 or 4 days instead of 7 days

- Extended-cycle low-dose estrogen (≤20 µg of ethinyl estradiol) COC continuously for 12 weeks, followed by 7 days of 10 µg of ethinyl estradiol[58,59]
- Contraception containing only progestin[53]

Progestin-only contraception, which inhibits ovulation, modulates the surge and rapid decline of estrogen in the luteal phase of the menstrual cycle. Desogestrel, 75 µg daily, is associated with modest reductions in migraine frequency and duration, and use of analgesics and triptans after 180 days is reduced in most patients.[53] Appropriate options may be found at the following Web site: https://www.straighthealthcare.com/ocp-formulations.html.

Anticipatory premedication (which extends through the usual duration of the previous migraine pattern) can significantly reduce or prevent the previously occurring menstrual migraine.[58] A tremendous benefit is the ultimate conversion of CMs to an episodic pattern correlating with a significant reduction in medication use, by resolving the menstruation-related migraines with hormonal manipulation.[59]

Pharmacologic Treatment of Migraine

Basic migraine pharmacologic treatment goals are:

- To abort headache development and provider pain relief in the acute phase, and
- To provide headache prophylaxis in patients experiencing:
  - Frequent headaches (>3–4 attacks per month), and/or
  - Disabling headaches

With input from the AAN and the American Headache Society (AHS), the 2019 clinical practice guidelines support over-the-counter analgesics or migraine-specific hydroxytryptamine receptor agonists (triptans) as abortive treatments for migraines.[60] The 2019 guidelines on the acute treatment of, and on the pharmacologic prevention of, migraines in children and adolescents are endorsed by the Child Neurology Society and the American Academy of Pediatrics (AAP)[56,60] (**Table 1**). Naproxen alone and ergotamines have not been studied in pediatrics.[60]

Prompt medication administration when the pain remains mild in adequate doses for restoring the patient's ability to function is imperative.[47,52,60,61] The therapeutic dose for migraines often is higher than that to reduce fever, and gastric stasis in migraineurs can obviate a higher dose.[49] Alternatives to oral formulations forego the stasis and have a more rapid onset of action.[49,60,61] Triptans are to be avoided in pregnancy, hypertension, when there is a history of ischemic vascular disease, and concomitantly with monoamine oxidase inhibitors or ergots. Patients with auras should be informed that triptans may be more effective when taken at the onset of headache, rather than during the aura.[45,60] One triptan failure does not eliminate the efficacy of another triptan.[60] Zolmitriptan, and sumatriptan with naproxen, help with photophobia and phonophobia.[60] Separately treating the accompanying symptoms is suggested, including antiemetics,[45,52,60,61] even without clinical studies substantiating antiemetic effectiveness in the nausea and vomiting related to migraines.[60]

When lifestyle modification, nonpharmacologic interventions, and abortive measures are not optimal, patients should be educated to remain adherent to short-term migraine preventive therapy for a trial of at least 2 months.[56] The long-awaited, updated practice guidelines disappointingly enumerate that little evidence supports pharmacology to prevent recurrences of migraines in adolescents. As the committee states it, there is insufficient evidence to confidently recommend the only US Food and Drug Administration (FDA)–approved medication for migraine prevention (in adolescents aged 12–17 years), topiramate, as a known efficacious preventive intervention.[56]

Table 1
Acute migraine treatment of adolescents

FDA Approval	Drug	Route	Age Approval	Usual Dosage	Max Dosage	Cost
—	Ibuprofen[a]	Oral	—	10 mg/kg Every 4–6 h PRN	400–800 mg q 6 h 3000 mg/d	—
—	Acetaminophen[a]	Oral	—	10–15 mg/kg/dose 1000 mg every 4–6 h PRN	4000 mg/d if >45 kg (100 lb)	—
—	Naproxen sodium[a] (Anaprox)	Oral	—	5–7 mg/kg Every 8–12 h PRN	250–500 mg q 8 h 1250 mg/d	—
✓	Almotriptan[b] (Axert)	Oral	>12 y	6.25 mg; 12.5 mg[d]	25 mg/d	$$$
—	Eletriptan[b] (Relpax)	Oral	>18 y	20 mg; 40 mg[c,d]	80 mg/d	$$
✓	Rizatriptan[b] (Maxalt, Maxalt-MLT)	Oral (tablet or ODT)	>5 y	5 mg (20–39 kg)[c] 10 mg (>40 kg)[c]	15 mg/d	$ $
✓ Only nasal approved	Zolmitriptan[b] (Zomig, Zomig-ZMT)	Oral (also melt) Nasal[e]	>12 y	2.5 mg; 5 mg[c,d] 2.5 mg; 5 mg[c,d]	10 mg/d	$–$$ $–$$
—	Sumatriptan[b] (Imitrex)	Oral Nasal[e] Subcutaneous	>12 y	25 mg; 50 mg; 100 mg 5 mg; 20 mg (>12 y 10–20 mg) 0.06 mg/kg; 4 mg; 6 mg >12 y)	200 mg/d 40 mg/d 12 mg/d	$–$$ $$ $$($$)
✓	Sumatriptan and naproxen sodium (Treximet)[c]	Oral	>12 y	10/60 mg; 30/180 mg;85/500 mg	85/500 mg/d	$$

AAN 2019 guidelines doses of level B recommendations[60] excludes acetaminophen, naproxen, eletriptan, and only the 5 mg dose of nasal Zolmitriptan and only the 20 mg dose of nasal Sumatriptan are included.

Abbreviations: FDA, US food and drug administration; ODT, orally disintegrating tablet; PRN, as needed; q, every.

[a] Avoid overuse more than 13 days/month.
[b] Avoid overuse more than 8 days/month.
[c] Be aware propranolol increases Cmax. Use lower dose of triptan.
[d] May repeat 1 dose in 2 hours.
[e] Rapid onset of action within 15 minutes. Elimination half-life is 2 to 3 hours.

However, topiramate remains with propranolol, and amitriptyline in combination with cognitive behavior therapy (CBT), as the uncompelling recommendations[56] (**Tables 2 and 3**). Studying migraine treatment is most challenging in pediatric trials, because a high placebo effect exists, with 30% to 61% of children who received placebo having had a 50% or greater reduction in headache frequency.[60] The most commonly used agents in the United States include the tricyclic antidepressant amitriptyline and anti-epileptics such as divalproex sodium, topiramate, and levetiracetam.[47] When there is a risk for pregnancy, alternatives to topiramate, valproate, and dihydroergotamine should be used. Especially when sleep issues may contribute to migraines and/or

Table 2 Migraine preventive medications			
Medication	**AAN 2019 Guidelines[56]**	**Dosing**	**Common Side Effects**
Cyproheptadine	Not mentioned	0.25–1.5 mg/kg/d	Sedation Weight gain Dry mouth
Topiramate	Moderate confidence: decrease of migraine and frequency of headache days. Low confidence: decrease migraine-related disability. Very low confidence: at least 50% reduction in headache frequency[56]	100 mg/d or 2–3 mg/kg/d[56]	Sedation Appetite suppression Cognitive changes Paresthesias Weight loss Glaucoma Kidney stones Teratogenicity Offspring's developmental disorder At doses >200 mg/d potential to decrease efficacy of COC
Extended-release divalproex	Very low confidence: decrease headache frequency, and to have a 50% reduction in headache frequency[56]	250, 500 or 1000 mg/d[56]	Weight gain Hepatotoxicity Pancreatitis Polycystic ovary syndrome Teratogenicity
Amitriptyline	Insufficient evidence to evaluate by itself. With CBT, high confidence: decrease of headache frequency by at least 50% and moderate confidence to decrease migraine-related disability. Very low confidence: decrease migraine-related disability[56]	1–2 mg/kg/d 1 mg/kg/d combined with CBT[56]	Sedation May exacerbate cardiac conduction defects Weight gain Dry mouth Constipation Suicidal ideations
Propranolol	Low confidence: to have at least 50% reduction in headache frequency[56]	20–40 mg, 3 times a day[56]	Hypotension Sleep disturbance Depression Worsens asthma

Data from Oskoui M, Pringsheim T, Billinghurst L, et al. Practice guideline update summary: pharmacologic treatment for pediatric migraine prevention: Report of the guideline development, dissemination, and implementation subcommittee of the American Academy of Neurology and the American Headache Society. Neurology 2019;93(1):1-10.

Table 3 Preventive medication algorithm for children older than 12 years			
Girls		**Boys**	
Overweight	Underweight or Normal Weight	Overweight	Underweight or Normal Weight
Topiramate	Amitriptyline	Topiramate	Valproate
Propranolol	Propranolol	Valproate	Propranolol

From Gofshteyn JS, Stephenson DJ. Diagnosis and management of childhood headache. Curr Probl Pediatr Adolesc Health Care. 2016;46(2):46; with permission.

depression may be worsening the frequency and severity of migraines, families need to be informed about the black box warning for amitriptyline regarding adolescent risk of suicidal thoughts and behaviors.

Nutraceuticals, complimentary therapies, and devices, were not evaluated by the AAN. In a small study in children and adolescents, long-term riboflavin (200 mg daily) was shown to decrease headache frequency by greater than half in 68% of participants compared with placebo.[47] A neuromodulation device for treatment of acute migraines with aura and for prophylaxis met FDA approval in the winter of 2019 in patients 12 years of age or older.[62] Spring TMS (transcranial magnetic stimulation) by eNeura is available for home-treatment by prescription.

Tension-type Headache

Tension-type headache (TTH) is the most common form of headache, and an inciting emotional event or physical stress often is identified.[47] Tension headache, muscle contraction headache, and stress headache are other names describing this type, which has a lifetime prevalence in the general population between 30% and 78%,[51] although some investigators believe it approaches 100%.[47] TTHs are bilateral, often in the suboccipital area; have a pressing, tightening, or squeezing quality that is nonpulsatile; and are of mild to moderate intensity.[47,51]

Unlike migraines, TTHs do not intensify with exercise, nor do they affect daily activities.[47] Gastrointestinal symptoms and dizziness are symptoms that may present in migraines, but they are not present in episodic TTH.[40,51] Dual presentation of photophobia and phonophobia can be present during a migraine, but, in episodic TTH, only 1 or the other exists.[51] Some people with TTH have tenderness on palpation of the jaw, neck, and/or shoulder muscle groups. TTH often coexists with migraines.[48]

Assistance in addressing as many life adversities affecting the adolescent may be a successful treatment. In a meta-analysis of both long-term follow-up data and controlled studies, the clinical improvement with thermal biofeedback and relaxation training reaches 80% in adolescent headache.[63] Acute treatments are generally less effective than those for migraines with different pathophysiologies.[63] Low-dose amitriptyline has been used for the prophylaxis of TTH in children.[63]

Trigeminal Autonomic Cephalalgia

Trigeminal autonomic cephalalgia (TAC), another type of primary headache disorder, is characterized by unilateral headache with prominent cranial parasympathetic autonomic features that are present on the side of the headache (**Box 3**).[48] The headaches are often severe and deserve neuroimaging to rule out a secondary headache, although most rule it out.[45] The frequency and duration distinguish the types[64]

Box 3
Cranial parasympathetic autonomic signs and symptoms

- Conjunctival injection
- Rhinorrhea
- Eyelid swelling
- Flushing
- Miosis and/or ptosis can be in cluster headache only

- Tearing
- Nasal congestion
- Forehead or facial sweating
- Sense of ear fullness

(Table 4). TACs are mentioned secondary to their unusual treatment of indomethacin, and not to imply that they are prevalent in adolescents.[64]

Cluster headaches (CHs) can begin at any age (but usually in older male patients, with a mean age of onset of 28 years) and have a strong familial predisposition.[64] Eighteen percent of patients with CH had their onset before 18 years of age, and 2% before age of 10 years.[64] Attacks are usually excruciating in a unilateral orbital or supraorbital area[48] and have been likened to a hot poker in the eye.[64] The pain may radiate to the temple, neck, jaw, or upper teeth, providing the perception of sinus or dental disease.[64] The attacks occur in groups or clusters, often with a seasonal preponderance, and then have a remission for weeks or months.[64] The attack's diurnal variability is usually limited to a specific time, which often is awakening from sleep.[54] One or more autonomic features occurring ipsilateral to the headache are timed in conjunction with the headache.[64] Often there is agitation and the patient feels worse when lying down.[48] Proven treatments include 100% oxygen at 8 to 10 L/min through a non-rebreather mask, sumatriptan, and dihydroergotamine.

Paroxysmal hemicranias (PHs) usually occur in adults but have been reported in children.[48] The unilateral pain is likely to be throbbing, boring, pulsatile, or stabbing in moderate to excruciating severity in the ocular, temporal, maxillary, and frontal regions but occasionally radiates to the ipsilateral shoulder and arm.[64] Unlike in CH, in which the patient may be pacing, during PH and hemicrania continua (HC), patients prefer to lie quietly.[64] HC, which is similar to PH but continuous, is more common in women.[65] Usually the onset is during the third decade of life, with a range from the first to the seventh decades.[65] It is particularly sensitive to indomethacin, unlike cluster headaches,[48] with some patients responding to doses as low as 25 to 50 mg daily (although up to 300 mg daily may be required).[65]

Other Primary Headaches

Primary stabbing headache is another less common primary headache mentioned because of its responsiveness to indomethacin.[45] Primary stabbing headache is not a TAC, because no cranial autonomic symptoms are present.[51] Patients experience

Table 4
Trigeminal autonomic cephalalgias

	Cluster Headache	Paroxysmal Hemicrania	Hemicrania Continua
Duration	15–180 min	2–30 min	>3 mo; with exacerbations
Frequency when active	QOD to 8/d	>5/d	Exacerbations occur every 20 min to several days
Indomethacin responsive?	No	Yes	Yes

Abbreviation: QOD, every other day.
Data from Headache Classification Committee of the International Headache Society. The international classification of headache disorders, 3rd edition. Cephalalgia 2018;38(1):1-211.

a stabbing sensation that lasts less than 3 seconds, once to a few times a day, in roving locations that, in 70% of affected individuals, are not in the trigeminal distribution. The irregular, severe, quick stabbing pain around the orbit, temple, and/or parietal regions can be experienced many times an hour or a few times in a week.[45] Neuroimaging is recommended.[51]

Another opportunity for neuroimaging is a new daily persistent headache (NDPH), in which the headache is persistent from the onset.[48] Within 24 hours, the pain becomes continuous and unremitting, and it often occurs in patients who normally do not have headaches.[51] NDPH seems more common in adolescents compared with adults,[48] and minor head trauma or surgery or minor illness can trigger NDPH.[52] The pain lacks characteristic features but may have a migraine or TTH phenotype, or elements of both, and must be present for 3 months before the diagnosis can be made.[51]

SUMMARY

Migraine is a common pain syndrome in adolescents, with postpubertal girls being at higher risk. A comprehensive history and physical examination are needed to differentiate primary from secondary headache in adolescents. A social history that takes into consideration lifestyle behaviors is important in determining modifiable risk factors. An understanding of primary headache disorders in adolescents is necessary to distinguish the various headache types and to determine appropriate management. Medication management includes both acute and prophylactic treatment strategies in conjunction with behavior modification. Appropriate treatment, diagnosis, and management of headache not only optimize headache outcomes during adolescence but may also decrease the likelihood of headache into adulthood.

DISCLOSURE

The authors have nothing to disclose.

REFERENCES

1. Walter S. Lifestyle behaviors and illness-related factors as predictors of recurrent headache in U.S. adolescents. J Neurosci Nurs 2014;46(6):337–50.
2. Eidlitz-Markus T, Zeharia A. Symptoms and clinical parameters of pediatric and adolescent migraine, by gender - a retrospective cohort study. J Headache Pain 2017;18(1):80.
3. Pesa J, Lage MJ. The medical costs of migraine and comorbid anxiety and depression. Headache 2004;44(6):562–70.
4. Perry MC, Yaeger SK, Toto RL, et al. A modern epidemic: increasing pediatric emergency department visits and admissions for headache. Pediatr Neurol 2018;89:19–25.
5. Slover R, Kent S. Pediatric headaches. Adv Pediatr 2015;62(1):283–93.
6. Mazzotta S, Pavlidis E, Cordori C, et al. Children's headache: drawings in the diagnostic work up. Neuropediatrics 2015;46(4):261–8.
7. Fearon P, Hotopf M. Relation between headache in childhood and physical and psychiatric symptoms in adulthood: national birth cohort study. BMJ 2001; 322(7295):1145.
8. Abend NS, Younkin D, Lewis DW. Secondary headaches in children and adolescents. Semin Pediatr Neurol 2010;17(2):123–33.

9. Walter SM. The experience of adolescents living with headache. Holist Nurs Pract 2017;31(5):280–9.

10. Walter SM, Parker RD, Wang K, Dai Z, Starcher M. Feasibility of a self-management intervention in adolescents with headache (SMI-AH). Appl Nurs Res 2019;151223.

11. Dowdell EB, Santucci ME. Health risk behavior assessment: nutrition, weight, and tobacco use in one urban seventh-grade class. Public Health Nurs 2004;21(2): 128–36.

12. Loughridge JL, Barratt J. Does the provision of cooled filtered water in secondary school cafeterias increase water drinking and decrease the purchase of soft drinks? J Hum Nutr Diet 2005;18(4):281–6.

13. Carmona RH. Healthy children: putting prevention first. J Am Diet Assoc 2006; 106(1):17.

14. Sheeler RD, Garza I, Vargas BB, et al. Chronic daily headache: ten steps for primary care providers to regain control. Headache 2016;56(10):1675–84.

15. Wober C, Wober-Bingol C. Triggers of migraine and tension-type headache. Handb Clin Neurol 2010;97:161–72.

16. Milde-Busch A, Blaschek A, Borggrafe I, et al. Associations of diet and lifestyle with headache in high-school students: results from a cross-sectional study. Headache 2010;50(7):1104–14.

17. Gelfand AA. Pediatric and adolescent headache. Continuum (Minneap Minn) 2018;24(4, Headache):1108–36.

18. Taheri S. Effect of exclusion of frequently consumed dietary triggers in a cohort of children with chronic primary headache. Nutr Health 2017;23(1):47–50.

19. Mitchell DC, Knight CA, Hockenberry J, et al. Beverage caffeine intakes in the U.S. Food Chem Toxicol 2014;63:136–42.

20. de Mejia EG, Ramirez-Mares MV. Impact of caffeine and coffee on our health. Trends Endocrinol Metab 2014;25(10):489–92.

21. Martin VT, Vij B. Diet and headache: part 1. Headache 2016;56(9):1543–52.

22. Orbeta RL, Overpeck MD, Ramcharran D, et al. High caffeine intake in adolescents: associations with difficulty sleeping and feeling tired in the morning. J Adolesc Health 2006;38(4):451–3.

23. Kenney EL, Long MW, Cradock AL, et al. Prevalence of inadequate hydration among US children and disparities by gender and race/ethnicity: national health and nutrition examination survey, 2009-2012. Am J Public Health 2015;105(8): e113–8.

24. Rosenberg L, Butler N, Seng EK. Health behaviors in episodic migraine: why behavior change matters. Curr Pain Headache Rep 2018;22(10):65.

25. Merison K, Jacobs H. Diagnosis and treatment of childhood migraine. Curr Treat Options Neurol 2016;18(11):48.

26. Rothner A. Chronic daily headache in adolescents are major medical family problem. 2016. Available at: https://consultqd.clevelandclinic.org/2014/12/chronic-daily-headaches-in-adolescents-are-major-medical-family-problem/. Accessed March 26, 2020.

27. Varkey E, Hagen K, Zwart JA, et al. Physical activity and headache: results from the Nord-Trondelag Health Study (HUNT). Cephalalgia 2008;28(12):1292–7.

28. Soderberg E, Carlsson J, Stener-Victorin E. Chronic tension-type headache treated with acupuncture, physical training and relaxation training. Between-group differences. Cephalalgia 2006;26(11):1320–9.

29. Nader PR, Bradley RH, Houts RM, et al. Moderate-to-vigorous physical activity from ages 9 to 15 years. JAMA 2008;300(3):295–305.

30. Gunner KB, Smith HD, Ferguson LE. Practice guideline for diagnosis and management of migraine headaches in children and adolescents: Part two. J Pediatr Health Care 2008;22(1):52–9.
31. Mack KJ, Gladstein J. Management of chronic daily headache in children and adolescents. Paediatr Drugs 2008;10(1):23–9.
32. Martin PR, MacLeod C. Behavioral management of headache triggers: avoidance of triggers is an inadequate strategy. Clin Psychol Rev 2009;29(6):483–95.
33. Messina E. Evaluation of the headache patient in the computer age. In: Diamond S, Cady R, Diamond M, et al, editors. Headache and migraine biology and management. Boston: Elsevier; 2015. p. 21–31.
34. Houle TT, Butschek RA, Turner DP, et al. Stress and sleep duration predict headache severity in chronic headache sufferers. Pain 2012;153(12):2432–40.
35. Paruthi S, Brooks LJ, D'Ambrosio C, et al. Consensus Statement of the American Academy of Sleep Medicine on the recommended amount of sleep for healthy children: methodology and discussion. J Clin Sleep Med 2016;12(11):1549–61.
36. Godsell S, White J. Adolescent perceptions of sleep and influences on sleep behaviour: a qualitative study. J Adolesc 2019;73:18–25.
37. Kira G, Maddison R, Hull M, et al. Sleep education improves the sleep duration of adolescents: a randomized controlled pilot study. J Clin Sleep Med 2014;10(7): 787–92.
38. Dooley J. The evaluation and management of paediatric headaches. Paediatr Child Health 2009;14(1):24–30.
39. Linder SL. Understanding the comprehensive pediatric headache examination. Pediatr Ann 2005;34(6):442–6.
40. Ohrbach R, Dworkin SF. The evolution of TMD diagnosis: past, present, future. J Dent Res 2016;95(10):1093–101.
41. Brouwer MC, Coutinho JM, van de Beek D. Clinical characteristics and outcome of brain abscess: systematic review and meta-analysis. Neurology 2014;82(9): 806–13.
42. Lewis DW, Ashwal S, Dahl G, et al. Practice parameter: evaluation of children and adolescents with recurrent headaches: report of the Quality Standards Subcommittee of the American Academy of Neurology and the Practice Committee of the Child Neurology Society. Neurology 2002;59(4):490–8.
43. Nissan GR. Screening and testing of the headache patient. In: Diamond S, Cady RK, Diamond ML, et al, editors. Headache and migraine biology and management. Waltham (MA): Academic Press; 2019. p. 33–9.
44. American Academy of Neurology. Five things patients and physicians should question. Choosing Wisely: An Initiative of the ABIM Foundation. 2014. Ref Type: Online Source. Available at: https://www.choosingwisely.org/societies/american-academy-of-neurology/. Accessed March 26, 2020.
45. Blume HK. Childhood headache: a brief review. Pediatr Ann 2017;46(4):e155–65.
46. Gelfand AA. Migraine and childhood periodic syndromes in children and adolescents. Curr Opin Neurol 2013;26(3):262–8.
47. Langdon R, DiSabella MT. Pediatric headache: an overview. Curr Probl Pediatr Adolesc Health Care 2017;47(3):44–65.
48. Gofshteyn JS, Stephenson DJ. Diagnosis and management of childhood headache. Curr Probl Pediatr Adolesc Health Care 2016;46(2):36–51.
49. Jacobs H, Gladstein J. Pediatric headache: a clinical review. Headache 2012; 52(2):333–9.

50. Szperka CL, VanderPluym J, Orr SL, et al. Recommendations on the use of anti-CGRP monoclonal antibodies in children and adolescents. Headache 2018; 58(10):1658–69.
51. Headache Classification Committee of the International Headache Society (IHS). The international classification of headache disorders, 3rd edition. Cephalalgia 2018;38(1):1–211.
52. Blume HK. Pediatric headache: a review. Pediatr Rev 2012;33(12):562–76.
53. Warhurst S, Rofe CJ, Brew BJ, et al. Effectiveness of the progestin-only pill for migraine treatment in women: a systematic review and meta-analysis. Cephalalgia 2018;38(4):754–64.
54. Curtis KM, Tepper NK, Jatlaoui TC, et al. U.S. medical eligibility criteria for contraceptive use, 2016. MMWR Recomm Rep 2016;65(3):1–103.
55. Watemberg N, Guidetti V. Headache and epilepsy. In: Guidetti V, Arruda M, Ozge A, editors. Headache and comorbidities in childhood and adolescence. headache. Cham (Switzerland): Springer; 2017. p. 115–24.
56. Oskoui M, Pringsheim T, Billinghurst L, et al. Practice guideline update summary: pharmacologic treatment for pediatric migraine prevention: report of the guideline development, dissemination, and implementation subcommittee of the American Academy of Neurology and the American Headache Society. Neurology 2019;59(8):1144–57.
57. Gelfand AA, Goadsby PJ. Treatment of pediatric migraine in the emergency room. Pediatr Neurol 2012;47(4):233–41.
58. Pakalnis A, Gladstein J. Headaches and hormones. Semin Pediatr Neurol 2010; 17(2):100–4.
59. Calhoun A, Ford S. Elimination of menstrual-related migraine beneficially impacts chronification and medication overuse. Headache 2008;48(8):1186–93.
60. Oskoui M, Pringsheim T, Holler-Managan Y, et al. Practice guideline update summary: acute treatment of migraine in children and adolescents: report of the guideline development, dissemination, and implementation Subcommittee of the American Academy of Neurology and the American Headache Society. Neurology 2019;93(11):487–99.
61. Lewis D, Ashwal S, Hershey A, et al. Practice parameter: pharmacological treatment of migraine headache in children and adolescents: report of the American Academy of Neurology Quality Standards Subcommittee and the Practice Committee of the Child Neurology Society. Neurology 2004;63(12):2215–24.
62. Dumas P. Latest device now FDA approved for teens with migraine. 2019. Ref Type: Online Source. Available at: https://migraineagain.com/stms-device-for-migraine/. Accessed March 26, 2020.
63. Grazzi L. Primary headaches in children and adolescents; B C Decker:Hamilton, Ontario. Neurol Sci 2004;25(Suppl 3):S232–3.
64. Newman L, Maytal J. Cluster and the trigeminal autonomic cephalalgias. In: Winner P, Lewis D, Rothner A, editors. Headache in children and adolescents. 2nd edition. Hamilton, Ontario: B C Decker; 2008. p. 147–61.
65. Evans RW. Migraine mimics. Headache 2015;55(2):313–22.

Selected Musculoskeletal Issues in Adolescents

Kevin Bernstein, MD, MMS, CAQSM[a],*, Paul Seales, MD, MS[b],
Alex Mroszczyk-McDonald, MD, CAQSM[c]

KEYWORDS

- Sports specialization • Resistance training • Patellofemoral pain syndrome
- Apophysitis • Relative energy deficiency in sports

KEY POINTS

- Early sports specialization does not increase an athlete's chance of obtaining scholarships or playing at elite levels. Exceptions to this are such sports as gymnastics, diving, dance, and figure skating, where athletes peak at young ages.
- With proper training and supervision, resistance training by adolescents is a safe and healthy activity that can be incorporated into a daily exercise routine.
- Apophysitis is a common and self-limiting condition that affects immature skeleture. Noncompliance to treatment can lead to significant further injury.
- Patellofemoral pain syndrome (PFS) is the most common cause of knee pain in adolescents, and is diagnosed without advanced imaging.
- Relative energy deficiency in sport (RED-S) is a new paradigm that expands the female athlete triad to include men, women, and para-athletes.

INTRODUCTION

It is commonly said that children are not just small adults, and this remains true when it comes to the care of their musculoskeletal system. By their nature, most athletes are at risk for acute injuries caused by trauma on and off the field, and overuse injuries associated with numerous activities, from video games to long-distance running. In this article, we highlight a growing epidemic toward early specialization in a single sport, two common musculoskeletal diagnoses (apophysitis and patellofemoral pain syndrome [PFS]), and areas with new and changing guidelines. These topics are all likely to be seen regularly by primary care physicians evaluating adolescents in emergent and nonemergent settings.

[a] Musculoskeletal Faculty, Naval Hospital Jacksonville Family Medicine Residency, 2080 Child St, Jacksonville, FL 32214, USA; [b] Fleet Surgical Team 4, 1084 Pocahontas Street, Suite 150, Norfolk, VA 23511, USA; [c] Kaiser Permanente Department of Family Medicine, 9961 Sierra Avenue, Fontana, CA 92335, USA
* Corresponding author.
E-mail address: kevin.bernstein@gmail.com

Prim Care Clin Office Pract 47 (2020) 257–271
https://doi.org/10.1016/j.pop.2020.02.005
0095-4543/20/© 2020 Elsevier Inc. All rights reserved.

EARLY SPORTS SPECIALIZATION

Engaging in physical activity and having an active lifestyle are important for people of all ages. For adolescents, participation in competitive sports can provide a multitude of benefits. Besides enhancing cardiovascular health, organized athletic programs can promote healthy socialization among peers, decrease stress, develop leadership and team-building skills, and improve self-esteem.[1] Organized team sports and athletic programs provide opportunities for adolescents to participate and compete in various sporting events. Many children and adolescents participate in organized sports throughout the country.

- A 2011 survey by the Sports and Fitness Industry Association found that 27 million, or more than 70%, of athletes ages 6 through 17 participated regularly in team sports in the United States.[2]
- A 2011 to 2012 National Federation of State High School Association survey found that more than 7.7 million athletes competed in high school sports across the United States.[3]

Despite the numerous benefits related to organized sports, competitive athletes with a history of success in a sport are subject to a variety of external stressors that can ultimately lead to overuse injuries, burnout, and cessation of physical activity.[1] One of the most alarming trends occurring in youth athletics contributing to these deleterious outcomes for young athletes is a continued increase in early sports specialization, or committing to playing a single sport nearly year-round while excluding participation in all other sports.[1] This early focus on a single sport typically occurs before adolescence and is at an all-time high.[4]

There are many factors that have contributed to this trend including: fear of falling behind peers, the desire to obtain a competitive edge for scholarships, college recruitment, membership on national and Olympic teams, potential professional contracts, and the recruitment by coaches to use higher-level athletes throughout each season to enhance their coaching resume.[5] Parents, guardians, scouts, coaches, and/or adolescents seek out additional out-of-season opportunities in a single sport to include elite travel teams, training camps, and other showcases without significant time off from this specific sport. The belief is that early specialization may increase the possibility of playing at an elite level, including collegiate athletics.[6] Of those who play high school sports, less than 2% of all high school athletes receive a college athletic scholarship.[7]

Few sports are known to have peak performance before full, skeletal maturity and complete growth. Exceptions, however, include gymnastics, figure skating, dance, and diving. Contrary to the belief that early sports specialization may result in better outcomes for young athletes, numerous studies continue to prove that diversification rather than specialization translates into a higher likelihood of being awarded collegiate athletic scholarships and continuing on to semiprofessional and professional careers.

- A 2019 survey of 303 athletes at 2 National Collegiate Athletic Association (NCAA) Division I programs found that 94.7% played multiple sports before college with 45% playing multiple sports up to age 16. The mean age for specialization was 14.9 years, with a statistically significant difference in time of specialization between team sports (15.5 years) and individual sports (14 years).[6]
- A 2017 survey by Post and colleagues[8] of 344 NCAA Division I male and female athletes at the University of Wisconsin found that specialization in a single sport increased each year during high school with 16.9% of 9th graders and 41.1% of 12th graders reporting specialization in their preferred sport. This study also

found that football athletes were less likely to be specialized than nonfootball athletes. There was no difference in specialization between genders at any level.

- A 2011 survey by DiFiori and colleagues[7] of 296 NCAA Division I male and female athletes at the University of California, Los Angeles found that 88% of their athletes averaged 3 to 4 sports as children. Seventy percent did not specialize until after age 12, and 38% did not specialize until they were older than age 14. Forty-five percent had a parent that competed at the professional or collegiate level, indicating that genetics may play a role in predicting future elite performance in sports.

In fact, multisport involvement is a predominant theme among the highest levels across most sports.

- A 2016 review by Rees and colleagues[9] of the world's best sporting talent found that elite international athletes began playing another sport as their first sport versus national-level athletes. They played more sports than those who peaked at the national ranks, continued participation in other sports at an older age, and did not specialize in their current sport until an older age.
- A 2016 analysis by Gullich[10] of Olympic and World Championship medalists versus nonmedalists confirmed all of the previously mentioned findings.

Year-round specialization in a single sport is much easier with the continued growth of elite traveling teams competing in regional and national leagues. Despite the significant growth of elite travel teams, early involvement in elite traveling and national teams may not result in long-term success.

- A 2014 study of 395 athletes found that approximately a third of international prejunior athletes were selected as senior athletes. More importantly, there were a statistically significant larger number of athletes that were not selected as prejuniors participating in senior squads compared with those that were members on prejunior teams.[11]

Overuse Injuries

According to an American Medical Society for Sports Medicine position statement on overuse injuries and burnout in youth sports, overuse injuries in adolescents are usually caused by "repetitive submaximal loading of the musculoskeletal system when rest is not adequate to allow for structural adaptation to take place."[1] Although any neuromusculoskeletal structure may be affected, adolescent athletes are unique in that they commonly suffer from apophyseal and physeal stress injuries in comparison with adult overuse injuries. Overall, studies are mixed as to whether early specialization in sport is an independent risk factor for injuries. Several studies show early specialization in sports as an independent risk factor for overuse injuries.[12–17] Other studies do not show this correlation.[18–20] However, a 2017 survey of 102 professional baseball players found that less than 50% specialized early. Those that specialized started playing baseball exclusively at a mean age of 8.9 years and reported more serious injuries during their professional career than those that did not. More than 64% of those surveyed did not believe that early specialization is necessary to play professional baseball.[21]

Burnout

Early specialization in sport may correlate with an increase in burnout: the cessation from a previously enjoyable sport or activity because of a variety of intrinsic and extrinsic factors including chronic stress from overreaching and overtraining.[1]

Overreaching is nonfunctional or functional, although both can completely resolve with adequate rest.[22] Functional overreaching is a decline in performance that an athlete can recover from quickly. Nonfunctional overreaching leads to a longer decrease in performance and may include psychological and/or neuroendocrine features. An extreme form of nonfunctional overreaching is known as overtraining syndrome.[22] Overtraining syndrome is a constellation of significant physical, psychological, and hormonal signs and symptoms that cannot be explained by another disease process with a significant decline in human performance that frequently lasts greater than 2 months. These symptoms often mimic a variety of mental health diagnoses including depression and anxiety, and medical conditions, such as thyroid disorders and relative energy deficiency in sport (RED-S).[23] A multidisciplinary treatment approach from clinicians is recommended to help adolescent athletes suffering from overtraining syndrome. The team should include, but is not limited to, their primary care physician and behavioral health specialist (eg, sports psychologist). If parental/guardian stressors are a significant causative factor driving overtraining and burnout, family counseling may also be beneficial.

It is worth noting that not all attrition from sport is caused by burnout.[24] In fact, a variety of other factors are more common for adolescents leading to cessation of sports including shifting interests in other activities, boredom, time conflicts with other activities, injury, minimal skill improvement in the current sport, lack of playing time, and lack of success.[25] Furthermore, if a teenager decides to temporarily discontinue a certain sport, they may elect to resume this sport in the future.

Sport Sampling

One way for adolescents to decrease the likelihood of attrition caused by burnout or other factors involves adequate personalized sampling of multiple sports with eventual specialization in the future.[1] This has several potential advantages. First, the teenager will be able to figure out what sports they like or do not like, which makes the ultimate decision their decision. This could potentially decrease the likelihood of burnout. Second, the teenager will be able to match their functional skill set to excel at one (or more) sport, which may also lead to increased personal satisfaction.

Organizational Guidelines

Several organizations have developed guidelines and recommendations for workload, rest, recovery, and diversification in sports.[1] This includes the American Medical Society for Sports Medicine,[1] the American Orthopedic Society for Sports Medicine,[26] the International Olympic Committee (IOC),[27] and the National Basketball Association.[28] The American Orthopedic Society for Sports Medicine states that early specialization in sport has been shown to be detrimental for high performance at the national, Olympic, or professional level and "identified as damaging for the future physical and mental health of the athlete."[26] For adolescents, most recommendations from various organizations advise that athletes take at least 1 rest day per week from all athletic activities. It is important to monitor training workload during adolescence, because injury risk is greater during growth spurts.[1] Adolescents should play as many sports as possible while gradually increasing time within their preferred sport and allowing for adequate time off. Significant specialization should not occur until at least the high school level for most sports that do not have peak elite performance during adolescence (Box 1). The maximum time they should play in an organized league within their preferred sport should be less than 9 to 10 months with a minimum of 2 months off from this sport. Participation in another sport is recommended during months that are not dedicated to their preferred sport.[28] Adolescents are also encouraged to get

---

Box 1
Recommendations regarding youth participation in, and diversification of, sport

- Adolescent participation in sports is encouraged for all healthy teenagers to promote active, healthy, physical and psychological lifestyles. This can include recreational and organized athletic leagues.

- Diversification in at least 2 different sports is recommended throughout grade school, especially for athletes with a strong desire to compete at elite levels of competition. Diversification in multiple sports is also recommended for those desiring collegiate athletic scholarships.

- Early specialization may be appropriate with early entrant sports where peak performance occurs before skeletal maturity (eg, gymnastics, diving, dance, and figure skating).

- To prevent burnout and overuse injury, avoid specialization in a single sport for more than 8 months of the year with less than 2 to 3 months away from that sport.

- Strength and conditioning programs, injury-prevention programs, skill development, and sport sampling are recommended.

- These recommendations should be discussed with adolescents and their parents or guardians during all preparticipation sports physicals and routine physical examinations.

- These recommendations should also be encouraged to grade school athletic directors, coaches, and other members of the community to prevent external pressures on adolescent athletes to specialize in a single sport.

---

an average of 9 hours of restful sleep to enhance recovery and optimize performance during sporting activities.[28]

WEIGHT TRAINING

Decades ago, there was concern that resistance training, which can include plyometrics, weight lifting, or other forms of resistance, might harm the growing body. Currently, however, it is understood that resistance training does not pose increased risks (eg, damage to growth plates or limitation on linear growth) compared with skeletally mature men and women. Importantly, resistance training has been linked to improved waist circumference, bone mineral density (BMD), and mental health. It is a prime avenue for increasing physical literacy and has also been shown to reduce risk of injuries in several sports settings.[29–32]

In 2008 the American Academy of Pediatrics released a statement on "Strength Training by Children and Adolescents," commenting that it is safe, and recommending it start no earlier than 7 to 8 years old, because this is when balance and postural control skills reach adult levels.[29] This is echoed in other studies that often cite 6 years as a reasonable age. Strength training actually helps with development of these movement skills, and stronger children and adolescents are less likely to incur preventable injuries related to physical activity.[31] Being physically unprepared for sports practice and competition is a risk factor for injury,[33] so the addition of structured resistance programs is one way to help prepare children for entry into sports.

Resistance training in childhood and adolescence should always begin with a focus on proper technique and weight room behavior. The idea of "training age" should be evaluated for each individual based on their general physical activity level and history of sports or motor skill–specific training.[33] Muscle strains are common injuries for all ages with resistance training, with adults actually being at higher risk than adolescents. However, adolescents and preadolescents are at higher risk of injuries related to improper use of weight, such as dropping or being pinched by them. Often these injuries are associated with training at home in unsupervised and unsafe manners. Proper technique and supervision reduce these injury rates to less than those seen in daily play at school.[29,30]

There is no clear consensus on the optimal resistance training routine. A reasonable approach would start with lower levels of resistance and higher repetitions as children become familiar with the techniques, and progress to heavier weights with lower repetitions over time if larger muscle mass is needed or desired. The literature reveals improvements in measured strength with both approaches, with some studies suggesting a medium number of repetitions with around 85% maximal weight may produce greatest results.[34] However, most gym equipment is geared toward adults and therefore is unlikely to provide opportunity for children to perform the movements properly. Therefore, consider free weights for adolescents who have not yet reached their full adult size. It is also important that exercises should allow for full range of motion to maintain flexibility. The current recommendation is to exercise at least 20 to 30 minutes per session, two to three times a week. More than four sessions per week does not seem to have added benefits. Eight to 15 repetitions seems to be a reasonable starting number of repetitions.[29,35]

Do not include movements considered to be "Olympic lifts" (eg, the "snatch" and the "clean and jerk") in routine weight training regimens geared toward gaining strength. These should only be undertaken by those well-trained in proper technique. Limited data do not point toward increased injury in these weightlifting competitions, but this is thought to be secondary to the emphasis on proper technique that these competitors maintain.[29]

Adolescent patients should inform their primary care practitioner of their interest in weight-lifting and undergo a medical evaluation before starting, because there are some precautions to keep in mind when recommending resistance training to adolescent patients. There is low-quality evidence that resistance training programs are safe for some specific conditions, such as cerebral palsy and spinal muscular atrophy, although evidence of true clinical benefit is still lacking.[35,36]

However, there are several conditions that require physician evaluation before starting a resistance training program. A pediatric cardiologist should be consulted before activity initiation in those with cardiomyopathy,[37] pulmonary hypertension, Marfan syndrome with a dilated aortic root, children with poorly controlled hypertension, children with a family history of early sudden cardiac death, and those who have received anthracyclines for chemotherapy. Those with a seizure disorder also need to have physician clearance before starting a weight-training program to discuss any exercises that should be avoided or modified based on physician judgment.[29]

Resistance training is an important aspect of healthy living and should begin at an earlier age. Physicians should feel confident in recommending this activity for children and adolescents of all ages.

APOPHYSITIS

Apophysitis is thought to arise from excessive forces applied to the insertions of a tendon at an apophysis, a normal bony protuberance that arises from an ossification center in growing bone. It can result from a specific traumatic event, as in the case with inversion injuries and proximal fifth metatarsal apophysitis (Iselin disease), or from chronic stress.[38] Factors contributing to the development of apophysitis vary depending on the site. Inflammation or stress injury to the upper limbs (eg, medial epicondyle apophysitis) are influenced mostly by repetitive trauma occurring while throwing,[39] whereas lower limb apophyses are more greatly affected by inappropriate foot and leg mechanics (eg, genu valgum, pronated feet, or elevated body mass index) in addition to overuse.[38,40,41]

Theoretically, apophysitis can come about in any area of bone growth and should be considered in most differentials of pediatric musculoskeletal complaints, including those affecting the groin and pelvis.[42] Close correlation between clinical examination and pertinent anatomy can help to narrow the diagnosis in each case. Three of the more common locations include the medial epicondyle (Little Leaguer's elbow), tibial tuberosity (Osgood-Schlatter disease), and the calcaneus (Sever disease).

Clinically, an affected apophysis presents with gradually worsening pain that specifically worsens when the associated muscle, and therefore the tendon, is activated. Often there is swelling, and the bony anatomy is usually tender to palpation. Care should be taken to expand the differential if anticipated bony tenderness is absent. However, it may not be possible to palpate some areas, such as the ischial tuberosity, in obese or muscular patients. Indirect tests are used in this situation (eg, hamstring stretching by straight leg raise for the ischial tuberosity, or the Ober test or hip abduction for the iliac crest).[38]

Radiographs are easily obtained and warranted to help narrow the differential, which includes avulsion fracture, stress fracture, fragmentation of the ossification center of the bone, and malignancy. Common findings include widening of the affected apophysis, fragmentation, and discontinuity between the anterior and posterior aspects of the apophysis.[38] Contralateral radiographs should be obtained for comparison in adolescents, because there are variations in appearance of the physes. It should be noted that different physes appear and ossify at different ages, determining when they can be seen on radiographs. Typically, the ischial tuberosity, iliac crest, and base of the fifth metatarsal are some of the last to ossify. Lack of appearance of an ossification center on plain films does not rule out apophysitis, and injuries should be treated as apophysitis injuries if clinically indicated.[38] Also, athletes (namely gymnasts) can lag behind 1 to 2 years in bone age.

Ultrasound may also be used and is more sensitive than plain radiography for making the diagnosis. It is also able to evaluate cartilage and tendon pathology.[43] MRI is more sensitive than ultrasound and is able to better characterize soft tissue swelling, bursitis, and bone marrow edema, but neither is required for diagnosis.[44] The convenience, accuracy, and lack of radiation with ultrasonography continue to increase its daily use, and in Japan, it is used to help detect changes of the apophyses of the humeral medial epicondyles of adolescent baseball players as part of their medical checkups. Study of this population has identified the high prevalence of changes at the medial apophysis, and a strong correlation with history of elbow pain.[45]

Technically these conditions are considered self-limiting, because all apophyseal sites eventually ossify. Nonetheless, lack of treatment and hasty return-to-play increase the risk of recurrent symptoms and progression to more severe conditions, such as avulsion fractures, physeal widening, premature closure of growth plates, and inappropriate ossification of tendons.[46] Because bony and cartilaginous structures are affected in apophysitis, treatment is guided by the same principles as those applied to stress fractures: rest the affected area through activity modification; apply ice; and, in some cases, immobilize the area. In youth who are prone to noncompliance, casting for 4 weeks is not unreasonable, although not necessary. Casting may also remove pressure placed on competitive athletes by parents and coaches to return to activity sooner than appropriate.[38] In weight-bearing areas, such as Sever disease, limited weight-bearing via use of crutches is warranted for 4 weeks. Short courses of nonsteroidal anti-inflammatory drugs are reasonable for more immediate pain relief. Corticosteroids do not play a role in pain management for this condition.

If conservative measures do not improve symptoms over the course of 4 weeks, further imaging or orthopedic or sports medicine consultation should be considered. Once pain has subsided, a stretching and strengthening program should be undertaken to avoid recurrent symptoms, with gradual return to sports and activity once symptoms have resolved.

PATELLOFEMORAL PAIN SYNDROME

PFS is the most common cause of knee pain seen by primary care, orthopedic, and sports medicine specialists.[47,48] It is often vague, anterior knee pain, without a single clear cause, and can be chronic and resistant to treatment. There are several terms that may be synonymous with PFS, including runner's knee, facet compression syndrome, and idiopathic anterior knee pain. Chondromalacia, however, is a true pathologic disorder characterized by softening of and wear and tear on the articular cartilage of the patellofemoral joint.[49]

PFS more commonly effects females in a ratio of 2:1 and accounts for up to 25% of all knee pain presenting for medical evaluation, and up to 40% of knee pain in sports medicine clinics.[50,51] It is most common in the second and third decades of life and affects up to 20% of adolescents.[52]

PFS may present insidiously, with minor trauma or with change in activity or training intensity. Pain is often poorly localized to the anterior knee or under the patella, and often described as an ache, but also may be sharp at times. Symptoms are often exacerbated by squatting, running, or prolonged flexion of the knee (often while riding in a car or watching a movie, historically referred to a theater sign).[53] Patients may present with crepitus or audible "popping" of the patellofemoral joint. Mechanical symptoms, such as intra-articular effusion, locking, or true instability, are absent; thus, this history suggests intra-articular pathology and not PFS.

A comprehensive clinical knee examination should include several maneuvers (discussed next). However, there is limited evidence on the sensitivity and specificity of these tests as they relate to the diagnosis of PFS.

- Observe active knee extension for "J-sign": With the patient sitting, ask them to actively extend the knee, as you observe the patellar motion. This sign is positive if, at the end of knee extension, there is a lateral shift of the patella, indicating relative weakness of vastus medialis quadricep muscle.
- Knee extension against resistance: This often loads the patellofemoral joint and can elicit pain.
- Patella facet/retinaculum tenderness: With the patient's knee in full extension and the quadriceps relaxed, displace the patella laterally and medially, and palpate the medial and lateral facet (undersurface). If there is tenderness, then this is a positive finding suggestive of PFS.
- Patella glide and apprehension: With the leg relaxed and slightly flexed to 30°, apply medial and lateral pressure with normal displacement reaching about one-third of the patellar width. More or less than that may indicate hypermobility or excessively tight patellar retinaculum. Apprehension is performed with lateral pressure applied to the patella while observing the patient's face. Winching or muscular guarding as the patella reaches maximal lateral displacement indicates a positive test. There have been some reports that the sensitivity of this test approaches 39%.[54]

- Bilateral and single leg squat: PFS is often exacerbated by squatting and is often worse with single leg squat. Ask the patient to face you and then to perform three to four single leg squats and observe the alignment of the hips, knee, and ankle. In the setting of PFS, there is often medial bowing with mild valgus collapse of the knee with internal femoral rotation, dropping of the contralateral hip, and difficulty with balance indicating weakness of the gluteus medius muscle. Additionally, in the setting of PFS, there may be pes planus, collapse of the arch of the foot, and overpronation of the ankle and valgus collapse of the ankle.[55]

PFS is a clinical diagnosis and radiographic imaging is not necessary to make the diagnosis; however, radiography can help to rule out other pathology.[56]

During the acute phase activity modification, ice, and nonsteroidal anti-inflammatory drugs (and possibly a patellar stabilization brace) are key to symptomatic relief.[57] However, long-term physical therapy and rehabilitation are integral in improving patellofemoral pain itself, although there is no high-quality evidence to support any specific protocol.[58] Unfortunately, almost half of patients continue to have some symptoms 1 year after rehabilitation therapy.

Physical therapy often focuses on increasing strength and mobility of key muscle groups and structures of the knee and hip,[59,60] most notably vastus medialis, gluteus medias, and iliotibial band. Patients should be started in rehabilitation therapy from an experienced physician or under the care of a trained physical therapist; however, a home rehabilitation program is reasonable to start in a limited-resource setting. It must be stressed to the patient that consistency with these stretches and exercises 5 to 6 days a week is critical for symptoms relief.

A sample rehabilitation program is as follows:

1. Strengthen hip abductors: clam shells, glut bridge, or "monster walks" with band.
2. Quadricep strengthening, emphasis on vastus medialis: straight leg raise and quadriceps activation.
3. Hamstring: hamstring curls and heel dig.
4. Pelvic/core stability training: single leg balance and single leg squats.
5. Flexibility: quadriceps, hamstring, and iliotibial band stretching.

There is some evidence that a subgroup of patients may benefit from patellofemoral bracing.[61] There is limited evidence that foot orthosis (orthotics) may benefit patellofemoral pain; however, this may only apply to a subset of patients.[62,63] There is little evidence to support corticosteroid or glucosamine injections for patellofemoral pain.[57,64]

PFS is the most common cause of knee pain presenting to primary care physicians. Diagnosis is reliably made based on history and physical examination without advanced imaging, and treatment can be initiated immediately without need for referral to a subspecialist. Strengthening and stretching of key knee and hip structure are the mainstay of treatment, with possible benefit from patella bracing or foot orthosis for a subset of patients.

RELATIVE ENERGY DEFICIENCY IN SPORT

The female athlete triad was first defined by the American College of Sports Medicine in 1992 in a "Task Force on Women's Issues." The female athlete triad was initially defined as disordered eating, amenorrhea, and osteoporosis in women. In 2007, the definition was updated by the American College of Sports Medicine to its current form: low energy availability (EA) with or without disordered eating, menstrual dysfunction, and low BMD. At the time, this was a significant advancement in monitoring of the health of female athletes.[65,66]

In 2014, the phrase "relative energy deficiency in sport" was coined by the IOC. This was caused by continued research that had shown that inadequate EA was associated with numerous other physiologic changes, such as changes in immunologic and psychological health, in addition to those listed in the female triad, and, furthermore, that these low EA changes affected men and para-athletes. As research continues, low EA is emerging as a significant factor in athlete illness and injury.[65,67] Unfortunately, studies have shown that only 50% of athletic coaches and trainers and 19% of high school nurses could identify all three components of even the female athlete triad, highlighting the need for further education.[66]

It is beyond the scope of this article to discuss calculations of EA. Indeed, it is exceedingly difficult to measure EA in clinical studies, and the ideal method has yet to be found. Generally speaking, adults need 45 kcal/kg of fat free mass per day. Symptoms of low EA occur at less than 30 kcal/kg of fat free mass per day.[68,69] Nonetheless, clinicians should be concerned for inadequate EA in athletes with a body mass index less than normal (ie, <18.5), signs of disordered eating (or known diagnosis of anorexia nervosa or bulimia), otherwise unexplained changes in menstrual cycle in females, and those in sports that place strong emphasis on body image and/or endurance.[65] For men, the IOC 2018 consensus statement cites cyclists, rowers, runners, jockeys, and sports where they must "make weight" (eg, wrestling) as at-risk individuals. In addition, lack of access to food, either secondary to financial means or cultural practices, can increase risk of low EA.[66,70] Other signs and symptoms may include mood changes, nutritional deficiencies, chronic fatigue, decreased athletic performance, lack of normal growth and development, recurrent injuries or illnesses, and infertility. Immunologic changes, gastrointestinal changes, cardiovascular changes, metabolic changes, and endocrine changes hypothesized by the RED-S model continued to be studied, but research continues to support their presence in athletes with low EA.[65,68,71]

It would be ideal to screen every athlete for RED-S at their yearly physical. The IOC recommends a yearly physical health examination that includes questions encompassing female athlete triad and eating disorder habits.[65] Some athletes are more likely to report symptoms when asked in an interview form as opposed to questionnaires.[68] In addition, there are several tools to help with this. When concerned for eating disorders in athletes, clinicians can choose from The Brief Eating Disorder in Athletes Questionnaire,[65] which is validated only in women; the Athletic Milieu Direct Questionnaire; the Female Athlete Screening Tool; and the Physiologic Screening Test for Eating Disorders Among Female Collegiate Athletes. For RED-S, the IOC developed the RED-S Clinical Assessment Tool, which divides athletes into low-, moderate-, and high-risk categories based on signs and symptoms related to RED-S. One can also use the Low Energy Availability in Females Questionnaire. Validated male screening questionnaires have yet to be created. The Sport-specific EA Questionnaire Combined With Clinical Interview is one option for male cyclists that has been able to identify low lumbar spine BMD.[66,67,71–73]

There is no required laboratory work-up for RED-S, but appropriate work-up for other causes of menstrual abnormalities and any other sequelae of RED-S should be performed, because RED-S is a diagnosis of exclusion.[68]

Treatment of RED-S can often be difficult, because there can be marked pressure to continue in sport from a variety of entities, and fear of negative impacts on performance can hinder deviation from long-held training methods.[72] The correction of the energy deficiency, either by increased caloric intake or decreased exercise, is essential to ensuring return of normal physiologic function. Weight gain in college athletes is the best predictor of return of menses. It also improves BMD, but even with this treatment, it is not guaranteed to return to normal. Measurement and correction of low 25-hydroxy vitamin D levels (<30 ng/mL) are reasonable.[66] It is not recommended to use oral contraceptives to help with return of menses, however, because this can mask their spontaneous return (the lack of which indicates ongoing pathology) and has not been shown to improve BMD. Estradiol (E_2) patches with oral progesterone for uterine protection are used as a short-term treatment in more extreme cases of bone mineral loss. Bisphosphonates should not be used with reproductive age women because they are teratogenic and stored in bone for extensive periods of time. In athletes resistant to treatment, an athletic contract citing return to play only after improvement of symptoms may be necessary.[65,66]

The clinician is encouraged to be knowledgeable regarding the female athlete triad, and look for similar situations that may occur in other specific patients. Referral to a nutritionist or sports medicine clinician familiar with these conditions is reasonable when the patient requires further evaluation beyond the comfort level of the general practitioner.

DISCLOSURE

The authors have nothing to disclose. Dr K. Bernstein and Dr P. Seales are current, active duty of the United States Navy. The views expressed in this article are those of the authors and do not necessarily reflect the official policy or position of the Department of the Navy, Department of Defense, or the United States Government.

REFERENCES

1. DiFiori JP, Benjamin HJ, Brennan JS, et al. Overuse injuries and burnout in youth sports: a position statement from the American Medical Society for Sports Medicine. Br J Sports Med 2014;48:287–8.
2. Sporting Goods Manufacturers Association Research/Sports Marketing Surveys USA. U.S. Trends in Team Sports Report, 2011. Jupiter, FL. 2011. Available at: http://www.sfia.org/reports/280_2011-U.S-Trends-in-Team-Sports-Report. Accessed May 11, 2019.
3. National Federation of State High School Association. 2011-12 high school athletics participation survey. Available at: http://www.nfhs.org/. Accessed May 10, 2013.
4. Mostafavifar AM, Best TM, Myer GD. Early sport specialisation, does it lead to long-term problems? Br J Sports Med 2013;47:1060–1.
5. Myer GD, Jayanthi N, DiFiori JP, et al. Sports specialization, part II: alternative solutions to early sport specialization in youth athletes. Sports Health 2016;8:65–73.
6. Swindell HW, Marcille ML, Trofa DP, et al. An analysis of sports specialization in NCAA Division I collegiate athletics. Orthop J Sports Med 2019;7(1). 2325967118821179.
7. DiFiori JP, Gray A, Kimlin E. Sports participation history and early sports specialization in National Collegiate Athletic Association Division I athletes. Clin J Sport Med 2011;21(2):168.
8. Post EG, Thein-Nissenbaum JM, Stiffler MR, et al. High school sport specialization patterns of current Division I athletes. Sports Health 2016;9(2):148–53.
9. Rees T, Hardy L, Güllich A, et al. The Great British medalists project: a review of current knowledge on the development of the world's best sporting talent. Sports Med 2016;46(8):1041–58.
10. Güllich A. Developmental sports activities of international medalists and non-medalists: a matched-pairs analysis. J Sports Sci 2017;35(23):2281–8.

11. Barreiros A, Côté J, Fonseca AM. From early to adult sport success: analyzing athletes' progression in national squads. Eur J Sport Sci 2014;14(Supplement 1):S178–82.

12. Post EG, Trigsted SM, Riekena JW, et al. The association of sports specialization and training volume with injury history in youth athletes. Am J Sports Med 2017; 45(6):1405–12.

13. Pasulka J, Jayanthi N, McCann A, et al. Specialization patterns across various youth sports and relationship to injury risk. Phys Sportsmed 2017;45(3):344–52.

14. Bell DR, Post EG, Trigsted SM, et al. Prevalence of sport specialization in high school athletics: a 1-year observational study. Am J Sports Med 2016;44(6): 1469–74.

15. Jayanthi NA, LaBella CR, Fischer D, et al. Sports-specialized intensive training and the risk of injury in young athletes: a clinical case-control study. Am J Sports Med 2015;43:794–801.

16. Hall R, Barber Foss K, Hewett TE, et al. Sport specialization's association with an increased risk of developing anterior knee pain in adolescent female athletes. J Sports Rehabil 2015;24(1):31–5.

17. Visnes H, Bahr R. Training volume and body composition as risk factors for developing jumper's knee among young elite volleyball players. Scand J Med Sci Sports 2013;23(5):607–13.

18. Kahlenberg CA, Nair R, Monroe E, et al. Incidence of injury based on sports participation in high school athletes. Phys Sportsmed 2016;44(3):269–73.

19. Fabricant PD, Lakomkin N, Sugimoto D, et al. Youth sports specialization and musculoskeletal injury: a systematic review of the literature. Phys Sportsmed 2016;44(3):257–62.

20. Beese ME, Joy E, Switzler CL, et al. Landing error scoring system differences between single-sport and multi-sport female high school-aged athletes. J Athl Train 2015;50(8):806–11.

21. Wilhelm A, Choi C, Deitch J. Early sport specialization: effectiveness and risk of injury in professional baseball players. Orthop J Sports Med 2017;5(9). 2325967117728922.

22. Meeusen R, Duclos M, Gleeson M. Prevention, diagnosis and treatment of the overtraining syndrome. Eur J Sport Sci 2006;6:1–14.

23. Merrigan B, Leggit JC. Broadening the female athlete triad: relative energy deficiency in sport. Am Fam Physician 2019;99(2):76–7.

24. Gould D. Intensive sport participation and the prepubescent athlete: competitive stress and burnout. In: Cahill BR, Pearl AJ, editors. Intensive participation in children's sports. Champaign (IL): Human Kinetics; 1993. p. 19–38.

25. Malina RM. Readiness for competitive youth sport. Chapter 7. In: Weiss MR, Gould D, editors. Sport for children and youths. Champaign (IL): Human Kinetics Publishers, Inc; 1986. p. 45–50.

26. LaPrade RF, Agel J, Baker J, et al. AOSSM early sport specialization consensus statement. Orthop J Sports Med 2016;4(4). 2325967116644241.

27. Bergeron MF, Mountjoy M, Armstrong N, et al. International Olympic Committee consensus statement on youth athletic development. Br J Sports Med 2015;49: 843–51.

28. DiFiori JP, Güllich A, Brenner JS, et al. The NBA and youth basketball: recommendations for promoting a healthy and positive experience. Sports Med 2018;48(9): 2053–65.

29. American Academy of Pediatrics Council on Sports Medicine and Fitness, McCambridge TM, Stricker PR. Strength training by children and adolescents. Pediatrics 2008;121(4):835–40.
30. Myer G, Quatman C, Khoury J, et al. Youth versus adult "weightlifting" injuries presenting to United States emergency rooms: accidental versus nonaccidental injury mechanisms. J Strength Cond Res 2009;23(7):2054–60.
31. Zwolski C, Quatman-Yates C, Paterno M. Resistance training in youth: laying the foundation for injury prevention and physical literacy. Sports Health 2017;9(5): 436–43.
32. Bea J, Blew R, Hetherington-Rauth C, et al. Resistance training effects on metabolic function among youth: a systematic review. Pediatr Exerc Sci 2017;29(3): 297–315.
33. Myer G, Lloyd R, Brent J, et al. How young is too young to start training? ACSMs Health Fit J 2013;17(5):14–23.
34. Peitz M, Behringer M, Granacher U. A systematic review on the effects of resistance and plyometric training on physical fitness in youth: what do comparative studies tell us? PLoS One 2018;13(10):e0205525.
35. Lewelt A, Krosschell K, Stoddard G, et al. Resistance strength training exercise in children with spinal muscular atrophy. Muscle Nerve 2015;52(4):559–67.
36. Ryan J, Cassidy E, Noorduyn S, et al. Exercise interventions for cerebral palsy. Cochrane Database Syst Rev 2017. https://doi.org/10.1002/14651858. cd011660.pub2.
37. Zorzi A, Pelliccia A, Corrado D. Inherited cardiomyopathies and sports participation. Neth Heart J 2018;26(3):154–65.
38. Frush T, Lindenfeld T. Peri-epiphyseal and overuse injuries in adolescent athletes. Sports Health 2009;1(3):201–11.
39. Gregory B. Medial elbow injury in young throwing athletes. Muscle Ligaments Tendons J 2013. https://doi.org/10.11138/mltj/2013.3.2.091.
40. Alicia J, Cylie W, Terry H. Contributing factors in children who present with calcaneal apophysitis. J Foot Ankle Res 2015;8(S2). https://doi.org/10.1186/1757-1146-8-s2-o21.
41. Rodríguez-Sanz D, Becerro-de-Bengoa-Vallejo R, López-López D, et al. Slow velocity of the center of pressure and high heel pressures may increase the risk of Sever's disease: a case-control study. BMC Pediatr 2018;18(1). https://doi.org/10.1186/s12887-018-1318-1.
42. Sailly M, Whiteley R, Read J, et al. Pubic apophysitis: a previously undescribed clinical entity of groin pain in athletes. Br J Sports Med 2015;49(12):828–34.
43. Yanagisawa S, Osawa T, Saito K, et al. Assessment of Osgood-Schlatter disease and the skeletal maturation of the distal attachment of the patellar tendon in pre-adolescent males. Orthop J Sports Med 2014;2(7). https://doi.org/10.1177/2325967114542084.
44. Vaishya R, Azizi A, Agarwal A, et al. Apophysitis of the tibial tuberosity (Osgood-Schlatter disease): a review. Cureus 2016. https://doi.org/10.7759/cureus.780.
45. Otoshi K, Kikuchi S, Kato K, et al. Age-specific prevalence and clinical characteristics of humeral medial epicondyle apophysis and osteochondritis dissecans: ultrasonographic assessment of 4249 players. Orthop J Sports Med 2017;5(5). 232596711770770.
46. Midtiby S, Wedderkopp N, Larsen R, et al. Effectiveness of interventions for treating apophysitis in children and adolescents: protocol for a systematic review and network meta-analysis. Chiropr Man Therap 2018;26(1). https://doi.org/10.1186/s12998-018-0209-8.

47. Thomeé R, Augustsson J, Karlsson J. Patellofemoral pain syndrome: a review of current issues. Sports Med 1999;28:245.
48. Dixit S, DiFiori JP, Burton M, et al. Management of patellofemoral pain syndrome. Am Fam Physician 2007;75:194.
49. Cutbill JW, Ladly KO, Bray RC, et al. Anterior knee pain: a review. Clin J Sport Med 1997;7:40.
50. Witvrouw E, Callaghan MJ, Stefanik JJ, et al. Patellofemoral pain: consensus statement from the 3rd International Patellofemoral Pain Research Retreat held in Vancouver, September 2013. Br J Sports Med 2014;48:411.
51. Boling M, Padua D, Marshall S, et al. Gender differences in the incidence and prevalence of patellofemoral pain syndrome. Scand J Med Sci Sports 2010; 20:725.
52. Tállay A, Kynsburg A, Tóth S, et al. Prevalence of patellofemoral pain syndrome. Evaluation of the role of biomechanical malalignments and the role of sport activity. Orv Hetil 2004;145:2093 [in Hungarian].
53. Post WR. Clinical evaluation of patients with patellofemoral disorders. Arthroscopy 1999;15:841.
54. Malanga G, Nadler SF, editors. Musculoskeletal physical examination: an evidence-based approach. Philadelphia: Elsevier Mosby; 2006.
55. Rabin A, Kozol Z. Measures of range of motion and strength among healthy women with differing quality of lower extremity movement during the lateral step-down test. J Orthop Sports Phys Ther 2010;40:792.
56. Haim A, Yaniv M, Dekel S, et al. Patellofemoral pain syndrome: validity of clinical and radiological features. Clin Orthop Relat Res 2006;451:223.
57. Heintjes E, Berger MY, Bierma-Zeinstra SM, et al. Pharmacotherapy for patellofemoral pain syndrome. Cochrane Database Syst Rev 2004;(3):CD003470.
58. Collins NJ, Barton CJ, van Middelkoop M, et al. 2018 Consensus statement on exercise therapy and physical interventions (orthoses, taping and manual therapy) to treat patellofemoral pain: recommendations from the 5th International Patellofemoral Pain Research Retreat, Gold Coast, Australia, 2017. Br J Sports Med 2018;52:1170.
59. Crossley KM, Stefanik JJ, Selfe J, et al. 2016 Patellofemoral pain consensus statement from the 4th International Patellofemoral Pain Research Retreat, Manchester. Part 1: terminology, definitions, clinical examination, natural history, patellofemoral osteoarthritis and patient-reported outcome measures. Br J Sports Med 2016;50:839.
60. Oliveira VC, Henschke N. Multimodal physiotherapy is effective for anterior knee pain relief. Br J Sports Med 2013;47:245.
61. Chew KT, Lew HL, Date E, et al. Current evidence and clinical applications of therapeutic knee braces. Am J Phys Med Rehabil 2007;86:678.
62. Sutlive TG, Mitchell SD, Maxfield SN, et al. Identification of individuals with patellofemoral pain whose symptoms improved after a combined program of foot orthosis use and modified activity: a preliminary investigation. Phys Ther 2004; 84:49.
63. Collins N, Crossley K, Beller E, et al. Foot orthoses and physiotherapy in the treatment of patellofemoral pain syndrome: randomised clinical trial. BMJ 2008;337: a1735.
64. Kannus P, Natri A, Niittymäki S, et al. Effect of intraarticular glycosaminoglycan polysulfate treatment on patellofemoral pain syndrome. A prospective, randomized double-blind trial comparing glycosaminoglycan polysulfate with placebo and quadriceps muscle exercises. Arthritis Rheum 1992;35:1053.

65. Mountjoy M, Sundgot-Borgen J, Burke L, et al. The IOC consensus statement: beyond the female athlete triad—relative energy deficiency in sport (RED-S). Br J Sports Med 2014;48(7):491–7.
66. Mountjoy M, Sundgot-Borgen J, Burke L, et al. International Olympic Committee (IOC) consensus statement on relative energy deficiency in sport (RED-S): 2018 update. Int J Sport Nutr Exerc Metab 2018;28(4):316–31.
67. Heikura I, Uusitalo A, Stellingwerff T, et al. Low energy availability is difficult to assess but outcomes have large impact on bone injury rates in elite distance athletes. Int J Sport Nutr Exerc Metab 2018;28(4):403–11.
68. Robertson S, Mountjoy M. A review of prevention, diagnosis, and treatment of relative energy deficiency in sport in artistic (synchronized) swimming. Int J Sport Nutr Exerc Metab 2018;28(4):375–84.
69. Burke L, Lundy B, Fahrenholtz I, et al. Pitfalls of conducting and interpreting estimates of energy availability in free-living athletes. Int J Sport Nutr Exerc Metab 2018;28(4):350–63.
70. Burke L, Close G, Lundy B, et al. Relative energy deficiency in sport in male athletes: a commentary on its presentation among selected groups of male athletes. Int J Sport Nutr Exerc Metab 2018;28(4):364–74.
71. Ackerman K, Holtzman B, Cooper K, et al. Low energy availability surrogates correlate with health and performance consequences of relative energy deficiency in sport. Br J Sports Med 2018;53(10):628–33.
72. Keay N, Francis G, Entwistle I, et al. Clinical evaluation of education relating to nutrition and skeletal loading in competitive male road cyclists at risk of relative energy deficiency in sports (RED-S): 6-month randomised controlled trial. BMJ Open Sport Exerc Med 2019;5(1):e000523.
73. Melin A, Fahrenholtz I, Lichtenstein M, et al. Exercise dependence, eating disorder symptoms and biomarkers of relative energy deficiency among male endurance athletes. Med Sci Sports Exerc 2019;51(Supplement):728.

Providing Care for Transgender and Gender Diverse Youth

Kacie M. Kidd, MD[a],*, Caitlin Thornburgh, MSW, LSW[b],
Catherine F. Casey, MD[c], Pamela J. Murray, MD, MHP[d]

KEYWORDS

- Transgender • Adolescents • Primary care • Young adults • Gender diverse
- Gender-affirming • Mental health

KEY POINTS

- Transgender and gender diverse youths (TGDY) have higher rates of health and health-related disparities, including suicidality, bullying, and homelessness compared with cis-gender peers.
- TGDY are highly resilient and are most successful with family and school support.
- Primary care providers and clinic staff should be educated on the unique health needs of this population and take action to create an affirming office environment.
- Primary care providers should consider the provision of comprehensive gender care to reduce barriers to care and improve health outcomes.

INTRODUCTION

Transgender and gender diverse youths (TGDY) do not identify as the sex they were assigned at birth (eg, female, male) and have a different gender identity (eg, female, male, nonbinary, agender). Gender identity is different from sexual orientation, which refers to physical and/or romantic attraction (**Fig. 1**). **Table 1** provides additional definitions. According to the 2017 Youth Risk Behavior Survey (YRBS), nearly 2% of high school students surveyed identified as transgender, and this population faces significant health disparities compared with cisgender peers, including increased victimization, substance use, and suicidality.[1] The goal of health care providers should be to support this population and minimize these disparities through the provision of affirming care.

[a] Center for Adolescent and Young Adult Health, University of Pittsburgh School of Medicine, 120 Lytton Avenue, Pittsburgh, PA 15213, USA; [b] Center for Adolescent and Young Adult Health, UPMC Children's Hospital of Pittsburgh, 120 Lytton Avenue, Pittsburgh, PA 15213, USA; [c] Department of Family Medicine, University of Virginia, 1215 Lee Street, Charlottesville, VA 22908, USA; [d] Department of Pediatrics, West Virginia University, PO Box 9214, Morgantown, WV 26506, USA
* Corresponding author.
E-mail address: Kacie.Kidd2@chp.edu
Twitter: @Kacie_Kidd (K.M.K.)

Prim Care Clin Office Pract 47 (2020) 273–290
https://doi.org/10.1016/j.pop.2020.02.006
0095-4543/20/© 2020 Elsevier Inc. All rights reserved.
primarycare.theclinics.com

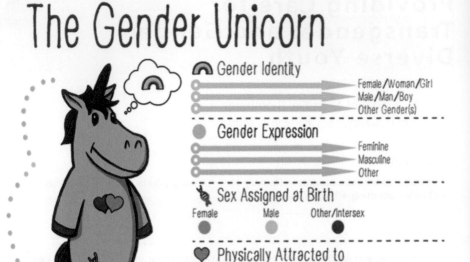

Fig. 1. The Gender Unicorn, used with permission from Trans Student Educational Resources. The authors recommend using this or similar imagery to help patients and families understand the differences between gender identity, gender expression, sex assignment at birth, and physical and emotional attraction. An interactive version of this figure is available at www.transstudent.org/gender.

NATURAL HISTORY OF GENDER IDENTITY

Children begin to display stereotypical gendered behaviors, such as playing with specific toys and preferring certain types of dress associated with perceived societal expectations, around ages 2 to 4 years, and this behavior continues through early school age.[2,3] Research with TGDY suggests that they often exhibit stereotypical behaviors associated with their gender identity.[2] Although many TGDY will persist in their gender identity and seek affirming medical, social, and/or legal intervention later in life, a small percentage of TDGY "desist" or begin to exhibit more traits aligned with their natally assigned gender.[4] Little is known about why some TGDY "desist" in their gender identity (ie, no longer identify as gender diverse) as opposed to those who "persist" (ie, maintain their gender diverse identity). Notably, the terms "desist" and "desisters" are controversial because of an association with the pathologization of the transgender experience based in prior medical guidelines as well as the use of conversion therapies, which have proven harmful.[5]

Supporting social transition for TGDY (using affirming name and pronouns, altering gender expression to better align with one's gender identity) is associated with improved health outcomes, including lower rates of depression and anxiety.[6] Some TGDY first present at puberty having had no stereotypical behaviors associated

Table 1 Brief terminology and definitions[a]	
Gender/gender identity	A person's sense of who they are through the perspective of masculine, feminine, neither, other, or a combination
Sex/natal sex	Typically refers to the assignment at birth following assessment of external genitalia, may also involve chromosomal testing
Gender expression	What a person displays externally, such as hairstyle, clothing, makeup, behavior, speech
Transgender	An umbrella term for a person whose gender identity and/or expression does not align with the sex assigned at birth
Cisgender	A person whose gender identity does align with the sex assigned at birth
Nonbinary/genderqueer	A person who does not identify as entirely masculine or feminine
Genderfluid	A person whose identity may vacillate from more masculine to more feminine or the reverse
Agender	A person whose identity is neither masculine nor feminine
Gender diverse	An umbrella term to include the range of gender identities with the exception of cisgender
Pronouns	A word that substitutes for a noun and either implies gender (eg, she/her, he/him) or gender neutrality (eg, they/them, zie/hir, zie/zir)
Misgendering	Using incorrect pronouns to describe a person, most often using the pronouns consistent with the patient's natal sex instead of their gender identity as well as misuse of honorifics (eg, sir, ma'am)
Misnaming/deadnaming	Using a person's birth name as opposed to their chosen name
Sexual orientation	Whom a person is attracted to, emotionally and/or physically
Passing	Not being easily identified as being transgender or gender diverse; note that this is not a goal for all transgender/ gender diverse persons
Puberty blockers/blockers	Medications that can temporarily halt puberty, often GnRH agonists
Gender-affirming hormone	Medications like testosterone and estradiol that can cause bodily changes sometimes desired by transgender and gender diverse people

[a] Note that these are brief definitions and that language changes and evolves geographically, culturally, and temporally. It is recommended that providers clarify what these words mean to the patient when used in the health care setting.

with their gender identity.[3] The distress associated with the incongruence of one's identity and pubertal expression of natal sex hormone-induced changes indicates the potential need for gender-affirming medical support in all TGDY, regardless of age of presentation.[4,7]

GENDER DYSPHORIA AND MENTAL HEALTH

Diagnostic criteria for experiences of incongruence between sex assigned at birth and gender identity were introduced in the third edition of the *Diagnostic and Statistical Manual of Mental Disorders* (*DSM-III*) in 1980.[8] As understanding of this incongruence evolved, criteria for the classification of gender identity-related conditions changed. Throughout this progression, diagnoses were categorized in the *DSM* as psychosexual disorders, disorders first evident in infancy, childhood, or adolescence, and sexual and gender identity disorders in the *DSM-III, DSM-III-R, DSM-IV,* and *DSM-IV-TR,* respectively.[8–11] Although these diagnoses were and are used to acquire medical and mental health services and insurance coverage, the classification of a mental health disorder can also be used to further stigmatize and marginalize this community by presenting their identities as pathologic.[12–14] In an effort to reduce stigma, *DSM-V* edits included changing the nomenclature of this diagnosis from "gender identity disorder" to "gender dysphoria." This change emphasizes that the distress experienced is related to gender incongruence, rather than deriving from the identity itself.[12,13,15]

DIAGNOSING GENDER DYSPHORIA

According to the *DSM-V*, an individual must meet specific criteria for the diagnosis of gender dysphoria. These criteria include experiencing incongruence between one's sex assigned at birth and one's true gender identity for a period of at least 6 months.[15] Full diagnostic criteria are available from the American Psychiatric Association (https://online.epocrates.com/diseases/99236/Gender-dysphoria-in-adults/Diagnostic-Criteria).

For some TGDY, gender dysphoria is felt and expressed early in childhood, and it may or may not continue throughout adolescence and adulthood. For others, it arises with the onset of puberty and the physical changes that occur in accordance with their sex assigned at birth.[16,17] Care of gender diverse prepubertal children is focused on mental health support and community referrals for the patient and their family. Providers can also support the concept of gender as a spectrum instead of a binary construct and validate the young person's experience. Practicing affirming language, including chosen name and pronouns, is important.

Gender dysphoria presents differently in each TGDY and is often, but not always, accompanied by dissatisfaction and discomfort with one's physical appearance.[16–18] Although individuals may be able to make changes to their behaviors, clothing, hairstyles, name, and pronoun use, they are often unable to change the physical presentation of their bodies without medical intervention.[16] In TGDY, gender dysphoria may present with internalizing symptoms associated with mood and anxiety disorders as well as externalizing symptoms, including behavioral problems and disruptive disorders, or symptoms leading to school, legal, or other problems.[19] Providers seeing these concerns should be mindful about the possibility of gender dysphoria and ask about gender identity.

HEALTH DISPARITIES

The 2017 YRBS survey found that nearly 35% of transgender-identifying youths had attempted suicide compared with 5% and 9% of cisgender male and female youths, respectively.[1] This population also experienced significantly higher rates of bullying (35% for transgender-identifying youths vs 15% for cisgender male youths and 21% for cisgender female youths) as well as higher rates of substance use and higher risk sexual activities (coitarche before age 13 years, lack of condom use, using substances before intercourse).[1] TGDY also have increased rates of homelessness and unstable housing often due to being forced out of homes because of their identity.[20] Current literature suggests that TGDY may be at higher risk of having an eating disorder than their cisgender peers, but there is little understanding of how presentations and best treatment practices may differ in this population.[21,22] Minority race or ethnicity can be additionally challenging for TGDY as compounded minority stress increases health disparities.[23,24]

RESILIENCE

Broader research on lesbian, gay, bisexual, transgender and questioning or queer (LGBTQ) youths shows that despite the significant health disparities and societal pressures they face, these young people are highly resilient in their ability to overcome adversity and excel.[25] Improved health outcomes are seen when youths had familial and school support.[25] Providers should strive to avoid seeing a patient's gender identity as an inherent risk factor or "high-risk behavior" because it is neither. It is the intersectionality of the patient's internal and external experiences associated with their gender identity that can be cause for poor health outcomes.

NONBINARY IDENTITIES

At least 20% of the transgender community feels that their gender that lies outside of or somewhere in-between the common societal construct that gender is binary (male or female gender).[26] Research that is inclusive of nonbinary gender identities is limited because historical data collection methods typically only allowed binary responses and the general notion that gender is fixed and aligned with sex assigned at birth.[27] As attitudes and representation of the transgender community are changing, more individuals express diverse identities.[27,28] The spectrum of transgender and nonbinary identities is vast. Affirming care includes sensitive questioning about terms that the individual prefers and mirroring that language.

The *DSM-V* includes a revision in the language of the diagnostic criteria, "of the other gender (or some alternative gender different from one's assigned gender)," which has been pivotal in helping nonbinary individuals gain access to gender-affirming medical care.[21] However, nonbinary individuals continue to experience additional barriers to care, poorer mental health, and additional stigma and experiences of invalidation in comparison to binary transgender individuals.[27,28] Nonbinary individuals have less comfort than their binary peers in expressing their health care needs with their provider and may feel pressured to misrepresent their true identity to align themselves with the gender binary in order to receive access to gender affirming care.[26,27] It is therefore important to use gender-neutral language, ask about gender identity after acknowledging that gender is a spectrum rather than a binary construct, and highlight the validity of nonbinary identities.[27]

TRANSGENDER-AFFIRMING MENTAL HEALTH CARE

TGDY experience disproportionately higher rates of clinical depression, anxiety, self-harm, and suicidality compared with their cisgender peers.[29] Because of stigma and bias, 33% of respondents in the 2015 US Transgender Survey experienced at least 1 negative interaction with a health care provider related to being transgender, including refusal of treatment and harassment.[30] In addition to discriminatory practices common in medical settings, there are added barriers to care for TGDY, such as provider inexperience, restrictive insurance coverage, lower socioeconomic status, and reduced access to transportation.[31] These barriers as well as historical pathologizing of gender dysphoria by the mental health community position TGDY to experience challenges in assessment and treatment of mental health conditions. It is important to keep in mind that mental health issues experienced by TGDY may or may not be related to their gender dysphoria.[32] Notably, many TGDY do not experience concerns requiring the assistance of mental health professionals.[32]

Previous standards of care outlined by the World Professional Association for Transgender Health (WPATH) required a letter written by a mental health clinician diagnosing gender dysphoria in order to access medical interventions, including hormone therapy or surgeries.[33] This requirement often exacerbated tensions already present between transgender individuals and mental health providers.[34] More recently, the WPATH standards of care were modified such that referral letters for hormone therapy are a recommended standard of care for mental health providers to offer to patients who have not established care with a medical provider, but are no longer required to access hormone therapy. The requirement for letters from mental health providers before obtaining surgical treatment persists because insurance providers adhere to antiquated guidelines.[35]

TGDY experience bias and disparity in a variety of life domains and thus have unique needs in accessing safe, effective, and restorative mental health care. Mental health providers working with TGDY require knowledge of transaffirming practices, including challenging interpretations of gender as a binary and encouraging TGDY to explore their identity in a safe, nonjudgmental space.[32,34,35] The opportunity for affirming relationships can serve to combat the stigma experienced by TGDY, and research indicates that feelings of being supported in their identity decreases mental health disparities between transgender and cisgender youths.[6,32,36,37]

FAMILY SUPPORT

Studies show that parental and family support improves mental health outcomes and increases the likelihood of parents providing consent and support to access gender-affirming medical care.[6,38] Supporting families who may be struggling with accepting their child's identity is critical. This support may include exploring and validating family members' emotions related to learning about the child's identity (potentially in a space or session separate from their child) and making recommendations to pursue individual and family support through referrals to gender-affirming therapists.[32] Additional recommendations include providing education about the impact of gender-affirming care and gender dysphoria on youths, referrals to support groups, resources to communicate with other families with TGDY and navigate concerns at school, and including families in the provision of gender-affirming care.[32]

INTERDISCIPLINARY CARE

Clinical practice guidelines from WPATH, the American Psychiatric Association, the Endocrine Society, and the American Academy of Child and Adolescent Psychiatry consistently recommend collaborative care provision with an interdisciplinary team when possible.[23] Care coordination and open communication between providers offer opportunities for a collaborative care plan and a more holistic approach to care.[23,32] For example, hormonal interventions may positively or negatively impact existing mood disorders.[32] Medical providers may rely on behavioral health providers to assist patients in coping with these changes in their mood and communicate with primary care providers about any concerns that may warrant an adjustment in medications or behavioral therapy.[32] Alternatively, medical providers may lean on behavioral health providers to conduct an additional assessment to support readiness for medical intervention in more complex patients or to provide additional therapy to build coping skills necessary to combat stigma, engage in further exploration of gender identity, and/or increase knowledge and understanding of safety and self-disclosure in a variety of spaces.[23]

WELCOMING OFFICE POLICIES & PROCEDURES

Staff that interacts with patients and families should receive training on both cultural humility (the understanding that our experiences in the world may not be similar to others and that similarity should not be assumed) and the potential causes of negative health care experiences for TGDY.[39] Providers are encouraged to examine their own implicit and explicit biases and realize that although we always learn from our patients, we must bring a level of medical competence to all interactions. Individuals should be welcoming and unassuming in their interactions with all patients. Nonaffirming interactions, such as assuming a patient's pronouns based on physical appearance or using a legal name based on the electronic medical record (EMR) or prior documentation, can be harmful for TGDY.

All members of the health care team, including front desk and scheduling staff, should be encouraged to privately ask patients what name and pronouns they would like to use during the visit. Young people report that using their chosen name and pronouns makes them feel seen and respected and can reduce mental health disparities.[37,40] In one recent study, the majority of TGDY endorsed wanting their affirmed names and pronouns documented in the EMR, and this is now an option for most systems.[42] Additional ways to address potential barriers are included in **Box 1**.

Box 1
Creating an affirming office space identifying social, setting, and system level interventions

Social level
- Training: Require training on gender-affirming care for all employees
- Advisory board: Consider creating a community advisory board to provide a voice for TGDY and their families

Setting level
- Check-in privacy: Ensure that patients are able to discretely discuss their pronouns and chosen name, or to mention wanting to speak to the provider or nurse about gender; consider offering ways this can be done via writing or online instead of out loud
- Patient forms: Use inclusive questions on forms to allow patients to indicate their gender identity and pronouns as well as the gender they were assigned at birth
- Affirming signage: Display rainbow or transgender pride flags or other insignia to indicate that the clinic space is affirming, use posters or pamphlets with images of gender diverse people, post your nondiscrimination policy
- Bathroom signage: Indicate that all single stall bathrooms are "All Gender" or that patients are encouraged to use the multiple stall bathroom most consistent with their identity

System level
- E-Record: Be mindful of how the EMR displays names and pronouns, and if possible, work to improve these interfaces so that all staff interacting with the patient is aware of how a patient should be addressed
- Inpatient policies: Be aware of the rooming and hormone management policies at the inpatient units in your area and advocate for individual rooms and continued hormone use whenever medically safe
- Institutional policies: Review institutional antidiscrimination policies and advocate for protection on the basis of gender identity and sexual orientation if not already outlined

PRIMARY CARE FOR TRANSGENDER AND GENDER DIVERSE YOUTHS

The provision of gender care can be done by primary care providers as well as endocrinologists, gynecologists, and others.[42] Even if the primary care provider is not prescribing hormones or puberty blockers, it is essential that TGDY have access to a supportive and affirming clinical space when seeking routine care. In a national survey of transgender adults, nearly 30% noted postponing medical care when sick or injured because of fear of discrimination, and 19% reported being refused care because of their gender identity.[43] In that same study, half noted feeling like they had to teach their providers how to care for them.[43] A typical gender-affirming primary care model is to "screen/treat" body parts and organ systems present. While this can be appropriate, it is important to note that feminizing or masculinizing therapies can impact this approach, including some cancer screenings (eg, consideration of breast cancer screening in patients on estrogen therapy).[35] At initial visits and periodically, organ and surgery inventories can categorize this information in a standard and accessible fashion, although it is important to explain why questions about specific organs are necessary for health maintenance instead of curiosity on the part of the provider.

The tracking of recommended screening interventions is often gender based in the EMR, further complicating care because a legal gender marker change alters provider reminders. Transmasculine patients are less likely to be up-to-date on cervical cancer screening than cisgender peers despite being more likely to have abnormal cells or inadequate samples.[44] Avoidance of this screening can be due to dysphoria associated with gynecologic care requiring an internal or speculum examination, but may also be due to providers and patients not recognizing the importance of this screening in those who appear masculine and whose gender marker may have been legally changed. There may be a role for human papillomavirus (HPV) self-swab, and this could help to screen patients who cannot tolerate speculum examination, particularly for those age ≥ 25 years.[45–47] Ultimately, providers must be comfortable discussing screening guidelines with patients and performing procedures such as cervical cancer screening where appropriate as well as maximizing prevention opportunities like HPV immunization, smoking cessation, and condom use.

Screening for sexually transmitted infections is important for all sexually active patients. It is important to ask open-ended questions, such as, "when you have sex, what body parts are involved for both you and your partner(s)?" These questions allow providers to determine if oral and/or rectal swabs should be obtained in addition to urine or genital swabs and serum studies in the workup for sexually transmitted infections.

Other health interventions may involve blood pressure screenings, particularly given the association between hormone use and increased blood pressure, or serial hemoglobin measurements owing to the risk of polycythemia when using testosterone.[39] Identified medical concerns should be treated as they would be in cisgender patients, that is, hyperlipidemia should be treated with a lipid-lowering drug, not discontinuation of testosterone. Given the significant mental health disparities associated with TGDY, routine conversations about mood and safety (at home, at school, and in the community) should also be standard in every visit. As some TGDY have unstable housing associated with lack of familial acceptance, as well as being at risk for sexual exploitation and survival/transactional sex in order to obtain basic essentials, food and housing security assessments are also important.[8]

Traditional methods of contraception may not be effective for or accepted by TGDY. Many patients assume that hormone blocking medications and testosterone/estradiol provide contraception, but this is not sufficient protection. Barrier methods are essential for any patients in a sexual relationship in which sperm and oocytes have the potential to meet. In addition, menstruation can be profoundly dysphoric for masculine-identifying patients, and these individuals may benefit significantly from measures that lessen or even stop menses via progestins (eg, levonorgestrel intrauterine devices [IUDs], medroxyprogesterone acetate) or gonadotropin-releasing hormone (GnRH) agonists (eg, leuprolide acetate, histrelin implant).

Primary care providers can identify local fertility centers that are affirming of TGDY and could serve as a resource to aid in fertility preservation efforts (gamete freezing) if having biological children is important to the patient. Current guidelines recommend having this discussion with patients and families before initiation of puberty blockers or hormones, although TGDY who have started a hormone blocker at Tanner (sexual maturity rating, SMR) stage 2 may not have developed functional gametes and may need to allow puberty corresponding to the sex assigned at birth to progress in the future to have viable gametes for preservation.[48,49] Research is ongoing to attempt to mature ovarian and testicular tissue in vitro.[49,50] Examples of affirming language for use in complex conversations like fertility preservation is presented in **Table 2**.

GENDER-AFFIRMING CARE

Medical interventions for affirming gender identity consist of 3 categories as delineated in the WPATH Standards of Care: reversible, partially reversible, and irreversible.[35] These categories can be further divided into masculinizing and feminizing interventions. Notably, written informed consent on the part of parents or guardians of minors (age < 18 years) and adult patients (age ≥ 18 years) is standard for partially reversible and irreversible interventions in the United States.

REVERSIBLE NONMEDICAL INTERVENTIONS
Feminizing

Reversible nonmedical feminizing interventions include vocal coaching (so as to have a more feminine-sounding voice); the use of breast prostheses, heavily padded bras, or tissue or fabric stuffed into a bra to simulate or enhance breast tissue; and "tucking" the genitals to allow for a more feminine silhouette. Tucking is the act of positioning the natal male genitalia between the legs and securing via a "gaff" or sling most often made of fabric. Tucking may also refer to the act of pushing the testicles up into the inguinal canals, which may increase risk for hernia.[42] Patients sometimes use tape to further secure their tucking, but this can cause significant skin irritation and is also associated with fungal infections and delayed urination.[42,51]

Masculinizing

Reversible nonmedical masculinizing interventions include chest binding and packing. Chest binding involves compressing breast tissue to achieve a more masculine silhouette, which can reduce dysphoria and improve mental health.[52] Although some sources recommend binding for no longer than 8 hours per day, taking regular days off from binding may be more likely to reduce adverse health outcomes.[52] It is essential that patients use items designed to be chest binders, as opposed to bandage wraps or tape. Negative sequelae from improper binding include but are not limited to chest, shoulder, back, and abdominal pain, rib injury or fracture, shortness of breath, and skin irritation.[42,52] Packing is the use of a prosthesis to either simulate the outline of male genitalia in clothing and/or to allow the user the ability to urinate while standing. Considerations when choosing a packing device include intended use or uses as well

Table 2 Affirming language for complex conversations	
Name and pronouns	Hello, my name is Dr X and my pronouns are she/her. What can I call you? What pronouns do you use?
Evolution of gender identity	When did you first understand or have words to describe your gender identity?[a]
Ways of affirming identity	We have talked about your name and pronouns. Are there other ways you have affirmed your identity, like in dress or hairstyle? How about binding/packing (transmasculine patients)? Tucking (transfeminine patients)?
Names for body parts	Some of my patients use different names to describe body parts that make them uncomfortable. Do you have different names for body parts that you would like me to use?
Sensitive examinations	Before we start a hormone blocker or hormones, we want to know where your body is in terms of puberty/development. We do this by examining chest tissue and your genital area. This kind of examination is very quick, but can be stressful for some patients. You can have a parent or other close support person with you. You can also wait to have this examination at our next visit before starting the medicine.
Reversibility/irreversibility	Hormone-blocking medication like GnRH agonists are fully reversible, so if you decide to stop the medication, your body will go back to making the same hormones it makes now. This gives you time to consider other medications, like testosterone, estradiol, spironolactone, and others, because they can have effects that will not go away even if you stop taking them. Some of these irreversible effects can involve your fertility or ability to have biological children
Fertility preservation	There are many ways to have a family. Have you thought about becoming a parent? Is having a biological child important to you? The medications you are interested in can impact your ability to have children (fertility) and/or be harmful to a pregnancy. Would you be interested in information about ways to preserve fertility by freezing eggs or sperm?
Addressing parental fears	Hearing about negative mental health outcomes in transgender youths can be really scary, and it's obvious that you want the best for your child. Research tells us that when transgender young people have affirming environments at home, school, and so forth, they can have mental health outcomes that look like their cisgender peers. One of the most important things you can do to be affirming is to use your child's chosen name and pronouns

[a] Note that this question is often seen by patients as challenging the validity of the patient's gender identity, so it is important to emphasize why this question is important:– it is needed to confirm a diagnosis of gender dysphoria, if present, and is often required on letters of medical necessity for insurance companies to approve medical or surgical interventions.

as budget. It is essential that devices are regularly cleaned and sized for a proper fit so as to limit skin irritation.[42,51]

Reversible Medical Interventions: Hormone-Blocking Medications

The most commonly used blocking medications are GnRH agonists, such as leuprolide acetate or histrelin implant. Leuprolide acetate can be administered as a monthly or every 3-month intramuscular (IM) injection. Histrelin acetate comes as an implant placed in the arm that lasts for at least a year, but possibly longer.[48] Although most commonly used in patients who are at least Tanner (SMR) 2, these medications can have benefit in halting further pubertal development in Tanner (SMR) 3 to 4 patients and in stopping menses (typically following a 1-time bleed after initiation) in those who have significant dysphoria with menses or may not be interested in or able to initiate hormones (ie, minors without parental support for testosterone/estradiol initiation).[53]

Additional Hormone-Blocking Medications for Masculine-Identifying Patients

Progesterone in the form of oral or IM medroxyprogesterone acetate or levonorgestrel IUD can be used in transmasculine-identifying individuals to inhibit the GnRH axis and create an atrophic endometrium.

PARTIALLY REVERSIBLE
Additional Hormone Blocking Medications for Feminine-Identifying Patients

Spironolactone and bicalutamide are hormone blocking medications used in patients desiring feminization that selectively block androgen receptors, creating a relatively

---

Box 2
Preinitiation and monitoring anthropometric measures, laboratory tests for hormone blockers, and affirming hormones[39,48]

Hormone blocking medications
GnRH agonists
- Before Initiation and quarterly
    Height, weight
    Tanner (SMR) staging
    Follicle-stimulating hormone (FSH), luteinizing hormone (LH), natal sex hormone (estradiol/testosterone)
    Calcium,[a] phosphorous,[a] alkaline phosphatase,[a] 25-hydroxyvitamin D[a]
- Before initiation and annually
    Bone age, Dual Energy X-ray Absorptiometry (DEXA) scan[a]
Spironolactone
- Before initiation and quarterly
    Potassium
    Blood urea nitrogen,[b] creatinine[b]

Affirming hormones (estradiol and testosterone)
- Before initiation and quarterly
    Height, weight, blood pressure
    Tanner (SMR) staging
    LH, FSH, estradiol,[c] testosterone
    Calcium,[a] phosphorous,[a] alkaline phosphatase,[a] 25-hydroxyvitamin D,[a] complete blood count, renal/liver function, fasting lipids,[d] glucose,[d] insulin[d]
- Before initiation and annually
    Prolactin (if on estradiol)[e]
    DEXA scan (if prior pubertal suppression)[a]
    Bone age (if prior pubertal suppression)[a]

[a] Alternative guidelines do not recommend these measures.[42]
[b] Alternative guideline recommendation.[42]
[c] Alternative guidelines recommend as needed estradiol monitoring for patients on testosterone.[42]
[d] Alternative guidelines do not recommend lipid or glucose monitoring.[42]
[e] Alternative guidelines recommend only if symptoms concerning for prolactinoma.[42]

estrogenic hormonal milieu. They induce development of breast tissue and decrease androgen-dependent terminal hair, often on the face and trunk. Spironolactone is taken in divided doses twice daily when used to block the effects of testosterone and to stimulate breast development.[48] Breast tissue resulting from this medication is unlikely to fully regress, making this intervention as well as a newer agent, bicaluta-mide, "partially reversible" interventions.

Bicalutamide has been described in a small sample as a possible alternative to GnRH agonists for patients desiring feminization.[54] This medication, like leuprolide and histrelin, has been used for precocious puberty.[54] There is notable breast tissue development with the drug and a theoretic risk of liver toxicity that was not found in the small (n = 13) sample studied.[54]

Further partially reversible feminizing interventions include estrogen, specifically 17-β estradiol, which comes in transdermal, sublingual, and parenteral formulations. Testosterone is a masculinizing intervention that comes in parenteral and transdermal formulations. A small study suggested testosterone administered subcutaneously achieved serum levels and desired effects similar to testosterone administered IM with the additional benefit of easier, less-painful self-administration by patients.[55] Consequently, subcutaneous administration is now commonly recommended. Prior recommendations suggested initiating gender-affirming hormonal therapy (estradiol or testosterone) at age 16, but this recommendation has softened to become more pa-tient specific, particularly for those whose dysphoria would likely benefit from medica-tion initiation at a younger age, more closely matching the puberty experienced by their cisgender peers.[53]

Recommended anthropometric and laboratory measures before initiation of these medications as well as for monitoring in addition to expected changes, possible side effects, and dosing guidelines are summarized in **Box 2** and **Tables 3 and 4**.

Table 3	
Anticipated changes, possible side effects from estradiol and testosterone[39,42]	
Anticipated Changes	**Possible Side Effects**
Estradiol	
Redistribution of body fat	Blood clots
Decrease in muscle mass	Stroke
Softening of skin	Macroprolactinoma
Decreased libido/erections	Breast cancer
Breast growth	Cholelithiasis
Decreased testicular volume	Mood changes/tearfulness
Decreased sperm production	Hypertriglyceridemia
Decreased terminal hair growth	Reduced fertility
Testosterone	
Redistribution of body fat	Erythrocytosis
Increased muscle mass	Liver dysfunction
Face/body hair growth	Stroke
Increased libido	Heart disease
Clitoral enlargement	Hypertension
Deepening of voice	Breast/uterine cancer
Menstrual suppression	Mood changes/tearfulness, male pattern baldness, vaginal atrophy, reduced fertility

Table 4
Formulations and dosing for hormone blockers and affirming hormone therapy[39,41,48]

Medication	Route	Frequency	Starting Dose	Maximum Dose
Hormone blockers				
Leuprolide acetate	IM injection	Every 3 mo	11.25–30 mg	11.25–30 mg
Histrelin acetate	SubQ implant	Every 1–3 y	50 mg	50 mg
Medroxyprogesterone acetate	IM injection	Every 3 mo	150 mg	150 mg
Medroxyprogesterone acetate	Oral	qd	2.5 mg	10 mg
Spironolactone	Oral	qd bid	25–50 mg qd	100 mg/d bid
Estradiol[a]				
Estradiol	Transdermal	Twice weekly	25 μg	100–400 μg
Estradiol	Sublingual	qd bid	1–4 mg qd	6–8 mg qd
Estradiol valerate	Parenteral	Every 2 wk	5-20 mg	40 mg
Estradiol cypionate	Parenteral	Weekly	2 mg	5-10 mg
Testosterone[a]				
Testosterone cypionate	IM or SubQ injection	Weekly or every 2 wk	20–50 mg	100 mg (weekly)
Testosterone enanthate	IM or SubQ injection	Weekly or every 2 wk	20–50 mg	100 mg (weekly)
Testosterone patch	Transdermal	Daily	1-2 mg	8 mg
Testosterone topical gel 1%	Transdermal	Daily	12.5 mg	100 mg
Testosterone topical gel 1.62%	Transdermal	Daily	20.25–60.75 mg	103.25 mg
Testosterone axillary gel 2%	Transdermal	Daily	30–60 mg	90–120 mg

Abbreviation: SubQ, subcutaneous.

[a] Note that if inducing puberty in a patient who was blocked at Tanner (SMR) 2, dosing starts lower and increases more gradually, see Hembree et al[39] for additional instruction.

Irreversible

Gender-affirming surgeries can be divided into masculinizing and feminizing procedures. Desires for and decisions to pursue surgery may evolve over time. Masculinizing surgeries include bilateral mastectomy, hysterectomy with bilateral salpingo-oophorectomy, and vaginectomy with construction of a neophallus (via metioidioplasty or phalloplasty) and scrotum.[35,56] Additional masculinizing procedures include dermatologic fillers, pectoral implants, and liposuction.[35]

Feminizing surgeries include breast augmentation, orchiectomy, vulvoplasty, and creation of a neovagina with labioplasty and clitoroplasty.[35,56] Additional feminizing procedures include facial feminization surgery and tracheal shave as well as hair removal, dermatologic fillers, and removal or redistribution of fat tissue.[35,56] Chest surgery (ie, mastectomy or breast augmentation) has been shown to significantly reduce gender dysphoria in teens and is often performed before age 18 years; however, further surgeries are typically done only after a patient reaches adulthood.[57,58]

Any surgery involving removal of gonadal tissue requires patients to be of legal age to consent. Further study is needed to better understand long-term outcomes and sexual function associated with current affirming genital surgery techniques. This care is often limited to specialized centers with surgeons having training and expertise in these types of procedures and with additional cost barriers when care is not covered by insurance.[56,59]

DISCUSSION

Although gender-affirming care has traditionally been siloed in urban medical centers, the shift into primary care creates opportunities for improved access for TGDY. The addition of transgender care to health care curricula (medical, nursing, pharmacy, physician assistant, counseling, and so forth) in the United States and around the world, as well as a focus on expanded sexual and gender minority health concerns in continuing education for providers, has begun to create a medical workforce able to support this population.[60–62] It is important to remember that delaying affirming care is not a neutral option and can lead to worsening mental health outcomes. Numerous training opportunities and resources are available and listed in **Box 3**. Everyone should strive to ensure that their medical setting reflects their desire for inclusivity through displays, language, and paperwork. Primary care providers in

---

Box 3
Additional resources

Emergency/Crises Mental Health Resources
Trans Lifeline: US (877) 565-8860/Canada (877) 330-6366, https://www.translifeline.org
The Trevor Project: (866) 488-7386, https://www.thetrevorproject.org

Parent and Family Resources
PFLAG: https://pflag.org
TransYouth Equality: http://www.transyouthequality.org/for-parents
Human Rights Campaign: https://www.hrc.org/resoureces/resources-for-people-with-transgender-family-members
Family Acceptance Project: familyproject.sfsu.edu
Seattle Children's Hospital: https://www.seattlechildrens.org/clinics/gender-clinic/patient-family-resources/

Legal Resources
Transgender Law Center: info@transgenderlawcenter.org, www.transgenderlawcenter.org
The Name Change Project, Transgender Legal Defense, and Education Fund: http://www.tldef.org
National Center for Lesbian Rights: info@nclrights.org, www.nclrights.org
Lambda Legal: www.lambdalegal.org/trans-toolkit
Whitman-Walker: https://www.whitman-walker.org/legal-services

School Resources
GLSEN: https://www.glsen.org/safeschools
Human Rights Campaign: Welcoming Schools: http://www.welcomingschools.org/resources
National Center for Transgender Equality: https://transequality.org/issues/youth-students
GenderSpectrum: Schools in Transition: https://www.genderspectrum.org/studenttransitions

Provider Resources/Training Opportunities
GenderSpectrum: https://www.genderspectrum.org
UCSF Center for Excellence for Transgender Health: http://transhealth.ucsf.edu
World Professional Association for Transgender Health: https//www.wpath.org
The Endocrine Society: https://www.endocrine.org
Fenway Health: https//fenwayhealth.org
Philadelphia Trans Wellness Conference: http://www.mazzonicenter.org/trans-wellness
Reproductive Health Access Project: https://www.reproductiveaccess.org/wp-content/uploads/2018/06/bc-across-gender-spectrum.pdf

particular have incredible potential to improve health outcomes in TGDY and are encouraged to ensure they are prepared to support these amazing young people.

ACKNOWLEDGMENTS

The authors thank Dr Elizabeth Miller, Dr Joanna Bailey, Dr Trina Peduzzi, Dr Linda Nield, Dr Gerald Montano, David Lewis, Dr Gina Sequeira, Dr Christine Burt Solorzano, Alicyn Simpson, and Ehren Emter for their review of this article.

DISCLOSURE

The authors have nothing to disclose.

REFERENCES

1. Johns MM. Transgender identity and experiences of violence victimization, substance use, suicide risk, and sexual risk behaviors among high school students— 19 states and large urban school districts, 2017. MMWR Morb Mortal Wkly Rep 2019;68(3):67–71.
2. Olson KR, Gülgöz S. Early findings from the transyouth project: gender development in transgender children. Child Dev Perspect 2018;12(2):93–7.
3. Steensma TD, Kreukels BP, de Vries AL, et al. Gender identity development in adolescence. Horm Behav 2013;64(2):288–97.
4. Steensma TD, Biemond R, de Boer F, et al. Desisting and persisting gender dysphoria after childhood: a qualitative follow-up study. Clin Child Psychol 2010;16(4):499–516.
5. Priest M. Transgender children and the right to transition: medical ethics when parents mean well but cause harm. Am J Bioeth 2019;19(2):45–59.
6. Olson KR, Durwood L, DeMeules M, et al. Mental health of transgender children who are supported in their identities. Pediatrics 2016;137(3):e20153223.
7. Wallien MS, Cohen-Kettenis PT. Psychosexual outcome of gender-dysphoric children. J Am Acad Child Adolesc Psychiatry 2008;47(12):1413–23.
8. American Psychological Association. Diagnostic and statistical manual of mental disorders. 3rd edition. Washington, DC: Author; 1980.
9. American Psychological Association. Diagnostic and statistical manual of mental disorders. 3rd edition, rev. Washington, DC: Author; 1987.
10. American Psychological Association. Diagnostic and statistical manual of mental disorders. 4th edition. Washington, DC: Author; 1994.
11. American Psychological Association. Diagnostic and statistical manual of mental disorders. 4th edition, text rev. Washington, DC: Author; 2000.
12. Beek TF, Cohen-Kettenis PT, Kreukels BP. Gender incongruence/gender dysphoria and its classification history. Int Rev Psychiatry 2016;28(1):5–12.
13. Olson-Kennedy J, Cohen-Kettenis PT, Kruekels BP, et al. Research priorities for gender nonconforming/transgender youth: gender identity development and biopsychosocial outcomes. Curr Opin Endocrinol Diabetes Obes 2016;23(2):172.
14. Vance Jr SR, Cohen-Kettenis PT, Drescher J, et al. Opinions about the DSM gender identity disorder diagnosis: results from an international survey administered to organizations concerned with the welfare of transgender people. Int J Transgend; 2010.12(1):1–14.
15. American Psychological Association. Diagnostic and statistical manual of mental disorders. 5th edition. Washington, DC: Author; 2013.

16. Cohen-Kettenis PT, Klink D. Adolescents with gender dysphoria. Best Pract Res Clin Endocrinol Metab 2015;29:485–95.

17. Leibowitz S, de Vries AL. Gender dysphoria in adolescence. Int Rev Psychiatry 2016;28(1):21–35.

18. Peterson CM, Matthews A, Copps-Smith E, et al. Suicidality, self-harm, and body dissatisfaction in transgender adolescents and emerging adults with gender dysphoria. Suicide Life Threat Behav 2017;47(4):475–82.

19. Skagerberg E, Davidson S, Carmichael P. Internalizing and externalizing behaviors in a group of young people with gender dysphoria. Int J Transgend 2013; 14(3):105–12.

20. Choi SK, Wilson BD, Shelton J, et al. Serving our youth 2015: the needs and experiences of lesbian, gay, bisexual, transgender, and questioning youth experiencing homelessness. California: UCLA: The Williams Institute; 2015.

21. Bell K, Rieger E, Hirsch JK. Eating disorder symptoms and proneness in gay men, lesbian women, and transgender and non-conforming adults: comparative levels and a proposed mediational model. Front Psychol 2018;9:2692.

22. Donaldson AA, Hall AL, Neukirch J, et al. Exploring multidisciplinary treatment approaches for gender non-conforming adolescents with eating disorders: a case series. J Adolesc Health 2018;S49.

23. Hendricks ML, Testa RJ. A conceptual framework for clinical work with transgender and gender nonconforming clients: an adaptation of the Minority Stress Model. Professional Psychology: Research and Practice 2012;43(5):460.

24. Chan CD. Families as transformative allies to trans youth of color: positioning intersectionality as analysis to demarginalize political systems of oppression. J GLBT Fam Stud 2018;14(1–2):43–60.

25. Levin DA. Office-based care for lesbian, gay, bisexual, transgender, and questioning youth. Pediatrics 2013;132(1):e297–313.

26. Koehler A, Eyssel J, Nieder TO. Genders and individual treatment progress in non-binary trans individuals. J Sex Med 2017;15:102–13.

27. Clark BA, Veale JF, Townsend M, et al. Non-binary youth: access to gender-affirming primary health care. Int J Transgend 2018;12(2):158–69.

28. Goldbert AE, Kuvalanka KA. Navigating identity development and community belonging when "there are only two boxes to check": an exploratory study of nonbinary trans college students. J LGBT Youth 2018;15(2):106–31.

29. Shumer DE, Nokoff NJ, Spack NP. Advances in the care of transgender children and adolescents. Adv Pediatr 2016;63(1):79–102.

30. James SE, Herman JL, Rankin S, et al. Executive summary of the report of the 2015 U.S. transgender survey. Washington, DC: National Center for Transgender Equality; 2016.

31. Gridley SJ, Crouch JM, Evans Y, et al. Youth and caregiver perspectives on barriers to gender-affirming health care for transgender youth. J Adolesc Health 2016;59(3):254–61.

32. American Psychological Association. Guidelines for psychological practice with transgender and gender nonconforming people. Am Psychol 2015;70(9):832–64.

33. Meyer IH. Why lesbian, gay, bisexual, and transgender public health? Am J Public Health 2001;91(6):856.

34. Austin A, Craig SL. Transgender affirmative cognitive behavioral therapy: clinical considerations and applications. Professional Psychology: Research and Practice 2015;46(1):21.

35. Coleman E, Bockting W, Botzer M, et al. Standards of care for the health of trans-sexual, transgender, and gender-nonconforming people, version 7. Int J Trans-gend 2011;13:165–232.
36. de Vries AL, McGuire JK, Steensma TD, et al. Young adult psychological outcome after puberty suppression and gender reassignment. Pediatrics 2014;134(4): 696–704.
37. Russell ST, Pollitt AM, Li G, et al. Chosen name use is linked to reduced depres-sive symptoms, suicidal ideation, and suicidal behavior among transgender youth. J Adolesc Health 2018;99(12):4379–89.
38. Riley EA, Sitharthan G, Clemson L, et al. The needs of gender-variant children and their parents: a parent survey. Int J Sex Health 2011;3:181–95.
39. Hembree WC, Cohen-Kettenis PT, Gooren L, et al. Endocrine treatment of gender-dysphoric/gender-incongruent persons: an Endocrine Society clinical practice guideline. J Clin Endocrinol Metab 2017;102(11):3869–903.
40. Turban J, Ferraiolo T, Martin A, et al. Ten things transgender and gender noncon-forming youth want their doctors to know. J Am Acad Child Adolesc Psychiatry 2017;65(4):275–7.
41. Sequeira GM, Kidd K, Coulter RW, et al. Affirming Transgender Youths' Names and Pronouns in the Electronic Medical Record. JAMA pediatrics; 2020.
42. Deutsch MB, editor. Guidelines for the primary and gender-affirming care of transgender and gender nonbinary people. San Francisco (CA): University of California; 2016.
43. Grant JM, Mottet L, Tanis J, et al. National transgender discrimination survey report on health and health care. Milwaukee, WI; 2010.
44. Gatos KC. A literature review of cervical cancer screening in transgender men. Nurs Womens Health 2018;22(1):52–62.
45. Tota JE, Bentley J, Blake J, et al. Introduction of molecular HPV testing as the pri-mary technology in cervical cancer screening: acting on evidence to change the current paradigm. Preventative Med 2017;98:5–14.
46. Wright TC, Stoler MH, Behrens CM, et al. Primary cervical cancer screening with human papillomavirus: end of study results from the ATHENA study using HPV as the first-line screening test. Gynecol Oncol 2015;136(2):189–97.
47. Huh WK, Ault KA, Chelmow D, et al. Use of primary high-risk human papilloma-virus testing for cervical cancer screening: interim clinical guidance. Gynecol On-col 2015;136(2):178–82.
48. Rosenthal SM. Approach to the patient: transgender youth: endocrine consider-ations. J Clin Endocrinol Metab 2014;99(12):4379–89.
49. Hudson J, Nahata L, Dietz E, et al. Fertility counseling for transgender AYAs. Clin Pract Pediatr Psychol 2018;6(1):84.
50. Mattawanon N, Spencer JB, Schirmer DA, et al. Fertility preservation options in transgender people: a review. Rev Endocr Metab Disord 2018;19(3):231–42.
51. Conard LE. Supporting and caring for transgender and gender nonconforming youth in the urology practice. J Pediatr Urol 2017;12(3):300–4.
52. Peitzmeier S, Gardner I, Weinand J, et al. Health impact of chest binding among transgender adults: a community-engaged, cross-sectional study. Cult Health Sex 2017;19(1):64–75.
53. Olson-Kennedy J, Forcier M, Geffner ME, et al. Management of transgender and gender-diverse children and adolescents. Waltham, MA: UpToDate; 2018.
54. Neyman A, Fuqua JS, Eugster EA. Bicalutamide as an androgen blocker with secondary effect of promoting feminization in male-to-female transgender ado-lescents. J Adolesc Health 2019;64(4):544–6.

55. Olson J, Schrager SM, Clark LF, et al. Subcutaneous testosterone: an effective delivery mechanism for masculinizing young transgender men. LGBT Health 2014;1(3):165–7.
56. Zurada A, Salandy S, Roberts W, et al. The evolution of transgender surgery. Clin Anat 2018;31(6):878–86.
57. Olson-Kennedy J, Warus J, Okonta V. Chest reconstruction and chest dysphoria in transmasculine minors and young adults: comparisons of nonsurgical and postsurgical cohorts. JAMA Pediatr 2018;172(5):431–6.
58. Marinkovic M, Newfield RS. Chest reconstructive surgeries in transmasculine youth: experience from one pediatric center. Int J Transgend 2017;18(4):376–81.
59. Weissler JM, Chang BL, Carney MJ, et al. Gender-affirming surgery in persons with gender dysphoria. Plast Reconstr Surg 2018;141(3):388e–96e.
60. Noonan EG, Sawning S, Combs R, et al. Engaging the transgender community to improve medical education and prioritize healthcare initiatives. Teach Learn Med 2018;30(2):119–32.
61. Vance SR Jr, Deutsch MB, Rosenthal SM, et al. Enhancing pediatric trainees' and students' knowledge in providing care to transgender youth. J Adolesc Health 2017;60(4):425–30.
62. Kauth MR, Shipherd JC, Lindsay JA, et al. Teleconsultation and training of VHA providers on transgender care: Implementation of a multisite hub system. Telemed E Health 2015;21(12):1012–8.

Health Care for Refugee and Immigrant Adolescents

Carina M. Brown, MD[a], Lalitha Swaminathan, MBBS[b], Nadia T. Saif, MD[b],
Fern R. Hauck, MD, MS[b],*

KEYWORDS

- Refugees • Immigrants • Adolescents • Health care • Migration
- Medical examination • Medical screening • Mental health

KEY POINTS

- Adolescents are migrating to the United States in record numbers, and have unique health care needs and vulnerabilities.
- Refugees, a subset of immigrants, undergo predeparture medical screening before departure to the United States and postarrival screening, as mandated by the Centers for Disease Control and Prevention.
- Adequate medical follow-up and continuity of care after initial screening are essential to ensure identification and appropriate management of medical conditions, and to provide preventive health care and education.
- New migrants suffer from a multitude of acute and chronic medical conditions compounded by mental health and developmental conditions that may affect long term health.
- Cultural sensitivity and use of interpreters when indicated are essential to ensure that adolescents receive comprehensive medical and preventive treatment in an atmosphere in which the patients feel safe and welcomed.

INTRODUCTION

By the end of 2017, 68.5 million individuals were forcibly displaced from their homes due to persecution, conflict, violation of human rights, or violence.[1] Refugees accounted for 25.4 million of these displaced persons, the highest number ever on record; asylum seekers numbered 3.1 million. Refugees are persons who have been forced to flee their country because of a well-founded fear of persecution for reasons of race, religion, nationality, political opinion, or membership in a particular social group.[2] They are recognized under United Nations conventions and protocols and the United Nations High Commissioner for Refugees statutes as deserving of

[a] Department of Family Medicine, UNC-Chapel Hill, Cone Health Family Medicine Residency, 1125 North Church Street, Greensboro, NC 27401, USA; [b] Department of Family Medicine, University of Virginia, PO Box 800729, Charlottesville, VA 22908, USA
* Corresponding author.
E-mail address: FRH8E@hscmail.mcc.virginia.edu

Prim Care Clin Office Pract 47 (2020) 291–306
https://doi.org/10.1016/j.pop.2020.02.007
0095-4543/20/© 2020 Elsevier Inc. All rights reserved.

primarycare.theclinics.com

protection. The process for resettlement includes applying for admission to the United States, typically from a transition country that is outside their home country. The president, in consultation with Congress, sets the number of refugees allowed entry to the United States annually. The United States has historically welcomed more refugees than all other countries combined, but with the Trump Administration, the US numbers have fallen below those of the rest of the world (**Fig. 1**).[3] It is difficult to define rates of English proficiency for new arrivals. Data collected by the University of Virginia's International Family Medicine Clinic (IFMC), which has cared for refugees since 2002, indicate that approximately one-third of new arrivals speak English on arrival (K.O. Tanabe, personal communication, May 2, 2019).

Special Immigrant Visa (SIV)-holders are people who worked with US government agencies in Afghanistan or Iraq and who have been granted special status to leave their country because of fear of harm as a result of their employment. Laws enacted by Congress authorized the Department of State to issue visas beginning in 2008 for Iraqis and 2009 for Afghans. Subsequently, Congress enacted several amendments and statutes into law governing extensions and numbers permitted to apply for visas.[4] The larger program for Afghans is still active, with 4000 additional SIVs and their immediate family members authorized in fiscal year 2019. However, the Iraqi program stopped taking new applications in September 2014. SIV principals (those who were employed by the US government) tend to speak relatively good English, and based on their experiences and backgrounds, their needs and expectations can be different from those of refugees. However, they receive the same services on arrival to the United States as refugees.

Immigrants are non–US-born individuals who move to the United States to seek residence, either permanent or temporary. Legal immigration consists of several categories, including family-based immigration, employment-based immigration, and the diversity visa program.[5] The number of immigrants in each of these categories is determined solely by Congress. In 2017, immigrants numbered more than 44.5 million. Together with their US-born children, immigrants currently number approximately 89.4 million, or 28% of the total US population.[6] Mexican individuals account for approximately 25% of immigrants, the largest group, followed by Indian and Chinese

Number of refugees resettled in the U.S. falls below total from the rest of the world for the first time in 2017

Number of resettled refugees worldwide, in thousands

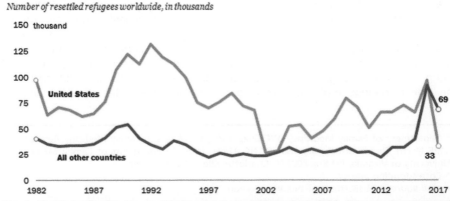

Fig. 1. Number of refugees resettled in the United States since 1992. (Source: Pew Research Center Analysis of United Nations High Commissioner for Refugees data, accessed June 27, 2018.)

individuals. The Pew Research Center estimates that, as of 2016, approximately one-quarter of the immigrants in the United States were undocumented.[7]

Asylees are persons already in the United States who seek protection on the same grounds as refugees. They may apply for asylum at their port of entry or within 1 year of arrival in the United States. There is no limit on the number of individuals who may be granted asylum in a given year. Refugees and asylees are eligible to become legal permanent residents after 1 year of arrival for refugees and after 1 year of receiving asylum.[5]

HEALTH EVALUATION OF REFUGEE AND IMMIGRANT ADOLESCENTS

The number of adolescents migrating to the United States has increased in recent years. They enter as refugees, asylum seekers, immigrants, student visa holders, and internationally adopted children. More than 40% of refugees are estimated to be <18 years old and approximately 30% of asylees are younger than 17.[8] Refugees and immigrants undergo mandatory medical screening before arrival to the United States through an organized system that is developed by the Centers for Disease Control and Prevention (CDC) and the Immigrant, Refugee, Migrant Health Branch of the Division of Global Migration and Quarantine. There is no standard medical screening for internationally adopted children or asylum seekers.[9] Adolescents who have migrated have unique health care needs and often are vulnerable to inequalities in health care caused by various factors, such as language and cultural barriers, underinsured parents, and limited awareness of school and vocational resources. It is important for health care providers to understand the overseas and postarrival medical screening of this population.

Overseas Medical Examination for Refugees

For refugees from most countries, a 3-step approach is applied for medical examination, as detailed in **Fig. 2**.

Visa medical examination

All US-bound refugees and immigrants applying for a visa undergo mandatory medical examination, which is performed according to CDC Technical Instructions.[10] Medical examinations are conducted by the local panel physicians appointed by US embassies in most countries. The purpose of the visa medical examination is to determine whether an applicant has a Class A or Class B condition. A Class A condition is a medical or psychiatric disorder, such as a communicable disease or substance use disorder, that precludes granting US entry. A Class B condition is a physical or mental disorder that may not prevent entry to the United States, but requires significant medical intervention, or may interfere with the applicant's ability to care for themselves, work, or attend school. This medical examination includes a full medical history, physical examination, mental status examination, screening for infections,

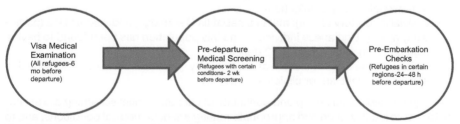

Fig. 2. Overseas medical examination process for refugees.

and appropriate immunizations. Unlike immigrant visa applicants, routine vaccination of refugees is not legally required at the time of initial admission to the United States. However, a vaccine program developed by the CDC for US-bound refugees encourages routine age-appropriate vaccination.[11]

Predeparture medical screening

Refugees with Class B1 conditions such as sputum-negative tuberculosis (TB) undergo history and physical examination by panel physicians, approximately 2 weeks before departure.[12] The process for tuberculosis screening is detailed separately.

Pre-embarkation checks

Only refugees from certain countries undergo preflight fitness checks and receive antihelminthic treatments, approximately 24 to 48 hours before travel.[12]

Postarrival Domestic Medical Screening

The CDC recommends medical screening for refugees within 30 days of arrival in the United States. Although medical screening is recommended for all migrants, many immigrants, students, and undocumented immigrants do not routinely receive this service. Internationally adopted children often receive medical evaluation on arrival through adoption clinics or primary care providers of the adoptive parents. Prearrival health evaluations are not comprehensive for refugee and immigrant children and provide limited information to the health care providers who see the children after arrival. These children often present with significant underlying medical or psychiatric conditions. Therefore, in-depth initial health screening is mandatory after arrival in the United States. The CDC has developed a comprehensive Domestic Screening Checklist, which has been implemented by local and state health departments and used by health care providers specializing in refugee care.[13,14]

The initial health screenings are specific to each state and are usually completed by health care providers in conjunction with the local health department and resettlement agencies. Initial refugee health screenings consist of review of available overseas health records, thorough medical history, physical examination, routine and specific laboratory tests, immunizations, and appropriate referrals. A general outline of the initial screening is summarized as follows:

- Medical: general history, physical examination (including vision and hearing), developmental and growth parameters, and immunizations
- Mental health screening for depression, anxiety, and posttraumatic stress disorder (PTSD)
- Routine laboratory testing: complete blood count with differential, urinalysis, chemistry panel, thyroid panel, hepatitis B serology, lead (6 months through 16 years of age), tuberculosis screening, human immunodeficiency virus (HIV), and syphilis and gonorrhea testing ($\geq$15 years of age unless there is suspicion or personal history of infection)
- Special laboratory testing: malaria, hepatitis C serology, and vitamin B12 (particularly among Bhutanese individuals, as this population has been found to have a high prevalence of vitamin B12 deficiency)
- Referrals as needed: vision, hearing, dentistry, psychiatric and behavioral health, specialists, dietician, or clinical pharmacist

Adequate medical follow-up and continuity of care after initial screening are essential to ensure identification and appropriate management of medical conditions, and to provide preventive health care and education. Primary care providers often work closely with a complex maze of support services, such as local health departments, resettlement agencies, volunteer organizations, and community and school support services while managing the health care needs of this special population. Providers also should be aware of the limited time that family benefits are available to new-comers, including stipends, vocational training, and health insurance, which usually lapse after 8 months of resettlement for refugees. Children younger than 19 years continue to receive health insurance coverage through the Children's Health Insurance Program, based on household income. Early interventions and referrals are recommended because of this problem of health care access and availability.

SPECIAL CONSIDERATIONS WHEN CARING FOR REFUGEE AND IMMIGRANT ADOLESCENTS

Refugee and immigrant adolescents have unique health needs as compared with those born in the United States. Refugee adolescents have been displaced from their homeland and suffer considerable repeat stress. Preflight, the time period before escaping an unstable home environment, often results in exposure to trauma and a disrupted education and social structure. Flight to a new location is often fraught with physical and psychological stressors as families escape their home country or region. Adolescents frequently miss months, or even years, of schooling due to war and lack of infrastructure. Finally, resettlement in a new country forces adolescents to learn a new system of beliefs and values.[15]

For both refugee and immigrant adolescents, acculturation includes 4 steps: initial contact, conflict, crisis, and adaptation.[14] Acculturation stress, defined as the stress emerging within the 4 steps of acculturation, can contribute to both physical and mental health conditions of adolescents.

For many immigrant and refugee families, the family unit serves as the basis for social support. Although this family dynamic can be disrupted as children and adolescents adopt new values and culture, in the initial immigration period, families provide emotional support for children and adolescents. In fact, the United Nations proposes that the single best way to promote the well-being of children is to support their family.[16] Although adolescence is a time of growing independence, supporting the family unit can ensure a happy, healthy teen.

For both adolescents and their families, health care services likely differ considerably from those available in their country of origin. Although some have access to acute care services, preventive services are frequently limited. The concept of preventive care and the complex network of health care providers can be difficult to manage and navigate. Families may overwhelm providers with concerns during initial visits, as they fear health care may be only seldom available. Finally, some families have unrealistic expectations of the health care provider or system, oftentimes expecting curative therapy for chronic or congenital conditions. Listening, asking, and then recognizing these perceptions of the health care system can help clinicians provide high-quality care for these patients.

COMMON MEDICAL CONDITIONS AMONG IMMIGRANT AND REFUGEE ADOLESCENTS

Before migration, many immigrant and refugee children and adolescents do not receive standard screening and preventive health services that most US citizens receive throughout childhood. Many children and adolescents experience limited access to food and safe water, as well as exposure to communicable diseases.

Infectious Diseases

Helicobacter pylori

Helicobacter pylori is a common bacterial infection among refugees and immigrants, predisposing adults to peptic ulcer disease and gastric cancer. The association of childhood and adolescent infection with gastric cancer has not been established. For refugees, there is no evidence of benefit of routine screening.[17] Most adolescents with *H pylori* remain entirely asymptomatic; a smaller proportion may develop abdominal pain, dyspepsia, and anorexia. Among adolescents with these symptoms, laboratory assessment with either a stool antigen test or urea breath test should be used rather than serologic testing, as this remains positive even after eradication of the organism.[18] The first-line therapy includes high-dose proton pump inhibitors in divided dosing, amoxicillin, and clarithromycin.

Hepatitis B

It is estimated that 3.5 million refugees worldwide have chronic hepatitis B infection, accounting for more than 700,000 cirrhosis-related deaths each year. Many immigrants and refugees come from areas of intermediate prevalence (2%–7% prevalence within the population) or high prevalence ($\geq$8%) of chronic hepatitis B infection.[19] Children and adolescents in endemic areas are commonly infected through perinatal transmission. Although many countries have implemented vaccination campaigns, acute and chronic infections continue to be identified.

Many countries now offer screening for hepatitis B with hepatitis B surface antigen (HbsAg) before departure.[19] For SIV holders and immigrants, no predeparture screening is performed. Those refugees with a positive HBsAg undergo further testing at the domestic medical examination. Those with negative HBsAg have the option to receive 2 doses of the hepatitis B vaccine before departure.[19]

On arrival, those adolescents without documented testing before departure should undergo serologic testing (**Table 1**). Those with 2 documented vaccinations should complete the series, whereas those with no documented vaccinations but nonimmune status should be offered vaccination.

For those with chronic hepatitis B infection, family members should receive 3 doses of the hepatitis B vaccine. Blood spills within the house should be cleaned with bleach and water (1 part bleach: 10 parts water) while wearing gloves. **Table 1** reviews serologic interpretation for hepatitis B along with appropriate management actions.

Mycobacterium tuberculosis

The prevalence of *Mycobacterium tuberculosis* infection among US citizens is falling, but the disease is seeing an increasing prevalence worldwide, with higher rates of extrapulmonary and drug-resistant infections. For adolescents undergoing predeparture refugee health examination, strict protocols are followed. For SIV holders and asylum seekers, no rigorous testing is performed. Adolescence represents a time of increased tuberculosis incidence and those ages 12 to 24 are most likely to be infected, as teens have a wide range of social contacts, often engage in risk-taking behavior, and may not adhere to therapy.[20]

Predeparture screening varies by the prevalence of *M tuberculosis* infection in the country of origin. In countries with fewer than 20 cases per 100,000 people, adolescents up to age 14 undergo testing if they have documented HIV infection or symptoms of active tuberculosis infection. Those with positive cultures must complete directly observed therapy before immigration. Children ages 2 to 14 years old in high-prevalence countries ($\geq$20 cases per 100,000) undergo interferon gamma release assay testing. Adolescents ages $\geq$15 years old undergo a detailed history and

Table 1
Interpretation and evaluation of hepatitis B serologies

HBsAg	Anti- HBc	Anti-HBs	Interpretation	Management
−	−	−	Never exposed, nonimmune to infection	Offer 3-dose vaccine series
−	+	+	Previously exposed ("natural infection"), immune	No further steps
+	+	−	Current infection	Obtain hepatitis B e-antigen, hepatitis B e-antibody, viral load, and refer to Pediatric Gastroenterology
−	−	+	Immune to hepatitis B due to vaccination	Complete vaccine series among those at risk for complications
−	+	−	Isolated positive hepatitis B core antibody 1. False positive 2. Early acute infection, resolving 3. Chronic infection with low-level viremia 4. Resolved infection (most common in refugees)	

Abbreviations: anti-HBc, hepatitis B core antibody; anti-HBs, hepatitis B surface antibody; HBsAg, hepatitis B surface antigen; +, positive result; -, negative result.

physical and receive a chest radiograph. Those adolescents with latent tuberculosis receive a waiver for travel and should be to be treated within 6 months of testing.[20]

Immigrants and refugees without prior testing overseas should be tested for tuberculosis (**Fig. 3**). The CDC provides guidance on treatment of both latent and active tuberculosis, which requires working with local health officials and infectious disease specialists.[21]

Hematologic Conditions

Anemia is common among refugees of all ages and ethnicities, with prevalence ranging from 19% among African refugees resettling in Australia to 37% among Southeast Asian refugees resettling in the United States.[22] Although iron-deficiency anemia is usually dietary, infectious diseases such as malaria and hookworm are also possible causes in refugee youth. Iron deficiency increases absorption of lead, so the CDC recommends lead testing of all refugees ages 6 months to 16 years on arrival to the United States and again 3 to 6 months later for children 6 months to 6 years old.[22] If initial complete blood count reveals a microcytic anemia, clinicians should obtain iron studies. If iron studies are normal or the anemia does not respond to therapy, the clinician should then obtain a hemoglobin electrophoresis to identify thalassemias or hemoglobinopathies.

Thalassemias are more prevalent in Southeast Asia (particularly the Philippines, Indonesia), India, Pakistan, the Middle East, Eastern Europe, and Africa and should be considered in cases of microcytic anemia.[14] Glucose-6-phosphate dehydrogenase deficiency is the most common inherited enzyme deficiency worldwide. It has a geographic distribution similar to the thalassemias but is particularly prevalent in Southeast Asia. Patients are usually asymptomatic until exposed to oxidizing medications, of which sulfa drugs, primaquine (for malaria), and dapsone (for leprosy) can be of particular concern in refugees. During acute hemolysis, laboratory tests show normocytic anemia, increased reticulocyte count, normal liver enzymes, and an elevated indirect bilirubin. Eosinophilia in a newly arrived refugee or immigrant (eosinophils >5% or an absolute eosinophil count >400 eosinophils/mm^3) can indicate parasitic infections, although allergies and drug reactions can cause this as well. One of the many possible causes of thrombocytopenia is infection, such as those that cause hypersplenism (eg, malaria, brucellosis, schistosomiasis, or visceral leishmaniasis). A careful history and examination along with tailored laboratory evaluation can aid clinicians in identifying the underlying etiology of such conditions.

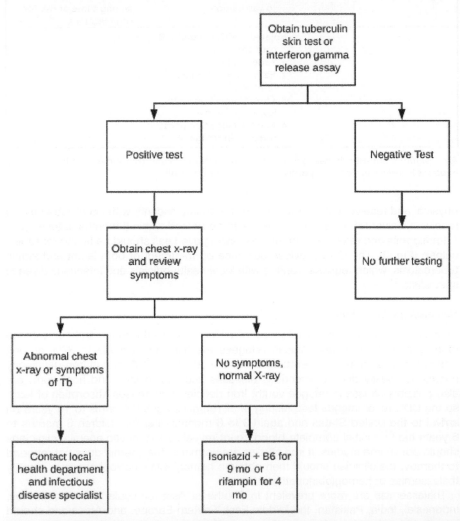

Fig. 3. Evaluation of newly arrived immigrants and refugees without documented tuberculosis testing. Tb, tuberculosis.

Nutrition Concerns

Overweight and obesity

Significant research has uncovered the pattern termed "the immigrant paradox," in which first-generation immigrants have lower prevalence of overweight and obesity than their native-born counterparts (cultural and linguistic isolation being a contributing factor). However, increased time of residency in the United States equalizes their rates of overweight and obesity to the native population due to the acculturation and adaptation process.[23] This pattern does not appear to apply uniformly to all immigrant youth necessarily: nationally representative data have shown that Asian immigrant children and adolescents have the lowest prevalence of obesity compared with other groups and the native-born population, whereas Latino youth have the highest.[24] The rising rates of worldwide overweight and obesity, along with changing socioeconomic status of immigrants to the United States, could affect the immigrant paradox trend. Interventions targeting sedentary behaviors to reduce obesity risk in immigrant youth are critical, as adolescence is a crucial period of transition and can affect health behaviors that persist into adulthood.

Nutritional deficiencies

Nutritional deficiencies are common among refugees and certain immigrant groups (**Table 2**).[25] In the dietary and social history, it is important to ask about prior periods of food insecurity and/or economic duress; intake of fruits, vegetables, and meat (cultural or religious exclusions may heighten suspicion for micronutrient deficiencies); and history of supplemental intake of specific micronutrients (vitamin A and/or zinc supplementation are provided in many settings in the developing world, making current deficiencies less likely).[25] An issue that may specifically affect immigrant nutritional status is that depending on immigration status, some families may be less likely to have access to federal assistance programs such as Temporary Assistance for Needy Families or Supplemental Nutrition Assistance Program, formerly known as the Food Stamp program.

Asthma and Allergic Conditions

Global findings from the International Study of Asthma and Allergies in Childhood show that migration from less affluent, lower-prevalence countries to more affluent, higher-prevalence Westernized countries is a protective factor for the development of asthma, rhinoconjunctivitis, and eczema.[26] Among adolescents specifically, migration after age 10 is protective, highlighting the protective effect of fewer years spent in the host country. Longer duration of residence in the Westernized country ultimately leads to immigrants acquiring similar rates of allergic diseases and asthma as those born in the host country.[27]

Mental Health Conditions

Previously published literature regarding immigrant children and adolescents cited lower rates of mental health conditions and behavioral health conditions, as well as higher rates of self-rated well-being.[28] This healthy immigrant hypothesis proposes that those immigrants with resilience and psychological well-being are more likely to immigrate. Others propose that the deeply rooted "familialism," represented by strong family values and bonding, results in lower rates of mental health conditions. Finally, immigrants and refugees may be less likely to report mental health conditions because of cultural differences in descriptions as well as stigma surrounding the disease in some cultures.[28] There are limited studies documenting the prevalence and incidence of mental health conditions among refugee teens. Although overall the prevalence of

Table 2
History and physical examination findings in children and adolescents and associated nutritional deficiencies

Nutrient Deficiency	Pertinent History	Signs and Symptoms
Severe undernutrition	Low food availability, change in behavior, chronic diarrhea	Emaciated appearance, marasmus (characterized by low body muscle mass, low body fat, thin hair), kwashiorkor (characterized by pitting peripheral edema)
Iron deficiency	Consumption of teas and phytates, low iron consumption	Low-grade cardiac flow murmur, pallor
Thiamine	Diet high in white rice, history of recurrent diarrhea	signs/symptoms of heart failure (S3 or S4, cardiomegaly, dyspnea, cough, edema)
Vitamin D (if severe can result in rickets)	Dark skin pigmentation, use of veil	Bone pain/tenderness, history of fractures or skeletal deformities, retarded growth, muscle weakness, craniotabes (thinning/softening of the skull in infants and children), costochondral swelling, dental problems
Zinc, niacin	Diet low in meat, fish, and nuts; high in corn	Dermatitis, diarrhea, stomatitis
Vitamin A	Vision change complaints, lack of vitamin A supplementation in refugee facility	Xerosis, Bitot spots (superficial buildup of keratin in the conjunctiva), poor night vision
Thiamine, niacin/tryptophan, B12	Bhutanese descent (B12 deficiency), limited access to fortified foods, limited intake of animal products, history of *Helicobacter pylori* infection	Neurologic issues: loss of proprioception, loss of deep tendon reflexes, ataxia, peripheral neuropathy
Iodine	Developing country without iodized salt	Palpable goiter

mental health conditions among refugee adolescents is unknown, small studies report markedly elevated rates of mental health conditions among refugee teens.[29]

For refugee teens ≥14 years old, the refugee health screener-15 has been validated to detect anxiety, depression, and PTSD. This can be performed at the initial domestic health screen, with sensitivity ranging from 81% to 95% and specificity ranging from 86% to 89%.[30]

Posttraumatic stress disorder and anxiety disorders
PTSD is a condition defined by exposure to a traumatic event with resulting distress and symptoms such as mood changes, hyperarousal, and sleep disturbance. PTSD and anxiety disorders commonly affect refugee teens. Trauma exposure can occur preflight, such as witnessing a family member's injury or death, while living in a refugee camp, or on arrival in a new country. In each instance, studies demonstrate a strong

relationship between the number of traumatic events and resulting PTSD symptoms.[29] Adolescents are more likely to be exposed to trauma, as they tend to venture outside the home frequently and may have persistent symptoms for many years after exposure. Symptoms of PTSD can vary considerably among patients. Some manifest more depressive symptoms (eg, sadness), whereas others demonstrate somatic symptoms, hyperarousal, or avoidance of triggers.

Effective treatment of PTSD includes a multidisciplinary approach, often involving the family, therapists, psychiatrists, primary care physicians, and school counselors. Successful components of PTSD care for refugees have been found to include care coordination, cultural sensitivity, and a multidisciplinary approach.[31]

Other common mental health conditions
Immigrants and refugees experience higher rates of depression, generalized anxiety, and somatic symptoms (**Table 3**).[29,31–33]

PREVENTIVE CARE

Immigrant and refugee families, depending on their background, may not be familiar with the concept of preventive care. Providers should use initial visits to familiarize them with this concept. When indicated, providers should tell adolescent patients and their parents to expect more frequent visits initially to catch up on routine care, as well as to follow up on chronic issues. During these visits, providers also can work to connect families with social safety-net services as necessary. Sports physicals can be an important tool and opportunity to address follow-up of chronic concerns and provide anticipatory guidance for youth who do not regularly present to care otherwise.

As with nonrefugee and nonimmigrant patients, primary care providers should review all previous immunization records and provide age-appropriate vaccinations and catch-up vaccinations as recommended by the CDC. In most cases, if records are unavailable, it is more cost-effective to vaccinate rather than obtain titers, except in the case of varicella zoster virus and hepatitis B. Varicella immunoglobulin G and hepatitis B serologies should be obtained before vaccinating.[34]

DENTAL CARE

Dental problems in refugees may be related to dietary issues, poor access to oral health services, or a history of torture or trauma. Limited access to dental care is

Table 3
Common mental health conditions among adolescent refugees and immigrants

Mental Health Condition	Signs and Symptoms	Treatment Approach
Major depressive disorder	Low mood, poor sleep, sense of worthlessness, suicidal ideation	Multidisciplinary approach, involving medications, therapists, family, and psychiatry
Generalized anxiety disorder	Poor sleep, panic symptoms, constantly worrying	Cognitive behavioral therapy, medication, family support
Somatic symptom disorder	Six months of a multitude of bodily symptoms associated with significant distress	Close coordination of care and frequent visits with primary care provider to limit overtesting, behavioral therapy

widespread among immigrants in general, especially those lacking health insurance. Poor dentition can indicate consumption of refined sugars and betel nuts (consumed across many age groups and cultures worldwide, especially Southeast Asia), poor oral care, and possibly vitamin D deficiency.[34] Primary care physicians should ask whether an adolescent has a dental home at every well-child visit, and have information available for referrals to local dentist offices that accept Medicaid or provide low-cost services.

ANTICIPATORY GUIDANCE
Bullying

Both first-generation immigrant and refugee adolescents experience far higher rates of bullying than native counterparts. One study found a strong family unit, diverse school population, and sense of safety at school were associated with lower rates of bullying.[35] Providing anticipatory guidance during initial visits and well-child checks, as well as discussing positive parenting skills, can help reduce the physical and emotional stress of bullying.

Substance Abuse

Although most research has been focused on Latino adolescents, it can be useful for providers to understand adolescent immigrant trends in substance abuse more generally. Researchers have cited the immigrant paradox to explain why foreign-born Latino adolescents tend to report lower rates of cigarette, alcohol, and drug use than their native-born peers.[36] Protective factors against substance abuse within Latino immigrant families include family-oriented cultural values and respect for elders, values that are prominent in other immigrant groups as well, such as Asian American families.[37,38] The process of acculturation and adaptation to the United States in adolescence can introduce stressors, which can undermine the protective effect of immigrant families' parenting practices.[36] For example, perceived discrimination is thought to be a risk factor for immigrant adolescent substance abuse, but the intricacies of this relationship are unclear. Clinicians should inquire about substance use and engage adolescents and families in a discussion about the harms of substance use.

Sexual Behavior

Most research, which again has been focused on Latino adolescents, shows that foreign-born youth have a lower rate of sexual initiation than native-born youth.[39] Some immigrant families, depending on cultural or religious beliefs, may hold conservative sexual values and strongly discourage sex outside of marriage. Some families may be particularly strict regarding gender relations for their daughters. In a diverse sample of 200 low-income immigrant youth in the United States, perception of a supportive community was associated with lower odds of intentions to have sex and sexual experience. This is consistent with prior research on neighborhood context; unsurprisingly, neighborhood poverty is associated with risky sexual behavior among youth.[39]

INTERPRETER USE

Title VI of the Civil Rights Act mandates all physicians who accept patients with federal payers (except certain small practices) to provide professional interpretation services to those patients with limited English proficiency (defined as individuals who do not speak English as their primary language and have limited ability to read, write, or understand the language).[40] Recommendations for appropriate use of interpreters include seating the interpreter next to or slightly behind the patient, addressing the patient directly, and using sentence-by-sentence interpretation with short statements.

Despite the legal requirement for interpreter services, services may not be available, or patients may decline using them. Parents and providers may rely on adolescents to serve as the interpreter for parents during the adolescent's visit. This may be tempting, but providers should avoid this whenever possible because it places undue burden on the adolescent when the focus of the visit should be on them. In addition, the adolescent may not thoroughly relay all aspects of the conversation to their parents, preventing parents from meaningfully participating in their child's care. For these reasons, families should be encouraged to accept interpreter services for all office visits.

PREDICTORS OF SUCCESS

Refugee and immigrant adolescents face a number of barriers to success after resettlement, including lack of academic support at home, acculturation stress, and limited proficiency in the dominant language. Some studies have demonstrated that different groups of adolescent refugees achieve differing levels of academic success.[41] One such study found Vietnamese teens were more likely to achieve academic success than those from Lao, Khmer, or Hmong backgrounds.[41] Being female, and having better English proficiency and lower baseline levels of psychological stress correlate with later academic success.[41] School safety, a sense of security, and school connectedness also have been postulated to predict academic success. Providing families and adolescents with community-based services to reduce acculturative stress may also increase the likelihood of academic success and improved health outcomes.

MODELS OF CARE

Given the complexity of immigrant and refugee health care, a number of models of care have been described. Primary health care remains a cornerstone of these models of care, often with other key features, such as easy access to services, readily available interpretive services, and coordination of care with the health care team and other services. We describe the current model of care at the IFMC as one example of the many successful models of primary care.[42]

The IFMC has served refugees and special immigrants of all ages since 2002. The clinic is located within the outpatient Family Medicine practice and includes family physicians, psychiatrists, psychologists, nurse practitioners, a nurse care coordinator, a social worker, a pharmacist, nursing staff, and access staff working together to provide comprehensive care to all patients. The IFMC works closely with the local health department and local relocation organization, the International Rescue Committee. Each newly arrived refugee and special immigrant undergoes a health assessment at the local health department within 30 days of arrival, followed by a full primary care evaluation by a family physician or nurse practitioner in the IFMC clinic, who then continues to provide ongoing primary health care. The IFMC approach to care involves a wide variety of team members to provide comprehensive, high-quality care to this vulnerable population.

DISCLOSURE

The authors have nothing to disclose.

REFERENCES

1. United Nations High Commissioner for Refugees. Refugee statistics. Available at: https://www.unrefugees.org/refugee-facts/statistics. Accessed May 23, 2019.
2. United Nations High Commissioner for Refugees. Refugee facts. Available at: https://www.unrefugees.org/refugee-facts/what-is-a-refugee. Accessed May 23,2019.
3. Connor P, Krogstad J. For the first time, U.S. resettles fewer refugees than the rest of the world. Pew Research Center. Available at: https://www.pewresearch.org/fact-tank/2018/07/05/for-the-first-time-u-s-resettles-fewer-refugees-than-the-rest-of-the-world. Accessed June 3, 2019.
4. United State Department of State. US visas for Iraqi and Afghan translators/interpreters. Available at: https://travel.state.gov/content/travel/en/us-visas/immigrate/siv-iraqi-afghan-translators-interpreters.html. Accessed May 23, 2019.
5. American Immigration Council. Fact sheet: how the United States immigration system works. 2016. Available at: https://www.americanimmigrationcouncil.org/research/how-united-states-immigration-system-works. Accessed May 23, 2019.
6. Migration Policy Institute. Frequently requested statistics on immigrants and immigration in the United States. 2019. Available at: https://www.migrationpolicy.org/article/frequently-requested-statistics-immigrants-and-immigration-united-states#Now. Accessed May 23, 2019.
7. Passel J, Cohn D. U.S. unauthorized immigrant total dips to lowest level in a decade. Pew Research Center. 2018. Available at: https://www.pewhispanic.org/2018/11/27/u-s-unauthorized-immigrant-total-dips-to-lowest-level-in-a-decade. Accessed May 23, 2019.
8. Department of Homeland Security, Office of Immigration Statistics. Annual flow report refugees and asylees 2017. 2019. Available at: https://www.dhs.gov/sites/default/files/publications/Refugees_Asylees_2017.pdf. Accessed June 5, 2019.
9. Hostetter MK. Medical evaluation of internationally adopted children. N Engl J Med 1991;325:479–85.
10. Centers for Disease Control and Prevention. Technical instructions for panel physicians. 2017. Available at: https://www.cdc.gov/immigrantrefugeehealth/exams/ti/panel/technical-instructions-panel-physicians. Accessed June 5, 2019.
11. Centers for Disease Control and Prevention. Vaccination program for US-Bound refugees. 2019. Available at: https://www.cdc.gov/immigrantrefugeehealth/guidelines/overseas/interventions/immunizations-schedules.html. Accessed June 5, 2019.
12. Centers for Disease Control. Refugee health guidelines. 2012. Available at: https://www.cdc.gov/immigrantrefugeehealth/guidelines/refugee-guidelines.html. Accessed June 5, 2019.
13. Center for Disease Control. Summary checklist for domestic medical examination of newly arrived refugees. 2012. Available at: https://www.cdc.gov/immigrantrefugeehealth/pdf/checklist-refugee-health.pdf. Accessed June 5, 2019.
14. Stauffer W. Medical screening of immigrant children. Clin Pediatr 2003;42(9):763–73.
15. Lustig SL, Kia-Keating M, Grant-Knight W, et al. Review of child and adolescent refugee mental health national center for child traumatic stress. J Am Acad Child Adolesc Psychiatry 2004;43(10):24–36.

16. United Nations Commissioner on Refugee Health. Refugee children: guidelines on protection and care preface. Available at: https://www.unhcr.org/protect/PROTECTION/3b84c6c67.pdf. Accessed March 24, 2019.
17. Morais S, Costa AR, Ferro A, et al. Contemporary migration patterns in the prevalence of *Helicobacter pylori* infection: a systematic review. Helicobacter 2017; 22(3):e12372.
18. Crowley E, Bourke B, Hussey S. How to use *Helicobacter pylori* testing in paediatric practice. Arch Dis Child Educ Pract Ed 2013;98(1):18–25.
19. Centers for Disease Control and Prevention. Screening for viral hepatitis during the domestic medical examination of newly arrived refugees. 2019. Available at: https://www.cdc.gov/immigrantrefugeehealth/guidelines/domestic/hepatitis-screening-guidelines.html. Accessed March 17, 2019.
20. Centers for Disease Control and Prevention. Guidelines for screening for tuberculosis infection and disease during the domestic medical examination for newly arrived refugees. 2019. Available at: https://www.cdc.gov/immigrantrefugeehealth/guidelines/domestic/tuberculosis-guidelines. Accessed March 24, 2019.
21. Borisov AS, Bamrah Morris S, Njie GJ, et al. Update of recommendations for use of once-weekly isoniazid-rifapentine regimen to treat latent *Mycobacterium tuberculosis* infection. MMWR Morb Mortal Wkly Rep 2018;67(25):723–6.
22. Centers for Disease Control and Prevention. Complete blood count with red blood cell indices, white blood cell differential, and platelet count. 2016. Available at: https://www.cdc.gov/immigrantrefugeehealth/guidelines/domestic/general/discussion/complete-blood-count.html. Accessed June 5, 2019.
23. McCullough MB, Marks AK. The immigrant paradox and adolescent obesity. J Dev Behav Pediatr 2014;35(2):138–43.
24. Singh G, Yu S, Kogan M. Health, chronic conditions, and behavioral risk disparities among U.S. Immigrant children and adolescents. Public Health Rep 2013; 128(6):463–79.
25. Centers for Disease Control and Prevention. Guidelines for the evaluation of the nutritional status and growth in refugee children during the domestic medical screening examination 2012. Accessed June 5, 2019. Available at: https://www.cdc.gov/immigrantrefugeehealth/pdf/nutrition-growth.pdf.
26. Garcia-Marcos L, Robertson CF, Anderson HR, et al. Does migration affect asthma, rhinoconjunctivitis and eczema prevalence? Global findings from the international study of asthma and allergies in childhood. Int J Epidemiol 2014;43(6): 1846–54.
27. Silverberg JI, Simpson EL, Durkin HG, et al. Prevalence of allergic disease in foreign-born American children. JAMA Pediatr 2013;167(6):554–60.
28. Filion N, Fenelon A, Boudreaux M. Immigration, citizenship, and the mental health of adolescents. PLoS One 2018;13(5):e0196859.
29. Reavell J, Fazil Q. The epidemiology of PTSD and depression in refugee minors who have resettled in developed countries. J Ment Health 2017;26(1):74–83.
30. Hollifield M, Verbillis-Kolp SWB, Farmer B, et al. The Refugee Health Screener-15 (RHS-15): development and validation of an instrument for anxiety, depression, and PTSD in refugees. Gen Hosp Psychiatry 2013;35(2):202–9.
31. McColl H, McKenzie K, Bhui K. Mental healthcare of asylum-seekers and refugees. Adv Psychiatr Treat 2008;14(6):452–9.
32. McCann TV, Mugavin J, Renzaho A, et al. Sub-Saharan African migrant youths' help-seeking barriers and facilitators for mental health and substance use problems: a qualitative study. BMC Psychiatry 2016;16:275.

33. Rohlof H, Knipscheer J, Kleber R. Somatization in refugees: a review. Social Psychiatry Psychiatr Epidemiol 2014;49(11):1793–804.
34. Mishori R, Aleinikoff S, Davis D. Primary care for refugees: challenges and opportunities. Am Fam Physician 2017;96(2):112–20.
35. Pottie K, Dahal G, Georgiades K, et al. Do first generation immigrant adolescents face higher rates of bullying, violence and suicidal behaviors than do third generation and minority born? J Immigr Minor Health 2015;17(5):1557–66.
36. Vega WA, Alderete E, Kolody B, et al. Illicit drug use among Mexicans and Mexican Americans in California: the effects of gender and acculturation. Addiction 1998;93(12):1839–50.
37. Germán M, Gonzales NA, Dumka L. Familism values as a protective factor for Mexican-origin adolescents exposed to deviant peers. J Early Adolesc 2009; 29(1):16–42.
38. Wang M, Kviz FJ, Miller AM. The mediating role of parent-child bonding to prevent adolescent alcohol abuse among Asian American families. J Immigr Minor Heal 2012;14(5):831–40.
39. Coleman-Minahan K, Chavez M, Bull S. Immigrant generation and sexual initiation among a diverse racial and ethnic group of urban youth. J Immigr Minor Heal 2017;19(6):1412–9.
40. Juckett G, Unger K. Appropriate use of medical interpreters. Am Fam Physician 2014;90(7):476–80.
41. Wong CWS, Schweitzer RD. Individual, premigration and postsettlement factors, and academic achievement in adolescents from refugee backgrounds: a systematic review and model. Transcult Psychiatry 2017;54(5):756–82.
42. Elmore CE, Tingen JM, Fredgren K, et al. Using an interprofessional team to provide refugee healthcare in an academic medical centre. Fam Med Com Health 2019;7:e000091.

Human Trafficking in Adolescents
Adopting a Youth-centered Approach to Identification and Services

Julia Einbond, JD[a],*, Angela Diaz, MD, PhD, MPH[b],
Anastasia Cossette, BA[a], Rosalyn Scriven, JD[a],
Silvia Blaustein, MD[b], Martha R. Arden, MD[b]

KEYWORDS

- Human trafficking • Adolescents • Youth-centered approach
- Trauma-informed care • Resilience • Primary care

KEY POINTS

- A majority of trafficked individuals access medical care during their victimization, but they rarely are identified by health care providers or hospitals.
- Using a youth-centered approach to serve clients in nontraditional primary care settings, 2 organizations—Mount Sinai Adolescent Health Center and Covenant House New Jersey—illustrate the ways in which this approach succeeds at identifying and serving youth who have experienced human trafficking.
- The 2 central features that characterize these agencies' youth-centered approach to service delivery are immediacy and relationships, and these are sustained by privacy and choice.
- Primary care providers adopt youth-centered approaches have the opportunity to remove obstacles to safety and treatment of survivors of human trafficking, who already have remained invisible for too long.

INTRODUCTION

Commercial sexual exploitation and sex trafficking of children are major global public health issues,[1] which has been increasingly recognized as also occurring domestically in the United States. Recent research has shown that a majority of human trafficking survivors interact with medical providers while they are being victimized,[2] and approximately half of survivors who were seen by medical providers were seeking primary care services.[2] Adolescents, in particular those who have been homeless, sexually

[a] Covenant House New Jersey, 330 Washington Street, Newark, NJ 07102, USA; [b] Department of Pediatrics, Icahn School of Medicine at Mount Sinai, Mount Sinai Adolescent Health Center (MSAHC), 320 East 94th Street, New York, NY 10128, USA
* Corresponding author.
E-mail address: jeinbond@covenanthouse.org

Prim Care Clin Office Pract 47 (2020) 307–319
https://doi.org/10.1016/j.pop.2020.02.008

abused, or exposed to other childhood trauma, have increased risk of human trafficking.[3] Health care professionals have reported a lack of training or resources for identifying trafficking, and lack of knowledge and training on how to assess and treat victims of trafficking, as major barriers to supporting patients who are victims of trafficking.[4]

Trained or not, and ready or not, providers who are treating adolescent patients who are experiencing human trafficking, are uniquely positioned to connect survivors to existing protection and treatment resources. By sharing the experiences of the Mount Sinai Adolescent Health Center (MSAHC) and Covenant House New Jersey (CHNJ), the authors hope to further the conversation on how the primary care community can adapt these interventions for adolescent patients who have experienced human trafficking and become key personnel on the frontline of recovery and prevention.

Definition of Human Trafficking

The United States Trafficking Victim Protection Act of 2000, reauthorized multiple times, including most recently 2017, defines human trafficking as

- The recruitment, harboring, transportation, obtaining, and/or provision of a person or persons, by the use of force, fraud, and/or coercion, for the purpose(s) of labor and/or sexual exploitation.
- The "force, fraud, and/or coercion" element is de facto satisfied if the victimized is under the age of 18 and engaged in commercial sexual activity.[5]

Human trafficking, sometimes referred to as "modern slavery," is not a new crime in the United States but it has remained largely invisible, because traffickers use force, fraud, and/or coercion to make victims too fearful of reporting their abuses. Sensational media coverage focuses primarily on global trafficking rings, shaping public perception of trafficking as a distant problem. In reality, human trafficking takes many forms and victims span all genders, ages, ethnicities, and nationalities. Labor trafficking occurs in legal fields, including the agriculture and food service industries, as well as illicit industries, such as drug trafficking. Commercial sex acts that may constitute sex trafficking may involve a third-party pimp or may be a forced sex act in a 1-on-1 encounter. An experience that may begin as consensual sex acts (a form of grooming) can be transformed into forced encounters by the trafficker. The commercial aspect of trafficking is not limited to monetary payment; a victim may be compensated by food, clothing, shelter, drugs, or something else of value.

A comprehensive typology of the 25 forms of human trafficking that are known to occur in the United States is a useful reference available on the Polaris Web site.[6] The US government provides tools to apply the federal definition of human trafficking, including the Action-Means-Purpose Model (**Table 1**).[7] Ultimately, the determination that a person is trafficked is made by law enforcement or another expert trained to identify human trafficking. The role of the medical profession is to become familiar enough with the definition of human trafficking and the common ways in which it presents so as to refer or report suspected survivors to appropriate providers. The National Human Trafficking Hotline (1-888-373-7888 or https://humantraffickinghotline.org/), operated by Polaris, is a first-line response available 24/7 to assist in identification and support.

Primary health care of adolescent human trafficking survivors and under-identification by health care providers

A majority of trafficked individuals access medical care during their victimization, while these victims are by and large still unknown to other helping professionals, including

Table 1
Action-means-purpose model

Action	Means	Purpose
Recruiting includes proactive targeting of vulnerability and grooming behaviors *Harboring* includes isolation, confinement, and monitoring. *Transporting* includes movement and arranging travel. *Providing* includes giving to another individual. *Obtaining* includes forcibly taking or exchanging something for ability to control. *Soliciting* includes offering something of value.[a] *Patronizing* includes receiving something of value.[a]	*Force* includes physical restraint, physical harm, sexual assault, and beatings. Monitoring and confinement often are used to control victims, especially during early stages of victimization to break down a victim's resistance. *Fraud* includes false promises regarding employment, wages, working conditions, love, marriage, or better life. Over time, there may be unexpected changes in work conditions, compensation or debt agreements, or nature of relationship. *Coercion* includes threats of serious harm to or physical restraint against any person, psychological manipulation, document confiscation, and shame-inducing and fear-inducing threats to share information or pictures with others or report to authorities.	*Commercial sex act* is any sex act on account of anything of value given to or received by any person. *Involuntary servitude* is any scheme, plan, or pattern intended to cause a person to believe that, if the person did not enter into or continue in such condition, that person or another person would suffer serious harm or physical restraint; or the abuse or threatened abuse of the legal process. *Debt bondage* includes a pledge of services by the debtor or someone under debtor's control to pay down known or unknown charges (eg, fees for transportation, boarding, food, and other incidentals; interest, fines for missing quotas, and charges for bad behavior). The length and nature of those services are not respectively limited and defined, where an individual is trapped in a cycle of debt that he or she can never pay down. *Peonage* is a status or condition of involuntary servitude based on real or alleged indebtedness. *Slavery* is the state of being under the ownership or control of someone where a person is forced to work for another.

[a] Only for sex trafficking.
Does Not Need to Be Present in a Situation of Sex Trafficking of Minors

law enforcement.[8–10] In a study conducted by Chisolm-Straker and colleagues,[2] 73% of survivors wanted to receive medical care while being trafficked and 68% of survivors actually visited a medical provider during their trafficking experience. Nearly half of those, or 44.4%, who saw a medical provider, sought primary care.[2] This high percentage is not surprising: trafficking survivors experience many health needs and adverse health outcomes, including "unintended pregnancies and sexually-transmitted infections, physical pain and injury, a wide range of mental and behavioral health problems, and chronic diseases."[11] Kaplan and colleagues[12] highlight the needs for underage domestic sex trafficking survivors to get medical care including comprehensive physical examination, sexually transmitted infection (STIs) testing and treatment, and pregnancy prevention.

Unfortunately, trafficking survivors rarely are identified by health care workers or hospitals. In research conducted by and Covenant House New Jersey (CHNJ) between 2015 and 2017, almost one-third (30.1%) of homeless youth who had a prior trafficking experience had received medical care, mainly from hospitals and clinics—but none of those youth disclosed facts that would have led a professional to determine that they were trafficked.[13]

The problem of under-identification can be attributed to multiple causes, including the lack of knowledge and training among health care professionals about human trafficking, the reluctance of victims to spontaneously disclose their experiences to professionals, and the limited use of validated screening tools to aid in identification. Without identification, survivors lack access to treatment and protection needed to escape or recover from trafficking experiences, and professionals lack the information needed to bring more victims to safety. Two specialized clinical settings, MSAHC and CHNJ, have vast experience using a youth-centered approach to identify and serve once-invisible survivors.

NONTRADITIONAL MODELS
Mount Sinai Adolescent Health Center Service Model

The MSAHC opened in 1968, with a part-time physician and a social worker providing integrated medical and behavioral health services 1 day per week. Over the years, the program has grown into a very large, youth-specific, full-time program open 6 days per week. The youths have access 24/7 to a physician on call. The services provided are holistic, comprehensive, and integrated medical care; sexual and reproductive health; dental, optical, and health education; and behavioral and mental health services. More than 12,000 young people ages 10 to 24 (and their children, if they have children) received services in 2018. Most youth connect with services by word of mouth from other youth or social media, but many are referred by parents, schools, and community organizations. The services are confidential and at no cost to the young people.

Covenant House New Jersey Service Model

Serving homeless youth for 30 years, CHNJ works with youth collaboratively and holistically. CHNJ, along with Covenant Houses in 31 cities across the United States, Central America, and Canada, provides wraparound services, including housing, clothing, food, legal aid, mental health counseling, and basic health care to youth ranging from ages 13 to 24. In the 2018 fiscal year (FY), Covenant House International served approximately 34,000 youth in residential and nonresidential/drop-in programs. Young people commonly find Covenant House through Covenant House Street Outreach efforts; drop-in center contacts; referrals from community partners, community members, and Covenant House alumni; foster care systems; and Internet searches. On any given night, CHNJ serves more than 200 youth and their infants with overnight beds. Newark and Atlantic City, in New Jersey, jointly care for more than 500 youth annually in the main Crisis Centers.

SUCCESS OF A YOUTH-CENTERED APPROACH

The developmental needs of adolescents are central considerations in the youth-centered approach to care at MSAHC and CHNJ.[14,15] These programs also recognize the needs of trauma survivors, building on their strengths and resiliency when addressing the long-term consequences of trauma (eg, anger, depression, fearfulness, hopelessness, poor self-image, distrust of the environment, and difficulty maintaining healthy interpersonal relationships).[16–18] Traumatic experiences can alter the brain in ways that cause inherent distrust of others, specifically those in a helper role, and youth who have experienced this trauma are likely to experience resentment toward systems for failing to protect them.[19] Trauma-informed care, or trauma-informed approaches, is used to reframe programs and systems to address trauma survivors from a perspective of what happened to them, instead of what is wrong with them, and is seen as essential to quality care.[20,21] For the authors, this means meeting young people where they are: removing barriers to entry into services, responding quickly to needs, respecting them, welcoming them, and helping them feel connected, safe, and not judged. In tailoring services to youth affected by trauma, the authors always are alert to the possibility of a trauma history and are sensitive to the effects that trauma history can have on the utilization of and reaction to health care services. This includes giving youth choices of which services they accept when, allowing friends to join them for parts of their visit, talking them slowly through more invasive parts of the examination, and, in general, letting them be in control of their care whenever possible.

The 2 central features that characterize the authors' agencies' youth-centered approach to service delivery are immediacy and relationships, and these are sustained by privacy and choice. The authors recognize that each client, and each interaction with each client, presents both short-term and longer-term needs. These needs must be addressed immediately and sensitively in order to build trust, and trust is dependent on the development of relationships.

The provider has the challenge of creating a trusting relationship with a client who may have learned to withhold trust as a survival strategy in interactions with new systems and adults in positions of power. Trust is the cornerstone of work in any field, medical or otherwise, with adolescent clients who have been chronically exposed to unsafe environments and experienced trauma. Without trust, trafficked clients do not disclose their experiences that permit discovery of medical risks. Lack of trust also contributes to not adhering to recommended testing, treatments, and follow-up appointments. The authors' 2 organizations follow the 2 universal principles of privacy and choice, to build trust.

Immediacy

In general, trafficking survivors do not present asking for help to escape trafficking. They often seek medical attention for a condition directly or indirectly caused by their trafficking experience, which could be anything from an STI to a sprained ankle. Their immediate need is known and specific, and it is the first opportunity for a primary care provider to engage the client.

A successful first interaction provides the client with the experience of having at least one instance of having been heard and having their needs immediately addressed. By establishing reliability and credibility from the beginning with clients, this interaction can be used as a gateway to identify other concrete and immediate needs and to provide more solutions clients may not have known were available, such as food, clothing appropriate for weather, safety, and shelter. This is key to being youth centered: making young clients feel welcome and letting them see that their expressed needs are important, even if they are not what providers might think they need. Young people are incredibly intuitive and direct—they can sense if staff can provide them with what they need, and if they do not, they will leave and find someone else who will.

Not all programs need this breadth of services to provide immediacy. Many aspects of immediacy can be built into the design of primary care centers. For the authors' programs, access to immediacy begins with the location and physical spaces of the centers:

- Easily identifiable buildings at street level with signage bearing their names
- Locations in urban areas close to public transportation
- Open walk-in and phone lines for same-day services, even for new clients
- Young clients can come alone or bring an adult to accompany them
- 24/7 availability of shelter or physician call assistance
- Outreach teams
- Safe spaces, with interior doors that are accessible only with permission of entry
- Options to leave at any time with the possibility of returning for services at a later time

Immediacy also is supported by no-cost services. MSAHC and CHNJ are 100% free of cost to clients. Health insurance is not required. The ability to provide free services avoids delays caused by preauthorization and conversations about ability to pay, factors that survivors identify as causes for their not seeking care.[22] Additionally, the 2 organizations cover indirect costs that may be barriers to receiving services, such as transportation (eg, bus and subway fare cards). The ability to provide no-cost services is achieved through a mix of public and private funding. Increasingly, funders are interested in supporting antitrafficking services, including, notably, the federal government, which, in FY2018, made more than $30 million available to service providers through Department of Justice grants alone.[23]

Co-located services—services covering multiple needs in the same building—expand the availability of immediacy for each young person's unique mix of needs.[24] Because the authors' services are centralized and integrated, clients can see the health educator, nutritionist, dentist, lawyer, and/or a mental health provider, if they have the time and desire. Survivors of human trafficking often can have their mental health and substance use treatment needs addressed in the same place.[25] Integrating all these services, especially mental health, into primary care makes it easier for survivors of human trafficking to avail themselves of needed services, interventions, and treatment. With few exceptions, the programs also try to avoid limiting programs to specific days or times—the goal is to have all services available at all times. When colocated services are not an option for providers, which often is the case due to cost and space challenges, providers can accomplish a similar goal through cross-agency collaborations.

Relationships

Relationships are necessary to learn more (or in some cases, any) information about trafficking experiences in order to provide access to interventions. Relationships with caring adults are now known to be the most predictive factor for resilience in children.[26] CHNJ's research on human trafficking among homeless youth identified having at least 1 caring adult relationship as the sole protective factor against human trafficking for traumatized youth.

Relationships also are necessary to support survivors to follow through with trafficking interventions, medical and otherwise, which often take time.[27] Even after a client has been freed or has decided to leave a trafficker, the client may be just beginning medical treatment or engagement with law enforcement as a witness. During these longer-term interventions, where progress can be slow and the future can seem uncertain, many trafficking clients are at high risk of returning to their traffickers.

A trauma-informed screening and assessment procedure creates an emotionally safe environment for the client where the goal is not disclosure of details, but identifying the health impacts of past experiences. Use of structured tools and open-ended questions has shown success in identifying prior lifetime human trafficking experiences. Identification by these methods support the primary care provider's ultimate goal of providing services that will be accepted in the short term and long term, as opposed to gathering detailed stories and losing touch with patients before treatment impacts are realized.[28,29]

There are several screening tools for sex trafficking, but few are scientifically validated, and none identifies labor trafficking. CHNJ created the first validated short screening tool for identification of human trafficking among homeless youth, called the Quick Youth Indicators for Trafficking (QYIT).[13] QYIT are composed of 4 dichotomous, destigmatizing questions that can be administered by nonexperts who have not had training in the application of the definition of human trafficking (**Fig. 1**). A positive score of 1 to 4 indicates the possibility of a lifetime experience of human trafficking. With a sensitivity of 86.7% and specificity of 76.5%, QYIT are successful at identifying a majority of human trafficking survivors, with only a small incidence of over-identification.[13] To confirm a human trafficking experience, QYIT-positive youth should be assessed by an expert in the definition of human trafficking.

Although QYIT have not yet been validated for use with younger adolescents (<18 years old) in noncrisis center settings (such as primary care clinics), a related

Covenant House New Jersey: Quick Youth Indicators for Trafficking (QYITs)

1. It is not uncommon for young people to stay in work situations that are risky or even dangerous, simply because they have no other options. Have you ever worked, or done other things, in a place that made you feel scared or unsafe?

   ☐ Yes   ☐ No   ☐ Refuse to Answer   ☐ Don't Know

2. Sometimes people are prevented from leaving an unfair or unsafe work situation by their employers. Have you ever been afraid to leave or quit a work situation due to fears of violence or threats of harm to yourself or your family?

   ☐ Yes   ☐ No   ☐ Refuse to Answer   ☐ Don't Know

3. Sometimes young people who are homeless or who are having difficulties with their families have very few options to survive or fulfill their basic needs, such as food and shelter. Have you ever received anything in exchange for sex (eg, a place to stay, gifts, or food)?

   ☐ Yes   ☐ No   ☐ Refuse to Answer   ☐ Don't Know

4. Sometimes employers don't want people to know about the kind of work they have young employees doing. To protect themselves, they ask their employees to lie about the kind of work they are involved in. Have you ever worked for someone who asked you to lie while speaking to others about the work you do?[*]

   ☐ Yes   ☐ No   ☐ Refuse to Answer   ☐ Don't Know

Fig. 1. QYIT.

tool that uses the same candidate questions—the Rapid Assessment for Trafficking—currently is being tested for use in emergency hospital settings.[30]

For settings that do not use a screening tool, such as QYIT, or for those that are using a screening tool and then assessing the positively screened clients, the use of open-ended assessment questions may be the first treatment intervention for the trafficked client. At MSAHC, the authors have come to realize that young people are not likely to come and spontaneously disclose sensitive issues that they have experienced or are experiencing. They are asked directly in simple language what they are thinking, what they are feeling, and how they are doing, not only physically but also emotionally and cognitively. Sometimes, especially if they have had bad experiences or have felt a sense of betrayal when they have shared personal information, they may not feel comfortable initially sharing certain things. According to a study conducted by Ashby and colleagues,[31] in situations where sex trade engagement was suspected but not acknowledged, disclosure of trafficking frequently required multiple conversations over a period of time. As trust is built, they may feel more comfortable and share what initially they were not able to share. Through experience, the authors often have found that young people who believe that there is real interest in getting to know them and being as helpful as possible are actually eager to share their stories.

At CHNJ, the authors have learned if they are able to positively engage clients who have been trafficked, the clients are more likely to want to stay or return for support. This means getting to know them beyond their wants, needs, and presenting problems and learning about their strengths, interests, talents, and hopes for the future. In order to accomplish these, youth participate in a series of assessments upon initial enrollment that contribute to staff and youth collaboratively creating an individualized case plan. This approach gives youth ownership over their goals and creates one positive relationship with a case manager where a youth can be more likely to build trust.[32] Youth who have experienced trafficking are most likely passing in and out of many systems, such as the foster care system, welfare systems, and juvenile justice system.[32] The case management relationship provides direct point persons for youth to work with for coordinating their many needs and helps the client acknowledge strengths and resiliency.

Choice

Health care settings can be composed of systems and environments that inherently remove autonomy and power from clients, and this is particularly troublesome for trafficked individuals who, by definition, have been in situations where they lacked control over their bodies and choices.[33] Providers must allow these patients to feel they have the ability to choose their health treatment and desired outcomes. Clinicians and care systems should closely examine where their systems can be retraumatizing, by making a client feel out of control or powerless, and where they can return power to the client.[20] A worthy challenge for any organization is to establish a culture of flexibility and responsiveness without becoming inconsistent or disorganized. Allowing clients to disengage and re-engage multiple times without judgment affirms youths' autonomy, and allows them to seek services when they are comfortable and ready, while keeping an open door for a positive relationship. A client may not get to choose many aspects of their treatment plan but can be offered choice of room and follow-up appointment times and can be asked if it is okay to close the door or if they want anyone to step out of the room. Making exceptions for no-show appointments, seeing patients regardless of how late they are for their appointment, following-up on missed appointments, reaching out to individuals directly to schedule appointments, maintaining continuity of care-provider, and providing patients with choices in their care whenever it may be possible further support patient choice in a trauma-informed system. This flexibility, of course, comes at the expense of efficiency, and it is not unusual for providers to have lulls and busy times in their schedule, sometimes with longer than desirable wait times for visits. The MSAHC handles long wait times by providing a comfortable environment with adequate seating, movies on wall-mounted screens, teen-friendly informational bulletin boards, simple snacks, and charging stations, and the authors find that many patients do not mind waiting. In addition, staff members are flexible about the order in which services are provided, sometimes having patients see health educators or getting bloodwork before they see the physician. Staff have plenty of work to do when patients do not show up on time for visits, including catching up on paperwork, doing outreach, and collaborating with other staff on clinical and administrative matters.

Privacy and Confidentiality

Privacy is important when serving young people.[34] Privacy and confidentiality regarding experiences of sex trafficking can be barriers for youth who have been trafficked to getting necessary services, especially health services.[35,36] The authors' agencies always spend part (or all) of the visits without people known to the young person in the room, allowing them the opportunity to ask questions and share important private information. It is critical to let clients know the purpose of these questions and exactly who will know the information that they disclose. The authors remind clients that, ultimately, they are the ones who get to decide what is shared. This can shift the youth's body language completely in the consultation room. Reminding them that they still have control and self-determination in disclosing their experiences matters. Victims of trafficking may choose not to disclose their experiences because they are afraid of repercussions from their trafficker, if they have one. They also worry about stigma from health care providers and may not trust what providers will do with their information. A major barrier for health care providers in providing confidential health care to youth who have experienced trafficking is understanding how to ask about experiences of trafficking, what to do with that information, and when it is mandatory to report.[4]

Learning How to Serve the Trafficked Client

MSAHC's and CHNJ's anti–human trafficking work developed through a commitment to being learning organizations. The authors continue to learn from the literature, follow the latest guidelines and best practices, and conduct their own research; but the young people themselves are the best teachers. Over the years, as new needs are identified, the programs have developed expertise to accommodate and provide services to individuals in these populations with the specific needs, such as survivors of human trafficking.

Since 2017, when CHNJ began administering QYIT to all new clients, CHNJ has been able to identify a significant minority of its clients as survivors of human trafficking—almost 10% in the first year the QYIT were used at the 2 crisis centers and increasing annually to greater than 14% in FY2018. At MSAHC, in 2018, 186 young people were identified as sex trafficking survivors, most of whom came by referrals from other youths, programs that work with survivors, and federal agencies.

Because human trafficking is both a federal crime and local crime, the authors' agencies provide the option for legal consultations for survivors to inform them of protections and resources that may be available to them. State and federal laws are survivor-focused, providing protections and rights for survivors if they choose to report, and survivors may seek criminal restitution or compensation in civil court.

Survivors may be able to obtain compensation for relocation, transportation, behavioral health, and mental health among many others among the comprehensive services offered by providers receiving federal funds for trafficking survivor services.[37] Survivors also can seek to expunge or vacate their criminal records associated with their trafficking experience, like prostitution.[38] For non–US citizen survivors, specialized immigration relief is available in the form of T visas.[39]

For the many trafficking survivors identified at the authors' organizations who choose not to report, the authors have drawn on lessons learned from their long histories of serving clients with emerging health, wellness, and social issues. They have realized the effectiveness of remarkably similar approaches to widely disparate health and social issues, whether it be sexual violence, human immunodeficiency virus/acquired immunodeficiency syndrome, or gender nonconforming youth. This is the ultimate value of the youth-centered approach: it is by definition adaptable and responsive to the client's needs, whatever they are, whether providers are already practiced experts or developing new competence. Using their models of providing immediacy and forming trusting relationships through privacy and choice, the authors have helped trafficked youth to find safety and treatment. For some, this has been accomplished by STI testing and treatment and psychiatric consultations; for others, it has been through peer leadership opportunities and positive youth engagement; for still others, it has been through employment and independent housing. For all, the youths' capacity for resilience is far higher than their experience of trauma. Awareness of human trafficking has increased solutions and creativity across the country for prevention of trafficking and for prosecution of traffickers who are investigated. Nonetheless, programs for the ongoing care of survivors remain necessary.

SUMMARY

Primary care providers who adopt youth-centered approaches have an opportunity to remove obstacles to safety and treatment of human trafficking survivors who already have remained invisible for too long. This article is a shared collaboration between MSAHC and CHNJ. It is a clear demonstration that through collaboration, more is learned and the practice model and care of young people are improved. The authors hope that their shared learning is helpful to primary care providers in their education about human trafficking and work. They invite primary care providers to join in improving and increasing the care for young trafficking survivors, who inspire with their courage and resilience.

DISCLOSURE

The authors have nothing to disclose.

REFERENCES

1. Goldberg A, Moore J. Domestic minor sex trafficking. Child Adolesc Psychiatr Clin N Am 2018;27(1):77–92.
2. Chisolm-Straker M, Baldwin S, Gaïgbé-Togbé B, et al. Health care and human trafficking: We are seeing the unseen. J Health Care Poor Underserved 2016; 27(3):1220–33.
3. Burke NJ, Hellman JL, Scott BG, et al. The impact of adverse childhood experiences on an urban pediatric population. Child Abuse Negl 2011;35(6):408–13.
4. Clawson HJ, Dutch N. Addressing the needs of victims of human trafficking: challenges, barriers, and promising practices. Department of Health and Human

Services, Office of the Assistant Secretary for Planning and Evaluation; 2008. Available at: https://aspe.hhs.gov/report/addressing-needs-victims-human-trafficking-challenges-barriers-and-promising-practices. Accessed April 10, 2019.

5. US Department of State. Victims of trafficking and violence protection act of 2000. 2000. Available at: https://www.state.gov/international-and-domestic-law/. Accessed June 12, 2019.
6. Polaris. The typology of modern slavery. Polaris. 2016. Available at: https://polarisproject.org/typology. Accessed June 14, 2019.
7. Office on Trafficking in Persons. What is human trafficking?. Available at: https://www.acf.hhs.gov/otip/about/what-is-human-trafficking. Accessed August 12, 2019.
8. Baldwin S, Eisenman D, Sayles J, et al. Identification of HT victims in health care settings. Health Hum Rights 2011;13(1):36–49.
9. Greenbaum J. Identifying victims of human trafficking in the emergency department. Clin Pediatr Emerg Med 2016;17(4):241–8.
10. Richie-Zavaleta AC, Villanueva A, Martinez-Donate A, et al. Sex trafficking victims at their junction with the healthcare setting—a mixed-methods inquiry. J Hum Traffick 2019. https://doi.org/10.1080/23322705.2018.1501257.
11. American Public Health Association. Expanding and coordinating human trafficking-related public health research, evaluation, education, and prevention. American Public Health Association; 2015. Available at: https://www.apha.org/policies-and-advocacy/public-health-policy-statements/policy-database/2016/01/26/14/28/expanding-and-coordinating-human-trafficking-related-public-health-activities. Accessed May 12, 2019.
12. Kaplan DM, Moore JL, Barron CE, et al. Domestic minor sex trafficking: medical follow-up for victimized and high-risk youth. R I Med J 2018;101(4):25–7. Available at: http://www.rimed.org/rimedicaljournal/2018/05/2018-05-25-cont-kaplan.pdf. Accessed April 6, 2019.
13. Chisolm-Straker M, Sze J, Einbond J, et al. Screening for human trafficking among homeless young adults. Child Youth Serv Rev 2019;98:72–9.
14. Somerville LH, Jones RM, Ruberry EJ, et al. The medial prefrontal cortex and the emergence of self-conscious emotion in adolescence. Psychol Sci 2013;24(8):1554–62.
15. Pattwell S, Casey BJ, Lee FS. The teenage brain: altered fear in humans and mice. Curr Dir Psychol Sci 2013;22(2):146–51.
16. Fortier MA, Dilillo D, Messman-Moore TL, et al. Severity of child sexual abuse and revictimization: the mediating role of coping and trauma symptoms. Psychol Women Q 2009;33(3):308–20.
17. Zerk DM, Mertin PG, Proeve M. Domestic violence and maternal reports of young children's functioning. J Fam Violence 2009;24(7):423–32.
18. Hopper EK, Bassuk EL, Olivet J. Shelter from the storm: trauma-informed care in homelessness services settings. Open Health Serv Policy J 2010;3(2):80–100.
19. Department of Justice. Report of the Attorney General's National Task Force on children exposed to violence. DOJ. 2012. Available at: https://www.justice.gov/defendingchildhood/cev-rpt-full.pdf. Accessed April 10th, 2019.
20. Substance Abuse and Mental Health Services Administration. SAMHSA's concept of trauma and guidance for a trauma-informed approach. HHS publication No. (SMA) 14-4884. Rockville (MD): Substance Abuse and Mental Health Services Administration; 2014.
21. Ginsburg K. Why be trauma-informed? Fostering resilience. Available at: https://fosteringresilience.com/professionals/why_be_informed.php. Accessed August 12, 2019.

22. Chisolm-Straker M, Miller C, Duke G, et al. A framework for the development of healthcare provider education programs on human trafficking park two: survivors. J Hum Traffick 2019. https://doi.org/10.1080/23322705.2019.1635333.

23. US Department of State. Trafficking in persons report. 2019:492. Available at: https://www.state.gov/reports/2019-trafficking-in-persons-report/. Accessed August 12, 2019.

24. Weiss M, Schwartz BJ. Lessons learned from a colocation model using psychiatrists in urban primary care settings. J Prim Care Community Health 2012;4(3): 228–34.

25. Cook MC, Barnert E, Ijadi-Maghsoodi R, et al. Exploring mental health and substance use treatment needs of commercially sexually exploited youth participating in a specialty juvenile court. Behav Med 2018;44(3):242–9.

26. Center on the Developing Child at Harvard University. Supportive relationships and active skill-building strengthen the foundation or resilience: working paper no. 13. 2015. Available at: https://developingchild.harvard.edu/. Accessed August 30th, 2017.

27. Chisolm-Straker M, Sze J, Einbond J, et al. A supportive adult may be the difference in homeless youth not being trafficked. Child Youth Serv Rev 2018;91: 115–20.

28. Machtinger EL, Davis KB, Kimberg LS, et al. From treatment to healing: inquiry and response to recent and past trauma in adult health care. Womens Health Issues 2019;29(2):97–101.

29. Leitch L. Action steps using ACEs and trauma-informed care: a resilience model. Health Justice 2017;5(1):5.

30. Chisolm-Straker M, Rotham E, Singer E. RAFT: rapid assessment for human trafficking. 2018. Available at: https://www.researchgate.net/project/RAFT-Rapid-Assessment-for-Human-Trafficking. Accessed June 14, 2019.

31. Ashby BD, Ehmer AC, Scott SM. Trauma-informed care in a patient-centered medical home for adolescent mothers and their children. Psychol Serv 2019; 16(1):67–74.

32. Gibbs DA, Hardison Walters JL, Lutnick A, et al. Services to domestic minor victims of sex trafficking: Opportunities for engagement and support. Child Youth Serv Rev 2015;54:1–7.

33. San Francisco Department of Public Health. Trauma informed systems initiative. Webinar released December 17, 2014.

34. Clawson HJ, Dutch N. Identifying victims of human trafficking: inherent challenges and promising strategies from the field. Department of Health and Human Services, Office of the Assistant Secretary for Planning and Evaluation; 2008. Available at: https://aspe.hhs.gov/system/files/pdf/75321/ib.pdf. Accessed April 10, 2019.

35. Britto MT, Tivorsak TL, Slap GB. Adolescents' needs for health care privacy. Pediatrics 2010;126(6):e1469–76.

36. Crane PA, Moreno M. Human trafficking: what is the role of the health care provider? J Appl Res Child 2011;2(1):1–27. Available at: https://digitalcommons.library.tmc.edu/childrenatrisk/vol2/iss1/7. Accessed April 10, 2019.

37. Office for Victims of Crime, Office of Justice Programs. Matrix of OVC/BJA-funded human trafficking services grantees and task forces. Available at: https://ovc.ncjrs.gov/humantrafficking/traffickingmatrix.html. Accessed August 12, 2019.

38. Castillo R. Vacatur laws: decriminalizing sex trafficking survivors. 2016. Available at: http://www.jgspl.org/vacatur-laws-decriminalizing-sex-trafficking-survivors. Accessed August 12, 2019.
39. US Department of State. Visas for victims of human trafficking. Available at: https://travel.state.gov/content/travel/en/us-visas/other-visa-categories/visas-for-victims-of-human-trafficking.html. Accessed August 12, 2019.

Crisis and Adolescents
Assessments and Initial Management

Patrice M. Leverett, PhD, NCSP[a],*, Stephanie D'Costa, PhD, LP[b,1],
Heather Cassella, MS[a], Manan Shah, MD[c]

KEYWORDS

- Adolescents • Crisis • Trauma-informed care • Collaboration • Mental health

KEY POINTS

- Adolescents experience high rates of trauma that can affect their mental, physical, and behavioral well-being. Medical providers can benefit from additional training in crisis response and trauma-informed care with these patients.
- Survey instruments are available to assess adolescents for indicators of traumatic experiences and crisis. These tools can provide insight on treatment directions or need for referrals.
- Community and school mental health providers are accessible for wraparound care for adolescents. The use of evidence-based interventions for the treatment of trauma in youth can have positive outcomes across multiple dimensions of adolescent patient health.
- Collaborations with community and school mental health providers can be a great asset in the reduction of symptoms related to crisis.

INTRODUCTION

Adolescence is a challenging time for most youth: they are negotiating the interplay of educational and work responsibilities, their home environments and social spheres, and their constantly changing bodies. Adolescence is a critical time, shaping the development of individuals' overall health and well-being in adulthood. In addition to general health concerns regarding healthy eating, sleeping, hygiene, and sexual health, young people may also face the complexities of trauma in their homes, schools, and communities, witnessing violence and/or experiencing it directly. These crises (defined as extremely negative, uncontrollable, and unpredictable events) may

[a] Counseling Education, School Psychology and Human Services, University of Nevada - Las Vegas, 4505 South Maryland Parkway, Box 453008, Las Vegas, NV 89154, USA; [b] Department of Education and Leadership, California State University - Monterey Bay100 Campus Center, Del Mar 110, Seaside, CA 93955, USA; [c] Child and Adolescent Day Hospital, Division of Child and Adolescent Psychiatry, Sheppard Pratt Health System, 6501 North Charles Street, Towson, MD 21204, USA
[1] Present address: 100 Campus Center, Del Mar 110, Seaside, CA 93955, USA.
* Corresponding author.
E-mail address: patrice.leverett@unlv.edu

Prim Care Clin Office Pract 47 (2020) 321–329
https://doi.org/10.1016/j.pop.2020.02.009
0095-4543/20/Published by Elsevier Inc.

primarycare.theclinics.com

result in physiologic or emotional symptoms.[1] Furthermore, the rates of mental health disorders such as depression and anxiety are increasing with the increasing demands of, and feelings of not belonging in, the school environment.[2] To fully address these issues, health practitioners must be able to assess, recognize, and identify appropriate treatment steps for adolescents who are combatting crisis and traumatic experiences.

Studies show that medical professionals may not think themselves competent in addressing mental health issues, including trauma.[3] This lack of confidence may be a result of physicians' deferring mental health trauma response to mental health professionals. Other barriers include lack of training and/or education; a lack of understanding regarding patients' unique symptoms and needs; provider discomfort in discussing issues of sexual assault, violence, and trauma; and lack of knowledge regarding available resources.[3,4] One study found that 48% of physicians rated themselves as not competent in providing information and psychoeducation on typical stress signs and reactions.[5] In addition, nearly half rated themselves as not competent in comprehending the factual evidence behind various assessment tools and evidence-based interventions for the treatment of traumatic stress and related disorders.[5] Although these findings were related to trauma following a physical injury, it can be argued that crisis that follows an emotional or psychological trauma can still be effectively treated with trauma-informed care (TIC). Another study found that primary care providers (PCPs) may be uncomfortable treating patients with trauma because of a lack of training in working with patients who have experienced violence, uncertainty on how to treat clients once they have been diagnosed, and their belief that these patients can be more difficult to work with than other patients.[6] More training for medical professionals in the assessment, diagnosis, and treatment of trauma is needed.

This article highlights current research on the assessment and intervention of crisis and trauma in youth in both community and home settings. It serves as an overview and offers possible resources that PCPs can use to help treatment of trauma. In addition, the article offers possible means of collaborating with school and community mental health providers to ensure wraparound care for adolescents who have experienced a traumatic event.

PREVALENCE OF CRISES IN ADOLESCENCE

According to the National Survey of Children's Exposure to Violence,[7] more than one-third of the 4000 youth participants experienced physical assault in the past year, with assaults occurring to boys more than girls (41.6% and 33%, respectively), whereas 16.4% of girls aged 14 to 17 years experienced a sexual offense and 4.6% experienced a sexual assault. In addition, several youth experienced multiple exposures to abuse, with 10.1% of the sample having greater than or equal to 6 exposures. Multiple exposures to violence are correlated with poorer health outcomes, with adolescents who reported greater than or equal to 5 forms of exposure to violence being 4.6 times more likely to report poorer health outcomes than adolescents who were not exposed to violence.[8]

McLaughlin and colleagues[9] (2013) found that approximately two-thirds of youth are exposed to trauma during childhood. By age 18 years, roughly 8% of traumatized youth are diagnosed with posttraumatic stress disorder (PTSD), and, in cases of sexual abuse and assault, the numbers are in excess of 40%, followed by kidnapping (37.0%), sexual assault (31.3%), physical assault by romantic partner (29.1%), and physical abuse by a caregiver (25.2%).[9] These outcomes were varied based on race and ethnicity. Witnessing domestic violence was more common among white non-Hispanic adolescents, witnessing the death of a loved one was more common among black non-Hispanics, and Hispanic adolescents more often reported more physical assault by a romantic partner.[8]

Trauma and particularly PTSD in adolescents can manifest in several ways, including lower academic success, loss of problem-solving skills, depression, disorganization, confusion, increased irrational behavior, and withdrawal.[10] Additional studies highlight the increased likelihood of suicidal ideation, suicide attempts, substance abuse, intentional self-injury/harm, impaired identity development, and immune system depression.[9,11,12]

Gun Violence in Schools

Over the last few decades, there has been an increasing concern about children's safety in primary and secondary schools and colleges, because school-based shootings seem to have become a perennial event. According to the US Naval Postgraduate School report, there were 94 school gun violence incidents and 55 deaths in 2018 alone.[13] The number of incidents more than doubled from 43 incidents in the preceding year. These incidents are defined as "each and every instance a gun is brandished, is fired, or a bullet hits school property for any reason, regardless of the number of victims, time of day, or day of the week."[13] Trends show that fatal shootings are more likely to occur in rural and suburban schools with younger students and a primarily white student body.[14] The psychological impact that these shootings have on adolescents can be devastating, including severe anxiety, anger, withdrawal, PTSD, sleep distortion, and desensitization.[15]

Suicide

According to the National Center for Health Statistics and the Centers for Disease Control and Prevention (CDC), suicide is the second leading cause of death of youth aged 15 to 24 years, after automobile accidents. Since 2010, the rates of suicide attempts and completion have increased among adolescents aged 13 to 18 years, particularly adolescent girls.[16] In addition, between 1991 and 2017, there was a 76% increase in reported suicide attempts among black youth.[17] Youth who identify as lesbian, gay, bisexual, transgender, and/or questioning have an increased rate of suicidal ideation and attempts compared with heterosexual youth.[18]

There are several factors that may contribute to the increase in suicide rates among youth and adolescents. Some studies suggest increased access to social media may contribute to feelings of loneliness and isolation,[19] whereas other studies suggest the bias against and lack of social support for youth who are ethnic, cultural, and/or sexual minorities account for some of the variations in outcomes.[20,21] There is also strong evidence that childhood maltreatment, such as sexual, physical, and emotional abuse, correlates directly with suicidal ideation and attempts. Screening for these factors in adolescents becomes even more important when concomitant mental health conditions, such as depression, are suspected.[18]

ASSESSMENTS

Based on the prevalence of crisis in the lives of adolescents, medical providers who see youth need to assess the impact of crises on the well-being of their patients to determine treatment options. There has always been a lack of universally accepted practice parameters or models of best practice in the assessment of adolescents presenting with crises. The guidelines for making decisions regarding disposition are also unclear. The American Academy of Child and Adolescent Psychiatry (AACAP) has published practice parameters for the assessment and management of suicidal behavior, which is a psychiatric emergency. However, these practice parameters do not address the assessment or disposition of other crisis presentations that do not involve suicide or suicidal ideation. Crises are often less specific and longer lasting than emergencies, and may or may not involve risk of danger to self or others. Consequently, they are likely to require a more thorough psychosocial and general psychiatric assessment compared with the more algorithmic approach for psychiatric emergencies such as suicidal ideation.[22]

Although there are a wide range of assessments for adults, the assessment of child related trauma and crisis is limited. Nonetheless, some assessments are available that may help physicians in daily practice. For example, the University of California, Los Angeles (UCLA) Child/Adolescent PTSD Reaction Index for Diagnostic and Statistical Manual of Mental Disorders, Fifth Revision (DSM-5)[23] and the Clinician-Administered PTSD Scale for DSM-5 – Child/Adolescent Version (CAPS-CA-5)[24] are physician-administered interviews to follow up on the frequency and severity of trauma-related issues. A potential downside of these assessments is that they can take up to an hour to complete, depending on the nature of the trauma. One of the most comprehensive tools in this regard is the Juvenile Victimization Questionnaire, which has been validated for ethnically diverse samples of children aged 2 to 17 years. As previously noted, because adolescents in crisis are potentially more likely to have co-morbid psychiatric disorders, assessing for the comorbidities and treating them in an integrated fashion is crucial. One example of such an integrated approach is the Seeking Safety model, which is an evidence-based treatment approach for PTSD and substance use.[25]

Alternatives to these assessments are trauma checklists, which can provide a brief overview of the needs of adolescent patients who have experienced trauma. Examples include the Beck Anxiety Inventory (BAI)[26]; the Child Stress Disorders Checklist (CSDC), which assesses for acute stress disorder and PTSD[27]; and the Primary Care PTSD Screen for DSM-5 (PC-PTSD-5),[28] which was developed by the National Center for PTSD in Washington, DC, and has 4 items to assess PTSD prevalence. These scales are shorter and easier to complete within a typical clinical encounter, but may lack the specificity that can help provide more tailored referrals or services.. **Table 1** summarizes these assessment tools.

In addition to scales and formal interviews, clinical assessment entails a personal interview with the adolescent and parents and can be aided by information from other sources (eg, teachers). The parent interview should clarify the nature, severity, and duration of the child's and family's stressor precipitating the crisis. An inventory of stressors should be made, and a thorough history should be taken of the spectrum of possible behavioral, mood, and anxiety symptoms and other psychological morbidities and somatic ills, including any unexplained physical symptoms. The developmental and medical history should be documented and any important contextual mediators (eg, social, religious, ethnic, or cultural factors) should be considered carefully. An assessment of resilience should also be performed in the context of risk and protective factors, because that dictates the ability of the adolescent to rebound from the crisis to the premorbid state.[29]

INITIAL MANAGEMENT

When encountering an adolescent with identified symptoms of a crisis, physicians can engage in several evidence-based practices for initial management. First, displaying empathy can allow teens in crisis to believe that whatever crisis they are going through

Table 1
Assessments for crisis response in adolescents

Title of Assessment	Description	For More Information
UCLA Child/Adolescent PTSD Reaction Index for DSM-5	A semistructured interview to assess trauma history and DSM-5 PTSD criteria in school-aged children and adolescents	https://www.ptsd.va.gov/professional/assessment/child/ucla_child_reaction_dsm-5.asp
CAPS-CA-5	An assessment of PTSD through a 30-item clinician-administered interview; ages 7 y and older	https://www.ptsd.va.gov/professional/assessment/child/caps-ca.asp
Juvenile Victimization Questionnaire	A 21-question scale with follow-up questions available as needed, assesses victimization, caregiver maltreatment, and exposure to domestic violence	https://www.lifepathsresearch.org/wp-content/uploads/Victimization-JVQ.pdf
Beck Anxiety Inventory	A 21-item anxiety scale for adolescents and adults; ages 17 y and older. Some evidence of effectiveness with those 12–16 y old	https://www.nctsn.org/measures/beck-anxiety-inventory
CSDC	An observer questionnaire of acute stress disorder and PTSD in children aged 2–18 y	https://www.nctsn.org/measures/child-stress-disorders-checklist
PC-PTSD-5	A 5-item screener designed for clinical settings based on the criteria for PTSD in the DSM-5	https://www.ptsd.va.gov/professional/assessment/screens/pc-ptsd.asp

is real and meaningful. This practice can be done effectively through the use of validation-based statements that speak to the underlying emotions that are being expressed and are less focused on the factualness of the content of the crisis. The use of validation has been found to reduce patients' feelings of being overwhelmed[30,31] and increase their willingness to engage in cognitive problem solving.[32]

Another important intervention strategy that medical providers can provide is information regarding crises. Providing further information around the clinician's understanding of the patient's medical concerns have been found to increase patient satisfaction.[33] Adolescents can benefit from understanding the medical aspects of stress hormones that get activated during a crisis and their impact on their cognitive and social-emotional functioning. In addition, conversations around the prevalence of teenagers experiencing crises can add to a sense of connectedness to their peers.

Considerations for Safety Planning

For many physicians, providing validation and psychoeducation may be sufficient in providing the initial steps toward managing adolescent crises. However, in serious cases of crisis, physicians may be required to create a safety plan with patients to reduce the risk of harm. A safety plan includes an identification of both the patient's access to lethal means and, separately, adults who can provide supervision and support.[34] In addition, an emergency contingency plan should be crafted in case the patient's mental health deteriorates.[35]

Stating the limits of patient confidentiality up front can be an essential component of working with adolescents. Research indicates that trust and confidentiality with physicians are of substantial import to adolescents,[36] and this can be especially important in moments of crisis, given that medical practitioners have both an ethical and legal obligation to report situations that put youth less than 18 years of age in danger. For instance, in some cases, treatment includes (psychiatric) hospitalization, either involuntarily or voluntarily.[34] Physicians need to be candid with adolescents about this possibility, so that damage to the relationship, if doctor-patient confidentiality must be broken, can be mitigated.

In addition, it can be important for physicians to recommend and cocreate a plan for treatment. Increased medical compliance by adolescents can be achieved by providing treatment choices.[37] Developmentally, the adolescent years are marked by the increasing need for autonomy and resistance to certain forms of compliance.[38]

Cultural Differences

Additional considerations around initial management must be made regarding cultural differences between medical providers and their patients. Research indicates that racial and cultural differences between physicians and their patients can lead to reduced information-giving on the part of the physician and less patient participation in the process,[15] which can affect the ways symptoms are presented to the provider and the patient's willingness to engage in treatment compliance. The American Psychological Association is encouraging providers to increase their racial and ethnocultural responsiveness as they engage in prescribed treatment.[39] When working with adolescents, it is vital to hold their intersectional identities in mind when providing initial crisis management.

COMMUNITY REFERRALS AND TREATMENT

Although many adolescents cope with crisis situations with support from stable adults in their lives, adolescents who experience chronic crises are at risk for developing more significant mental health disorders.[40] It is important for physicians to have a referral list on hand because further support may be warranted from mental health professionals. Research indicates strong evidence for collaborative practices between physicians and mental health providers.[35]

School-Based Mental Health

Because of the amount of time adolescents spend in school, school-based mental health practitioners (eg, school psychologists, school counselors, and social workers) and school nurses are often the first line of intervention for these students.[41] Through their certification body, the National Association of School Psychologists (NASP), school psychologists can be trained in school-based crisis response that addresses events ranging from natural disasters to school shootings.[42] School-based providers receive referrals from school staff about the educational achievement challenges, as well as difficulties in behavior, attention, and suspected mental health needs. From here, school-based providers conduct a preliminary assessment of student needs. In addition, certain school-based mental health providers are trained neuropsychologists who can integrate those assessments into their reports. School psychologists are then able to make recommendations about individual and group interventions available at school or make referrals to outside bodies such as community mental health providers and PCPs. The capacity of school psychologists in schools is limited by high demands and limited resources. NASP recommends a ratio of school psychologists to students of 700:1, although many school psychologists are working at ratios nearly twice that amount.[43] By facilitating a channel of communication between PCPs and school-based providers, PCPs can get more information about the manifestation of symptoms, duration, and impact on daily function, which could lead to better medical management of the needs of adolescent patients.

SUMMARY

Adolescents are already navigating many life events that affect their physical development, mental health, and academic achievement. These factors can be exacerbated by exposure to traumatic events. Depending on previous training experience, TIC and crisis response for adolescent youth may be limited for PCPs. Adolescents are witnessing and experiencing high rates of traumatic events in their homes, schools, and communities: domestic violence, school-based violence, and sexual assault. Assessment tools are available to glean more information about the well-being of these students, but the length of these assessments may be prohibitory.

It is important for physicians to receive additional training in trauma-informed practices to mitigate the risk of retraumatizing patients while also gathering information to make informed decisions about treatment and safety plans. By providing more training for physicians on adolescent trauma response, reduction in health-related issues can be anticipated.

Further training for medical providers is one way to improve the awareness, assessment, and initial management of adolescent crisis. Training in residency programs can help providers gain basic skills and also understand the limits of their practice. Brief training for physicians has been found to increase their awareness and confidence in engaging in conversations regarding the variety of crises that occur within adolescence.[44] In addition, more research on effective assessment of trauma in adolescents in primary care settings is needed.

DISCLOSURE

The authors have nothing to disclose.

REFERENCES

1. Brock SE. Crisis theory: A foundation for the comprehensive school crisis response team. In: Brock SE, Lazarus PJ, Jimerson SR, editors. Best practices in school crisis prevention and intervention. Bethesda (MD): National Association of School Psychologists; 2002. p. 5–17.
2. Anderman EM. School effects on psychological outcomes during adolescence. J Educ Psychol 2002;94(4):795.
3. Freedy JR, Brock CD. Spotting – and treating – PTSD in primary care. J Fam Pract 2010;59(2):75–80.
4. Green BL, Kaltman S, Frank L, et al. Primary care providers' experiences with trauma patients: A qualitative study. Psychol Trauma Theor Res Pract Policy 2011;3(1):37–41.
5. Bruce MM, Kassam-Adams N, Rogers M, et al. Trauma providers' knowledge, views, and practice of trauma-informed care. J Trauma Nurs 2018;25(2):131–8.
6. Polusny MA, Follette VM. Long-term correlates of child sexual abuse: Theory and review of the empirical literature. Appl Prev Psychol 1995;4:143–66.
7. Finkelhor D, Turner HA, Shattuck A, et al. Prevalence of childhood exposure to violence, crime, and abuse: results from the national survey of children's exposure to violence. JAMA Pediatr 2015;169(8):746–54.

8. Boynton-Jarrett R, Ryan LM, Berkman LF, et al. Cumulative violence exposure and self-rated health: longitudinal study of adolescents in the United States. Pediatrics 2008;122(5):961–70.

9. McLaughlin KA, Koenen KC, Hill ED, et al. Trauma exposure and posttraumatic stress disorder in a national sample of adolescents. J Am Acad Child Adolesc Psychiatry 2013;52(8):815–30.e14.

10. Pynoos RS. Traumatic stress and developmental psychopathology in children and adolescents. In: Oldham JM, Riba MB, Tasman A, editors. American Psychiatric Press review of psychiatry Vol. 12. Washington, DC: American Psychiatric Press; 1993. p. 205–38.

11. Ayaydin H, Abali O, Akdeniz N, et al. Immune system changes after sexual abuse in adolescents. Pediatr Int 2016;58(2):105–12.

12. Lawson D, Quinn J. Complex trauma in children and adolescents: evidence-based practice in clinical settings. J Clin Psychol 2013;69(5):497–509.

13. Riedman D, O'Neill D. "CHDS – K-12 School Shooting Database," Center for Homeland Defense and Security, US Naval Postgraduate School. Available at: www.chds.us/ssdb. Accessed December 20, 2019.

14. Livingston MD, Rossheim ME, Hall KS. A descriptive analysis of school and school shooter characteristics and the severity of school shootings in the United States, 1999–2018. J Adolesc Health 2019;64(6):797–9.

15. Gordon HS, Street RL Jr, Sharf BF, et al. Racial differences in doctors' information-giving and patients' participation. Cancer 2006;107(6):1313–20.

16. Lindsey MA, Sheftall AH, Xiao Y, et al. Trends of suicidal behaviors among high school students in the United States: 1991-2017. Pediatrics 2019;144(5) [pii: e20191187].

17. Shain B. Increases in rates of suicide and suicide attempts among black adolescents. Pediatrics 2019;144(5).

18. Cha CB, Franz PJ, M Guzmán E, et al. Annual research review: suicide among youth–epidemiology, (potential) etiology, and treatment. J Child Psychol Psychiatry 2018;59(4):460–82.

19. Twenge JM, Joiner TE, Rogers ML, et al. Increases in depressive symptoms, suicide-related outcomes, and suicide rates among US adolescents after 2010 and links to increased new media screen time. Clin Psychol Sci 2018;6(1):3–17.

20. Lanier Y, Sommers MS, Fletcher J, et al. Examining racial discrimination frequency, racial discrimination stress, and psychological well-being among Black early adolescents. J Black Psychol 2017;43(3):219–29.

21. Hatzenbuehler ML. The social environment and suicide attempts in lesbian, gay, and bisexual youth. Pediatrics 2011;127:896–903.

22. Goldstein AB, Findling RL. Assessment and evaluation of child and adolescent psychiatric emergencies. Psychiatric Times 2006;23(9):76.

23. Steinberg AM, Brymer M, Decker K, et al. The University of California at Los Angeles Post-Traumatic Stress Disorder Reaction Index. Curr Psychiatry Rep 2004;6:96–100.

24. Pynoos RS, Weathers FW, Steinberg AM, et al. Clinician-Administered PTSD Scale for DSM-5 - Child/Adolescent Version. Scale available from the National Center for PTSD 2015. Bethesda, Md. Available at: https://www.ptsd.va.gov/professional/assessment/child/index.asp. Accessed March 13, 2020.

25. Cohen JA, Bukstein O, Walter H, et al, AACAP Work Group on Quality Issues. Practice parameter for the assessment and treatment of children and adolescents with posttraumatic stress disorder. J Am Acad Child Adolesc Psychiatry 2010;49(4):414–30.

26. Beck AT, Epstein N, Brown G, et al. An inventory for measuring clinical anxiety: Psychometric properties. J Consult Clin Psychol 1988;56:893–7.

27. Saxe GN. Child stress disorders checklist (CSDC) (v.4.0-11/01. National Child Traumatic Stress Network and Department of Child and Adolescent Psychiatry, Boston University School of Medicine; 2001.

28. Prins A, Bovin MJ, Kimerling R, et al. The primary care PTSD screen for DSM-5 (PC-PTSD-5) 2015. *Scale available from the National Center for PTSD at.* https://www.ptsd.va.gov/professional/assessment/screens/pc-ptsd.asp. Accessed March 10, 2020. [Measurement instrument].

29. Pfefferbaum B, Shaw JA. Practice parameter on disaster preparedness. J Am Acad Child Adolesc Psychiatry 2013;52(11):1224–38.

30. Carson-Wong A, Hughes CD, Rizvi SL. The effect of therapist use of validation strategies on change in client emotion in individual DBT treatment sessions. Personal Disord Theor Res Treat 2018;9(2):165.

31. Huffman JC, Stern TA, Harley RM, et al. The use of DBT skills in the treatment of difficult patients in the general hospital. Focus 2005;44(2):421–60.

32. Lynch TR, Chapman AL, Rosenthal MZ, et al. Mechanisms of change in dialectical behavior therapy: Theoretical and empirical observations. J Clin Psychol 2006;62(4):459–80.

33. Ishikawa H, Son D, Eto M, et al. The information giving skills of resident physicians: relationships with confidence and simulated patient satisfaction. BMC Med Educ 2017;17(1):34.

34. Kostenuik M, Ratnapalan M. Approach to adolescent suicide prevention. Can Fam Physician 2010;56(8):755–60.

35. Zuckerbrot RA, Cheung A, Jensen PS, et al, GLAD-PC Steering Group. Guidelines for adolescent depression in primary care (GLAD-PC): Part I. Practice preparation, identification, assessment, and initial management. Pediatrics 2018; 141(3):e20174081.

36. Klostermann BK, Slap GB, Nebrig DM, et al. Earning trust and losing it: adolescents' views on trusting physicians: specific physician behaviors – particularly those implying an assurance of confidentiality – encourage trust-building among adolescents. J Fam Pract 2005;54(8):679–88.

37. McCabe MA. Involving children and adolescents in medical decision making: developmental and clinical considerations. J Pediatr Psychol 1996;21(4):505–16.

38. Spear HJ, Kulbok P. Autonomy and adolescence: a concept analysis. Public Health Nurs 2004;21(2):144–52.

39. American Psychological Association, APA Task Force on Race and Ethnicity Guidelines in Psychology. Race and ethnicity guidelines in psychology: promoting responsiveness and equity. Available at: http://www.apa.org/about/policy/race-and-ethnicity-in-psychology.pdf. Accessed Dec 13, 2019.

40. Cook A, Spinazzola J, Ford J, et al. Complex trauma in children and adolescents. Psychiatr Ann 2017;35(5):390–8.

41. Splett JW, Fowler J, Weist MD, et al. The critical role of school psychology in the school mental health movement. Psychol Sch 2013;50(3):245–58.

42. Brock SE, Nickerson AB, Reeves MA, Savage TA, Woitaszewski SA. Development, evaluation, and future directions of the PREP a RE school crisis prevention and intervention training curriculum. Journal of School Violence 2011;10(1):34–52.

43. Castillo JM, Curtis MJ, Tan SY. Personnel needs in school psychology: A 10-year follow-up study on predicted personnel shortages. Psychol Sch 2014;51(8):832–49.

44. Taliaferro LA, Borowsky IW. Perspective: physician education – a promising strategy to prevent adolescent suicide. Acad Med 2011;86(3):342–7.

Sexual Assault in Adolescents

Christine Banvard-Fox, MD[a,b,*], Meredith Linger, MSN, RN[c], Debra J. Paulson, MD[d], Lesley Cottrell, PhD[e], Danielle M. Davidov, PhD[f]

KEYWORDS

- Sexual abuse • Sexual violence • Sexual assault nurse examiner (SANE)
- Child advocacy center (CAC) • Multidisciplinary investigational team (MDIT)
- Expert medical review • Vulnerable populations

KEY POINTS

- Alarming numbers of US adolescents have experienced sexual violence, with 26.6% of 17-year-old girls and 5.1% of 17-year-old boys reporting having experienced sexual abuse.
- Other studies support the higher prevalence of victimization among lesbian, gay, bisexual, transgender, and queer adolescents, noting between 23% and 62% of this population reports bullying, sexual victimization, and child maltreatment.
- Undesired sexual experiences in adolescence may increase later physical and sexual violence experiences, and the victim may perpetrate physical or sexual violence in the future.
- Medical peer review, in addition to expert review, is invaluable to assure utmost quality of interpretation of questionable or findings interpreted indicative of sexual abuse.
- Prevention of adolescent sexual abuse would have a pronounced effect on public health and health economics.

INTRODUCTION

Pervasive sexual violence (SV) in the United States frequently affects youth under the age of 18. With the prevalence of sexual abuse/assault, medical providers of adolescents will see affected individuals, including many remaining silent of the one or more

[a] Department of Pediatrics, West Virginia University, 6040 University Town Center Drive, Morgantown, WV 26501, USA; [b] Department of Adolescent Medicine, West Virginia University, 6040 University Town Center Drive, Morgantown, WV 26501, USA; [c] Department of Emergency Medicine, WVU Medicine, 1 Medical Center Drive, PO Box 8220, Morgantown, WV 26506, USA; [d] Department of Emergency Medicine, West Virginia University, 1 Medical Center Drive, PO Box 9149, Morgantown, WV 26506, USA; [e] Department of Pediatrics, West Virginia University, 1 Medical Center Drive, PO Box 9214, Morgantown, WV 26506, USA; [f] Department of Social and Behavioral Sciences, West Virginia University, 1 Medical Center Drive, PO Box 9190, Morgantown, WV 26506, USA
* Corresponding author.
E-mail address: cbanvard@hsc.wvu.edu

Prim Care Clin Office Pract 47 (2020) 331–349
https://doi.org/10.1016/j.pop.2020.02.010
0095-4543/20/© 2020 Elsevier Inc. All rights reserved.

instances. Besides addressing potential pregnancy, infections, and physical/mental health concerns, when SV is disclosed to a health care professional, Child Protective Service (CPS) and law enforcement need to be involved. The age to consent, age set for statutory rape, and maximum age difference permissible for legal sexual activity among minors are legal determinations that vary among states. Practitioners should familiarize themselves with their jurisdiction's statutes (Appendix 1).

Even with appropriate trauma-informed interventions, SV during childhood can result in immediate and lifelong adverse consequences.[1,2] SV in childhood triples an individual's likelihood of suffering future sexual or physical abuse or may increase the chances of becoming a perpetrator later in life.[1,2] Engaging in unhealthy behaviors with substances, exercise, and sexual activity is more prevalent in survivors of sexual abuse, as are other negative symptoms and physical and psychological health outcomes[3,4] (**Table 1**). Some resilient survivors are spared of these.[4]

No culture, socioeconomic class, race, gender, sexual orientation, nor age is immune from SV. It is a serious public health problem that can be prevented, and efforts are best focused on stopping SV before it starts.[2,3]

DEFINITIONS OF SEXUAL VIOLENCE

"Child sexual abuse occurs when a child is engaged in sexual activities that he or she cannot comprehend, for which he or she is developmentally unprepared and cannot give consent, and/or that violate the law or social taboos of society."[5] The first revision

Table 1 Sequelae of adult survivors of child sexual abuse	
Gynecologic problems	Chronic pelvic pain Dyspareunia Dysmenorrhea Vaginismus Disturbances of sexual desire, arousal, and orgasm May seek little to no prenatal care/have Pap smears Early adolescent or unintentional pregnancy History of STI >50 intercourse partners Prostitution
Substance use	Alcohol and illicit drug use, 4 to 5× rate of general population Tobacco use, 2× as likely
Increased somatic complaints	Disproportionately use health care services Lower pain threshold Chronic and diffuse pain, especially abdominal or pelvic pain Gastrointestinal disorders
Mental health	Symptoms of posttraumatic stress Depression Anxiety Eating disorders
Miscellaneous	Self-neglect Victimized repeatedly Physically sedentary, 2× as likely Severe obesity, 2× as likely

Data from Adult manifestations of childhood sexual abuse. ACOG committee opinion No. 498. Obstet Gynecol 2011; 118:392-95.

to the 1927 definition of rape occurred in 2012 by The Department of Justice: "The penetration, no matter how slight of the vagina or anus with any body part or object, or oral penetration by a sex organ of another person, without the consent of the victim."[6] Physical resistance is not required on the part of the victim to demonstrate lack of consent[6] (**Table 2**).

EPIDEMIOLOGY OF SEXUAL VIOLENCE IN MINORS IN THE UNITED STATES

Exact statistics on the prevalence of SV are not available because many victims do not disclose abuse until adulthood, and it is common for instances to never be reported (**Table 3**). Between 40% and 60% of all rape victims are under the age of 18, and most are adolescents.[7] It is estimated that two-thirds of minors who have experienced sexual abuse were 12 to 17 years old when it first occurred.[8] Women aged 16 to 19 are 4 times more likely to be sexually assaulted than women in all other age groups.[9]

Finkelhor and colleagues[10] amalgamated 3 telephone surveys of 2293 fifteen to 17 year olds between 2003 and 2011. The lifetime experience of 17 year olds with sexual abuse and sexual assault was 26.6% for girls (being 16.8% for 15 year olds) and 5.1% for boys (being 4.3% for 15 year olds).[10] This study notes an increase in perpetrator types (adults, peers, family, acquaintances, and, rarely, strangers) over time.[11] Adult perpetration of sexual abuse and assault was revealed in 1 in 9 girls and 1 in 53 boys less than the age of 18.[10]

Emerson Hospital's Youth Risk Behavior Survey[12] (2018) reported 8% of the 11,018 subjects had unwanted sexual contact with someone. This percentage was higher for female subjects (11%) than for male subjects (3%). Four percent of all the students had this abuse greater than 12 months before the survey; 3% within the past 12 months of the survey, and 1% both before and during the past 12 months. Common traits in those reporting sexual contact against their will are listed in **Table 4**.

Minors who experienced attempted or completed rape were perpetrated by someone known to the victim 89.9% to 93% of the time.[2,13] Older adolescents are most commonly victims during social encounters with assailants. In younger adolescent victims, the assailant is more likely to be a member of the adolescent's extended family[11]

Table 2		
Forms of sexual violence		
Sexual assault • Nonconsensual sexual acts that occur in the context of physical force, psychological coercion, incapacitation, or impairment, and/or the inability of a victim to provide consent or understand their actions because of age, developmental limitations, or the influence of alcohol or drugs • May involve threatened or actual physical force in the use of coercion, intimidation, or weapons		
Contact	Abuser touching the child	Child being urged to touch the abuser
	Penetrative (eg, digital, penile, and object insertion into the vagina, anus, or oral cavity)	*Nonpenetrative* (eg, fondling of the victim's genitals, breast, groin, or anus; sexual kissing)
Noncontact	Exposure to exhibitionism, voyeurism, sexual harassment, and involvement in pornography (both filming and exposure)	
Other forms of SV	Being made (forced) to penetrate another	Verbal threats

Data from Refs.[1,19,54,55]

Table 3
Sexual violence experienced during youth[a]

	Rape		Made to Penetrate
Girls	**Boys**		**Boys**
Approximately 8% or an estimated 10 million experienced rape or attempted rape	0.7% or an estimated 791,000 experienced either rape or attempted rape		Almost 2% or an estimated 2 million were made to penetrate someone or there was an attempt to make them penetrate someone
About 6% or an estimated 7 million experienced	Rape 0.4% or an estimated 500,000 experienced rape		0.8% or an estimated 883,000 were made to penetrate someone
About 4% or an estimated 4 million experienced rape involving drugs or alcohol	X		1% or an estimated 1 million experienced being made to penetrate, involving drugs or alcohol
2% or an estimated 2.6 million experienced attempted rape	X		X

X, Estimates are not reported. Too few men and boys reported these forms of violence in 2012 to produce a reliable estimate.

[a] Adult women and men reported on their SV experiences, including those that occurred in youth (before the age of 18) on the National Intimate Partner and Sexual Violence survey. The authors use the terms "girls" and "boys" in this fact sheet to describe these experiences.

From National Center for Injury Prevention and Control Division of Violence Prevention. In: Sexual Violence in Youth Findings from the 2012 National Intimate Partner and Sexual Violence Survey. 2013.

Table 4
Emerson Hospital's youth risk behavior survey, 2018 (Massachusetts)

(6th, 8th, and 9th to 12th Graders)	N = 11,018
Youth who use illegal drugs	38–51%
Youth who smoke cigarettes	32%
Youth with grades in the "D-F" range	32%
Gender-nonconforming youth	28%
Youth who misuse others' or their own prescription medication	27–28%
Youth who chew tobacco	27%
LGBTQ youth	17%
Middle Eastern youth	16%
African American youth	15%

Data from Emerson Hospital 2018 Youth Risk Behavior Survey, www.emersonhospital.org.

(**Table 5**). In 88% of CPS-substantiated sexual abuse claims, the perpetrator is a man regardless of the sex of the victim; in 9% the perpetrator is a woman, and in 3% the sex of the perpetrator is unknown.[11,14]

EVALUATION OF THE ADOLESCENT PATIENT

Evaluation of the sexual assault patient can vary greatly based on details unique to the patient, such as age, gender identity; the assault itself, including the timeline; and what may be known about the perpetrator or perpetrators. Such evaluation can be greatly affected by the rapport developed between the examiner and the patient. One reason for delayed or lack of disclosures is the prevalence of SV inflicted by individuals known by the victim.[13] The provider should recognize that overcoming barriers to disclosure can be difficult for the child, and a safe place for the child to discuss their safety should be provided. Unless the patient objects, the adolescent should not have acquaintances present during the interview, allowing the victim to freely discuss safety, disclose information, discuss treatment, and ask questions that may not otherwise be addressed. The patient may require pain control. Local rape crisis centers have advocates who can be present for support during the sexual assault examination, should the patient desire. Other roles of advocates are discussed later.

PRIMARY CARE VERSUS EMERGENCY DEPARTMENT

The provider should be aware of signs, symptoms, and behaviors suggestive of abuse. Because indicators or symptoms of sexual abuse are often nonspecific and common complaints, the provider's observation of the victim's behavior during a physical examination is crucial[15] (**Box 1**). Primary care has a role in screening for teen dating violence; if any SV is present, they should ask about commercial sexual exploitation.[16]

The patient may acutely present to the primary care provider's office or to an emergency department (ED). The decision to perform forensic examinations in the office is preferably triaged before the arrival of the patient. For patients triaged for sexual assault concerns, avoid prolonged periods in the waiting room. Ask the patient to refrain from eating, drinking, rinsing his/her mouth, and to remain clothed so that evidence is not compromised. Alert the patient, if he/she needs to void, to obtain an *unclean*

Table 5 Perpetrators of sexual violence among victims who experienced sexual violence during youth	
Completed or Attempted Rape (Girls)	**Completed or Attempted Made to Penetrate (Boys)**
43.6% Acquaintance	35.1% Acquaintance
28.8% Current or former intimate partner	X
27.7% Family member	X
4.5% Person in a position of authority	X
10.1% Stranger	X

X, Estimates are not reported. Too few men and boys reported these forms of violence in 2012 to produce a reliable estimate for type of perpetrator.

From National Center for Injury Prevention and Control Division of Violence Prevention. In: Sexual Violence in Youth Findings from the 2012 National Intimate Partner and Sexual Violence Survey. 2013.

Box 1
Symptoms of sexual assault or abuse
Headaches
Stomachaches
Fatigue
Sadness
Withdrawal
Irritability
Difficulty sleeping
Outbursts of anger
Change in academic performance
Substance abuse
Risky sexual behaviors

Data from Hanson RF, Adams CS. Childhood sexual abuse identifications, screening, and treatment recommendations in primary care settings. Prim Care. 2016;43(2):313–26.

("dirty") specimen.[17] A patient with acute injuries or symptoms, such as pain on urination or anogenital bleeding, suggests a potential assault occurred within the past 72 hours. Even without a disclosure, this warrants further investigation of the child's safety and may indicate the need for a medical forensic examination.

Regardless of the timeframe since the abuse, the primary or initial care provider should evaluate the patient for injury, because assessing patient stability takes precedence over forensic evidence collection. If the contact was recent, referring to a protocolized sexual assault forensic examination (SAFE) for forensic assessment, documentation, evidence collection and preservation, and photography provides the patient with the best opportunity to investigate SV. If the patient is in the window for evidentiary collection, gloves should be worn during the entire physical assessment, taking care to avoid contamination of any evidence.

The primary care provider should educate the patient and parents/guardians on the medical forensic examination. The time-sensitive forensic examination often takes several hours to complete. Some clothing may be kept as evidence. Any items brought in from home as evidence should be stored in paper bags; plastic bags promote the growth of mold and degrade evidence. Only under certain circumstances whereby there is significant vaginal bleeding, suspicion for pelvic inflammatory infection, or a foreign body, would a victim experience a vaginal examination.[18,19] In a trauma-sensitive manner, the examiner will inquire if this is a first-time occurrence. Otherwise, a speculum or bimanual examination is rarely used.[20] If the provider defers conducting evidentiary examinations in their office, a listing of locations of local SAFE facilities should be accessed. Provided the patient and family desire this process, referral to a regional Child Advocacy Center (CAC) for medical evaluation may be appropriate.[21] If the patient's available option is a sexual assault nurse examiner (SANE) in the ED, contacting the nearest facility before patient transfer will confirm availability of an SANE to perform the SAFE.

Should the victim be identified outside of the timeframe for evidence collection, conducting a medical forensic examination is not appropriate. When an emergent physical examination is not required for a patient with ongoing symptoms (eg, genital pain, bleeding, discharge, or significant emotional duress), the most experienced practitioner should be sought in a scheduled appointment within a couple of days. Menstrual and contraceptive history, if ejaculate was near the genitals, or the last consensual contact should the adolescent be sexually active, may indicate the need for education on emergency and ongoing contraceptive. Pregnancy testing, safety, and mental-health assessments are appropriate at this visit.

Providers should limit documentation of the details of the assault if the detailed examination is anticipated by another examiner. It is more desirable to the patient to avoid retelling his/her experience and reduces possible discrepancies in the record. Refrain from words such as "normal," "alleged," "apparently," "story," "satisfactory," "positive," or "negative" in the documentation, because these imply judgment. The author should never document "no signs or symptoms of sexual assault" in the physical examination.

HISTORY AND PHYSICAL EVALUATION

Document open-ended questions and quote the patient's responses describing the timing, type of sexual contact, and any resultant symptoms for the purpose of learning the minimal facts to direct the medical evaluation and treatment. History and observations may raise suspicion for drug facilitation. Alcohol is the most common agent used in "date rape" and commonly accompanies SV within this age.[20,22] Benzodiazepines other than flunitrazepam are more commonly used than drugs suspected in sexual assault, for example, flunitrazepam (Rohypnol), gamma-hydroxybutyric acid, gamma-butyrolactone, and ketamine.[19,20,22] The latter 4 are not included in standard urine drug screen (UDS), but should be additions to the standard UDS to detect common benzodiazepines.

Physical evaluation includes a detailed assessment of the scalp, all skin surfaces, mucosa, conjunctiva, anogenital region, and airway for the following:

- Hair removal, bruises, contusions, abrasions, petechia, and bite marks
- Palatal petechia, torn frenulum, and other evidence of oral/dental trauma, ulcerations
- Genital evaluation for bleeding, bruising, swelling, lacerations, irritation, scarring, discharge, urethral inflammation, odor, warts, ulcerations, hymenal transections, adenopathy
- Anal swelling, bruising, tearing, scarring, spontaneous or immediate dilation (without the presence of stool), loss of sphincter tone, or loss of anal rugae pattern

Strangulation has been identified as a lethality indicator in interpersonal violence (IPV), and all victims of sexual assault should be assessed for the signs of neck/airway injury.[23] Symptoms include neck/throat pain, petechia, vocal changes, shortness of breath, and difficulty swallowing.[24] Nonfatal strangulation is often present with no external physical signs. A computed tomography angiogram (CTA) should be considered in those with a history of strangulation evaluating potential vascular injuries, despite lack of physical examination findings[24] (see Appendix 1). This CTA is in addition to the usual physical examination, and forensic evidence collection at the direction of the patient (see Appendix 1).

Injuries should be photographed and described in the record. Providers should be aware that patients presenting for sexual assault evaluation often have no obvious physical injuries. Having no obvious physical injuries does *not* mean that assault/abuse has *not* occurred. This fact, or an explanation of the findings, needs communicated with the patient.

SEXUAL ASSAULT NURSE EXAMINER

SANEs are registered nurses with additional training in trauma-informed care and evidence collection. They act as liaisons between the medical and legal fields. The International Association of Forensic Nurses dictates the educational guidelines and certifies SANEs.[18] The SANE's involvement, with their knowledge of the neurobiology of trauma and forensics, allows for a victim-centered methodology to the investigation.

Whereas health care providers evaluate the patient for acute medical needs, the SAFE is the process of obtaining the assault history, documenting examination findings, and collecting evidence. Although state forensic guidelines vary, research suggests that DNA evidence may still be present up to 7 to 10 days.[19,25] Informed consent is needed for each step (eg, physical examination, photo-documentation, evidence collection, presence of an advocate, and treatment). Regardless of their age, the patient may at any time withdraw consent for any part of the evaluation.

It is not the SANE's focus to discern nor investigate whether an assault occurred; rather, SANE should remain nonbiased while providing medical treatment. Because the SANE's medical forensic documentation is considered evidence, it is recommended that this documentation remain separate of the medical record and kept in a secured manner that protects the chain of custody. The evidence is transferred to law enforcement, often providing a starting point for the investigation. SANE evaluations result in improved evidence collection, expert testimony, and stronger cases for the prosecution.[26,27]

The SANE can educate on the trauma process and devise informed treatment plans while debunking myths surrounding sexual assault. The SANE may have suggestions, such as sexually transmitted infection (STI) prophylaxis and emergency contraception (EC), for the medical provider to be communicated before the patient's discharge.

MANAGEMENT OF POST–SEXUAL ASSAULT PREGNANCY AND SEXUALLY TRANSMITTED INFECTION RISKS AND FINAL DETAILS

All postpubertal patients are to be universally tested and presumptively treated for gonorrhea, chlamydia, and trichomonas in contrast to prepubertal patients, who do not receive empiric treatment.[16,19,28] If testing, with the patient's consent, is performed, nucleic acid amplification test (NAAT) is preferred for the diagnostic evaluation of postpubertal sexual assault survivors.[22,28] Urine specimens for chlamydia, gonorrhea, and trichomonas are suitable over vaginal or cervical specimens, or urethral specimens in men. Oropharynx and rectum specimens should be obtained if they are sites of penetration or attempted penetration.[28] A positive NAAT result warrants confirmatory testing, with an Infectious Disease Service consultation, which can be completed on the original specimen in adolescents with no history of consensual peer sexual activity (as is also imperative in prepubertal individuals). Serum samples for hepatitis B and syphilis should be obtained.[28] The baseline human immunodeficiency virus (HIV) *result* is not needed to expeditiously start the nonoccupational postexposure prophylaxis (PEP) if the risk-benefit ratio deems PEP initiation (see Appendix 1). PEP would then be changed to antiretroviral treatment if preexisting HIV infection is diagnosed. Empiric treatment and other considerations are listed in **Table 6**.[19,28] Admission of the survivor's previous sexual history into discovery is limited by laws in every state. These laws are meant to allow medical testing and treatment of STIs without demeaning the victim's credibility in court.[28]

The adolescent patient will need counseling regarding PEP and EC. The risk of pregnancy is higher than the 5% per sexual assault among women aged 12 to 45 quoted

Table 6
2015 Centers for Disease Control and Prevention guidelines for sexually transmitted infection prophylaxis after sexual assault

Gonorrhea	Ceftriaxone 250 mg IM (single dose)
Chlamydia	Azithromycin 1 g PO (single dose)
Trichomonas	Metronidazole 2 g PO or tinidazole 2 g PO (single doses)
Pregnancy	Levonorgestrel 1.5 mg PO or ulipristal acetate 30 mg PO or Cu IUD

Consider as indicated:
  HIV PEP ≤72 h exposure
  HPV vaccine, if ≥9 y and not fully immunized
  Tdap (tetanus, diphtheria, acellular pertussis) booster
  Hepatitis B vaccine and hepatitis B immune globulin (HBIG)
  Antiemetic avoiding ondansetron if susceptibility to prolongation of the QT interval exists

Adapted from Division of STD Prevention, National Center for HIV/AIDS, Viral Hepatitis, STD, and TB Prevention, Centers for Disease Control and Prevention. Sexual assault and abuse and STDs. In: 2015 sexually transmitted diseases: treatment guidelines 2015. Available at: https://www.cdc.gov/std/tg2015/default.htm

statistic because adolescents have higher fertility and lower rates of concurrent contraceptive use.[3] Levonorgestrel (Plan B One-Step) is most effective when taken within 72 hours.[29] If the patient's body mass index (BMI) is greater than 25 kg/m^2, or if the assault was between 72 and 120 hours, the likelihood of levonorgestrel providing effective prophylaxis for pregnancy is lessened considerably. As the BMI increases to greater than 25 kg/m^2, the efficacy decreases, and at a BMI over30 kg/m^2, the risk of pregnancy was 5.8% with levonorgestrel and 2.6% with ulipristal acetate (Ella). Therefore, Glasier and colleagues[30] recommend ulipristal acetate or a copper intrauterine device (IUD) as an alternative for pregnancy prophylaxis if the BMI is greater than 25 kg/m^2 with effectiveness up to 5 days after vaginal intercourse. In cases whereby the ulipristal acetate is given, hormonal birth control (progestin) should be avoided for 5 to 7 days following the progesterone receptor antagonist, ulipristal acetate, because it may decrease the progestin's effectiveness. Additional birth control measures should be used during those 7 days. Alternates to ulipristal acetate in those taking hormonal contraception should be considered.[29,31]

The risk of HIV in the United States for a women having receptive vaginal intercourse with ejaculation with an HIV-positive man is 1 in 1250, and the risk of HIV acquisition in the receptive partner via anal intercourse with an HIV-positive man with ejaculation is 1 in 70.[32–34] Decisions regarding PEP for HIV should be based on the individual's risk using the information provided by the victim and the examination, and if able, testing the assailant. PEP resources are provided (see Appendix 1). The patient should be informed that the cost of PEP medications can exceed $1000 to $2000. Although the cost of the medical forensic examination should be free to the patient in accordance with Violence Against Women Act, medical costs vary by facility.[18] Assistance, such as the Victim's Compensation Fund, may be available (see Appendix 1).

Recommended doses of azithromycin and metronidazole or tinidazole are likely to induce nausea and emesis. Because alcohol contributes to adolescent sexual assault, providers should be cognizant of the Antabuse-like reaction of the -idazoles with alcohol. A delay of several hours in administration of the empiric treatment of trichomonas will likely improve the patient experience.[19,28]

Before discharge, the patient should be offered the opportunity to clean up if desired. Because the patient's clothing items are often taken as evidence, a clothing bank in the office or ED may serve this purpose well. The mental health status of the patient should be assessed and the family provided with advice and resources to help their child through the process. Jenny and Crawford-Jakubiak's article is helpful in this regard (see Appendix 1). The patient should be educated on the symptoms of STIs, including acute retroviral syndrome, and instructed to return if symptoms present. Detailed written instructions should be given to the patient to share with the medical provider in follow-up.

SEXUAL ASSAULT REPORTING

In 42 U.S.C. § 13031 under the Victims of Child Abuse Act of 1990, it is required that all professionals report any suspicion of child abuse.[35] Any nonconsensual sexual act on an individual less than the age of 18 is considered child sexual abuse, and therefore, a mandatory reportable crime.[18] Law enforcement should be notified if the patient is less than 18 years of age or is a vulnerable adult (eg, has developmental or cognitive disabilities).[19] When in doubt, report to law enforcement and CPS or a similar agency in your state. The Rape, Abuse and Incest National Network provides a database on state laws (see Appendix 1).

FOLLOW-UP

The patient will need to follow up with his/her medical home or a specialty treatment center in 3 to 7 days to review the laboratory results, assess tolerance of medication, confirm, or clarify any initial positive findings on examination, and access healing. If the patient opted out of the recommended prophylaxis for sexually transmitted infections, 7 to 14 days after the event is an opportune time to retest for chlamydia, gonorrhea, trichomonas, and pregnancy. In addition, the patient has several distant laboratory studies and may need hepatitis B and human papilloma virus (HPV) vaccines to complete their series. Concerning behaviors may prompt referral for trauma-focused cognitive-behavioral therapy, possible psychotropic medication, or hospitalization (Table 7).

ADVOCACY RESOURCES

Advocacy centers can offer emergency shelter, counseling, support groups, advocacy, and education. In addition to crisis intervention and support to the patient and family during the examination, rape and domestic abuse advocates provide support during the law enforcement investigation and court proceedings. Rape crisis centers effectually decrease secondary distress and retraumatization that the victim may experience following a traumatic event.[36,37]

CACs are able to help facilitate the investigation of child sexual abuse in a safe, child-focused environment.[21] The victim may disclose to a trained forensic interviewer, who is able to communicate with the child in a developmentally appropriate manner. CACs, present in every state, offer courtroom preparation, victim advocacy, case management, and sometimes, individual and group therapy.[21] Providers should direct clients to their local rape crisis centers and local CACs (see Appendix 1) and have protocols with them and their local multidisciplinary investigative teams (MDITs) to determine the appropriate response method within their community.

VULNERABLE YOUTH

Certain subgroups of adolescents, for example, lesbian, gay, bisexual, transgender, and queer (LGBTQ) youth, sexually exploited children, victims of IPV, and individuals

Table 7
Follow-up

	SAFE or Initial Examination	3–7 d[a]	2 wk[a]	3–6 wk[a]	3 mo[a]	6 mo[a]
UDS if suspect drug facilitation	≤96 h					
Pregnancy	X	≥7 d				
Anogenital examination	X	Reevaluate any positive findings		Evaluate for warts; primary syphilis with dark field examination	if signs present	
Wet mount if discharge present	X		X			
Gonorrhea, chlamydia, trichomonas if negative initial test and no empiric treatment	X	≥7 d or, not initially tested	it signs present	[b]		
Medication tolerance/ adherence. Adjust medications accordingly		X	X			
ALT, AST, creatinine, complete blood count if taking PEP	X		X			
HIV combined antigen/ antibody, with confirmatory test as needed	X			X (4 wk if fourth generation; 6 wk if third generation)	X	In addition, only if third generation
Hepatitis B surface antibody	X					
Hepatitis C[c]	X					x
Nontreponemal syphilis (RPR or VDRL), with confirmatory test as needed	X			X	X	X
Psychiatric well-being	X	X	X	X	X	X

[a] Time from last suspected encounter.
[b] Retest sexually active women 2 wk to 3 mo after trichomonas treatment. Retest chlamydia and gonorrhea 3 mo after treatment in both genders for assessment of new infection if sexually active.
[c] Hepatitis C serology may be considered, but is not substantiated by research in the circumstance of sexual assault.

with intellectual or developmental disabilities, are at higher risk for sexual harassment, assault, and other forms of victimization. Unfortunately, data on prevalence rates are limited and vary between studies.

A longitudinal study among LGBTQ youth aged 16 to 20 demonstrates 45.2% were physically abused and 16.9% were sexually victimized by a dating partner.[38] Female LGBTQ youth were significantly more likely to experience victimization than male LGBTQ youth, and transgender youth were 2.4 times more likely to experience victimization than cisgender youth.[38] The prevalence of physical IPV declined over time as youth aged, but that of sexual victimization increased over time, particularly among men.[38] Others support the higher prevalence of victimization among LGBTQ adolescents, noting 23% to 62% of LGBTQ adolescents reported bullying, sexual victimization, and child maltreatment.[39]

The 4500 youth from the Child and Adolescent Twin Study reported a high prevalence of sexual victimization among youth with neurodevelopmental disorders, for example, attention-deficit/hyperactivity disorder (ADHD) and autism spectrum disorder (ASD).[40] They reported that youth with ASD were almost 3 times more likely to experience coercive sexual victimization; youth with ADHD had double the risk.[40] A literature review on sexual abuse involving children with intellectual disabilities confirmed a higher risk of both victimization and perpetration among youth with cognitive and communication impairments.[41] The risk of abuse also increased by 78% among individuals with both intellectual and developmental disabilities because of the nature of the disability, but also environmental factors, such as existing institutional services.[42] Youth with disabilities are less likely to receive appropriate sexual education or information regarding healthy sexuality, and the type of services and level of potential environmental control could contribute to the higher risk among this group for victimization.[43]

Clinical staff should be cognizant of any biases in working with vulnerable populations of youth and consider any additional service providers that are neededand/or received so that the individual understands the situation and the proposed treatment plan.[43] Trauma services may or may not be as effective if all needed services are not available. Vulnerable youth may also demonstrate trauma-related symptoms differently from other youth given previous experiences and/or the level of functioning. Clinicians should consider psychosocial factors the youth is experiencing and evaluate how these factors would influence the effectiveness of (and the youth's participation in) trauma-related services.[44]

Existing effective approaches for preventing adolescent (10 to 15years) IPV and SV were reviewed.[44] Overall, most studies available demonstrated short intervention periods, limited follow-up, and retention issues. Of those available, school-based dating violence interventions showed considerable success but were not being studied among low-income settings. Interventions focused on gender-equitable attitudes for boys and girls were equally successful targeting some factors that increase vulnerability for LGBTQ and male youth.

Trauma-related interventions, particularly for youth with disabilities, may also be overprotective and infantilized.[43] The individual's level of functioning should be considered, and this level incorporated into their care. Clinicians should ensure the individual understands the plan and has an opportunity to contribute to that plan when possible. Finally, clinicians should be aware of the level of sensory stimuli in the clinical setting, particularly when interviewing or examining youth with ASD.[43] Despite the current paucity of literature, select studies are available that could be used as resources for responding appropriately for youth representing these populations (see Appendix 1).

QUALITY ASSURANCE

Those working in this field should routinely review deidentified cases to review content completeness and to discuss the interpretation of findings with others. Medical peer review involves reviewing photo-documented findings of sexual abuse. This form of case review supports proficiency[45] and likely helps relieve compassion fatigue.

Expert review differs from peer review. Adams and colleagues[25] recommend practitioners have all abnormal cases reviewed by an expert provider. Participants may submit deidentified history and images securely to a board-certified child-abuse pediatrician for case review, or quality improvement projects (see Appendix 1). In addition to an independent assessment of clinical judgment, reviewers promote amelioration in written documentation and photographic proficiency, utilization of alternate diagnostic techniques, and interpretation of findings. It may even make one a more confident, credible witness. Medical providers who perform 5 or more sexual abuse examinations per month, remain current in the specialized literature, and regularly review cases with an expert demonstrate greater diagnostic accuracy in child sexual abuse evaluations.[45] Select educational opportunities are listed in Appendix 2.

PREVENTION EFFORTS

Sexual assault prevention programs for youth have historically relied on awareness campaigns and increasing risk-reduction behaviors among potential victims, for example, attending events with groups of friends, not traveling alone, and walking in well-lit areas. Given the failure of these individual-level approaches to produce meaningful reductions in rates of sexual assault, experts recommend prevention strategies that move beyond individual-level risk reduction techniques to target interpersonal, community, and societal level influences of sexual assault.[46] Approaches that aim to prevent SV perpetration are thought to hold greater promise than those solely promoting risk reduction practices for potential victims. There is ample evidence to suggest that endorsements of hostile masculinity, traditional gender roles, and dominating attitudes toward women are among the strongest predictors of violence perpetration.[47] In addition, rape-supportive attitudes and norms are strongly associated with violence perpetration across individuals, their peer groups, and within communities and society.[47] The bystander approach to sexual assault prevention, which targets entire communities as agents of change, as opposed to a sole focus on victims or perpetrators, has gained popularity in recent years. These programs aim to change social norms that promote violence by providing bystanders (ie, individuals observing risky or violent situations) with knowledge and skills to safely and effectively intervene instead of remaining silent.[47,48]

Bystander-based SV prevention programs, such as *Green Dot* and *Bringing in the Bystander*, have demonstrated effectiveness in reducing SV among college populations[49] (see Appendix 1). Because a substantial proportion of individuals who experience sexual assault do so before age 18, there is a need for violence prevention efforts that begin earlier, such as in middle and high school settings. Recently tested in a randomized controlled trial in 26 Kentucky high schools, the college-adapted *Green Dot* bystander intervention found a significant reduction in the frequency of sexual assault, sexual harassment, physical and psychological dating violence, and reproductive coercion.[50] Findings indicate that a high school version of *Bringing in the Bystander*, and many other college-based violence prevention programs, may be successfully adapted for younger populations. Pre-matriculation education is particularly important given emerging evidence for the "red zone," the timeframe shortly after college students' arrival on campus when most sexual assaults occur.[51]

Although many are familiar with the Title IX Education Amendment of 1972 and its involvement on college campuses, Title IX is essential in providing guidance for prevention and response to violence for any federally funded education program.[52] They can be a great resource to adolescents in primary-secondary schools. Organizations should also be aware of other SV resources, such as RAINN (Rape, Abuse and Incest National Network), the largest anti-SV organization in the United States, and Prevent Child Abuse America (see Appendix 1).

IT TAKES A TEAM

An MDIT comprises allied professionals who work to coordinate a victim-centered response to sexual assaults to minimize the ambiguity of the medical and legal processes for the victim and ensure medical, psychological, and emotional support to survivors and their families. MDITs encompass individuals involved in the care of a child, including CPS, law enforcement, criminal justice, medical providers, psychologists, and victim advocates. The coordinated effort prioritizes the needs of the sexual assault victim, works to minimize the trauma, and can increase the likelihood that a victim will attend wrap-around services, thus promoting actual healing. "Optimal management of adolescents who have been sexually assaulted can have a positive impact on these youth."[53]

ACKNOWLEDGMENTS

The authors thank Emma Mason, MS, RN; Melinda Sharon; Aisha Lawson; and Clare McMahon, PharmD for their assistance with the preparation of this article.

DISCLOSURE

The authors have nothing to disclose.

REFERENCES

1. Smith SG, Chen J, Basile KC, et al. The National Intimate Partner and Sexual Violence Survey (NISVS): 2010-2012 State report. Atlanta (GA): National Center for Injury Prevention and Control, Centers for Disease Control and Prevention; 2017. Available at: https://www.cdc.gov/violenceprevention/pdf/NISVS-State ReportBook.pdf. Accessed June 10, 2019.
2. Smith SG, Zhang X, Basile KC. The National Intimate Partner and Sexual Violence Survey (NISVS): 2015 Data brief – updated release. Atlanta (GA): National Center for Injury Prevention and Control, Centers for Disease Control and Prevention; 2018. Available at: https://www.cdc.gov/violenceprevention/pdf/2015data-brief 508.pdf. Accessed June 10, 2019.
3. Sexual assault. ACOG committee opinion No. 777. Obstet Gynecol 2019;133(4): e296–302.
4. Adult manifestations of childhood sexual abuse. ACOG committee opinion No. 498. Obstet Gynecol 2011;118:392–5.
5. Kellogg N. AAP Committee of Child Abuse and Neglect. The evaluation of sexual abuse in children. Pediatrics 2005;116(2):506–12.
6. An updated definition of rape. The United States Department of Justice. 2017. Available at: https://www.justice.gov/archives/opa/blog/updated-definition-rape. Accessed June 10, 2019.
7. English A, Kenney KE. State minor consent laws: a summary. 2nd edition. Chapel Hill (NC): Center for Adolescent Health & Law; 2003.

8. Greenfield LA. Department of Justice, Office of Justice Programs, Bureau of Justice Statistics. Sex offenses and offenders: an analysis of data on rape and sexual assault. 1997. Available at: https://www.bjs.gov/content/pub/pdf/SOO.PDF. Accessed August 27, 2019.
9. Rickert VI, Wiemann CM. Date rape among adolescents and young adults. J Pediatr Adolesc Gynecol 1998;11:167–75.
10. Finkelhor D, Shattuck A, Turner H, et al. The lifetime prevalence of child sexual abuse and sexual assault assessed in late adolescence. J Adolesc Health 2014;55:329–33.
11. Breiding MJ, Smith SG, Basile KC, et al. Prevalence and characteristics of sexual violence, stalking, and intimate partner violence victimization - national intimate partner and sexual violence survey, United States 2011. MMWR Surveill Summ 2014;63(SS-8):1–18.
12. Emerson Hospital 2018 youth risk behavior survey. Available at: https://www.emersonhospital.org/EmersonHospital/media/PDF-files/2018-Youth-Risk-Behavior-Survey-Final-Report.pdf. Accessed June 10, 2019.
13. The National Center for Victims of Crime Reports on Child Sexual Abuse. Available at: https://victimsofcrime.org/media/reporting-on-child-sexual-abuse. Accessed June 18, 2019.
14. United States Department of Health and Human Services. Administration for Children and Families, Administration on Children, Youth and Families, Children's Bureau (2018) child maltreatment 2016. Available at: https://www.acf.hhs.gov/cb/research-data-technology/statistics-research/child-maltreatment. Accessed April 30, 2019.
15. Vrolijk-Bosschaart TF, Brilleslijper-Kater SN, Teeuw ARH, et al. Physical symptoms in very young children assessed for sexual abuse: a mixed method analysis from the ASAC study. Eur J Pediatr 2017;176(10):1365–74.
16. Kaufman M, American Academy of Pediatrics Committee on Adolescence. Care of the adolescent sexual assault victim. Pediatrics 2008;122(2):462–70.
17. West Virginia Foundation for Rape Information & Services, Inc. West Virginia protocol for responding to victims of sexual assault Revised 2016 – 6th edition.
18. U.S. Department of Justice Office on Violence Against Women. A national protocol for sexual assault medical forensic examinations adults/adolescents. 2nd edition. 2013. NCJ 228119. Available at: https://cdn.ymaws.com/www.safeta.org/resource/resmgr/Protocol_documents/SAFE_PROTOCOL_2012-508.pdf. Accessed April 28, 2019.
19. Crawford-Jakubiak JE, Alderman EM, Leventhal JM. AAP Committee on Child Abuse and Neglect, AAP Committee on Adolescence. Care of the adolescent after an acute sexual assault. Pediatrics 2017;139(3):e20164243.
20. Mollen CJ, Goyal M, Lavelle J, et al. Evaluation and treatment of the adolescent sexual assault patient. Adolesc Med 2015;266(3):647–57.
21. National Children's Alliance annual report 2018. Available at: https://www.nationalchildrensalliance.org/cac-model/. Accessed June 5, 2019.
22. Danielson CK, Holmes MM. Adolescent sexual assault: an update of the literature. Curr Opin Obstet Gynecol 2004;16(5):383–8.
23. Crane J. Interpretation of non-genital injuries in sexual assault. Best Pract Res Clin Obstet Gynecol 2013;27(1):103–11.
24. Zilkens RR, Phillips MA, Kelly MC, et al. Non-fatal strangulation in sexual assault. A study of clinical and assault characteristic highlighting the role of intimate partner violence. J Forensic Leg Med 2016;43:1752–928.
25. Adams JA, Kellogg ND, Farst KJ, et al. Updated guidelines for the medical assessment and care of children who may have been sexually abused. J Pediatr Adolesc Gynecol 2016;29:81–7.

26. Kagan-Krieger S, Rehfeld G. The sexual assault nurse examiner. Can Nurse 2000;96(6):20–4.

27. Nugent-Borakove ME, Fanflik PL, Troutman D, et al. Testing the efficacy of SANE/ SART programs: do they make a difference in sexual assault arrest and prosecution outcomes? Alexandria, Virginia: American Prosecutors Research Institute; 2006.

28. CDC 2015 sexually transmitted diseases treatment guidelines. Sexual assault and abuse and STDs. Available at: https://www.cdc.gov/std/tg2015/sexual-assault.htm. Accessed June 15, 2019.

29. MedAsk Drug News. Interactions between Ella (ulipristal acetate) and hormonal contraception (Progestins). Available at: https://medask.usask.ca/documents/newsletters/35.2%20Ulipristal%20Intereactions.pdf.   Accessed June 11, 2019.

30. Glasier A, Cameron ST, Blithe D, et al. Can we identify women at risk of pregnancy despite using emergency contraception? Data from randomized trials of ulipristal acetate and levonorgestrel. Contraception 2011;84(4):363–7.

31. Ella monograph for professionals. Available at: https://www.drugs.com/monograph/ella.html. Accessed June 21, 2019.

32. NAM Aidmap HIV risk levels for the insertive and receptive partner in different types of sexual intercourse. Available at: http://www.aidsmap.com/HIV-risk-levels-for-the-insertive-and-receptive-partner-in-different-types-of-sexual-intercourse/page/1443490/. Accessed April 30, 2019.

33. CDC HIV risk behaviors. Available at: https://www.cdc.gov/hiv/risk/estimates/riskbehaviors.html. Accessed April 30, 2019.

34. Announcement. Updated Guidelines for Antiretroviral Postexposure Prophylaxis after Sexual, Injection-Drug Use, or Other Nonoccupational Exposure to HIV — United States, 2016. MMWR Morb Mortal Wkly Rep 2016;65:458. https://doi.org/10.15585/mmwr.mm6517a5external icon. Accessed March 26, 2020.

35. Duty to report suspected child abuse under 42 U.S.C. § 13031. Available at: https://www.justice.gov/file/20601/download. Accessed June 18, 2019.

36. Paulson D, Denny M, Sharon M. Sexual assault and the sexual assault nurse examiner in West Virginia. W Va Med J 2017;113(6):18–21.

37. Campbell R, Wasco SM, Ahrens CE, et al. Preventing the "second rape": rape survivors' experiences with community service providers. J Interpers Violence 2001;16(12):1239.

38. Whitton SW, Newcomb ME, Messinger AM. A longitudinal study of IPV victimization among sexual minority youth. J Interpers Violence 2016;34(5):912–45.

39. Sterzing PR, Gartner RE, Goldbach JT, et al. Polyvictimization prevalence rates for sexual and gender minority adolescents: breaking down the silos of victimization research. Psychol Violence 2019;9(4):419–30.

40. Gotby VO, Lichtenstein P, Langstrom N, et al. Childhood neurodevelopmental disorders and risk of coercive sexual victimization in childhood and adolescence–a population-based prospective twin study. J Child Psychol Psychiatry 2018;59(9):957–65.

41. Wilczynski SM, Connolly S, Dubard M, et al. Assessment, prevention, and intervention for abuse among individuals with disabilities. Psychol Sch 2014;51(1):9–21.

42. Sobsey D, Doe T. Patterns of sexual abuse and assault. Sex Disabil 1991;9(3):243–59.

43. Houdek V, Gibson J. Treating sexual abuse and trauma with children, adolescents, and young adults with developmental disabilities. A workbook for clinicians. Springfield, Illinois: Charles C Thomas Publisher; 2017.

44. Lundgren R, Amin A. Addressing intimate partner violence and sexual violence among adolescents: emerging evidence of effectiveness. J Adolesc Health 2015;56(1):S42–50.

45. Adams JA, Starling SP, Frasier LD, et al. Diagnostic accuracy in child sexual abuse medical evaluation: role of experience, training, and expert case review. Child Abuse Negl 2012;36:383–92.

46. Basile KC. A comprehensive approach to sexual violence prevention. N Engl J Med 2015;372(24):2350–2.

47. Cook-Craig PG, Millspaugh PH, Recktenwald EA, et al. From empower to green dot: successful strategies and lessons learned in developing comprehensive sexual violence primary prevention programming. Violence Against Women 2014;20(10):1162–78.

48. Coker AL, Bush HM, Fisher BS, et al. Multi-college bystander intervention evaluation for violence prevention. Am J Prev Med 2016;50(3):295–302.

49. Jouriles EN, Krauss A, Vu NL, et al. Bystander programs addressing sexual violence on college campuses: a systematic review and meta-analysis of program outcomes and delivery methods. J Am Coll Health 2018;66(6):457–66.

50. Coker AL, Bush HM, Cook-Craig PG, et al. RCT testing bystander effectiveness to reduce violence. Am J Prev Med 2017;52(5):566–78.

51. Cranney S. The relationship between sexual victimization and year in school in US colleges: investigating the parameters of the "Red Zone". J Interpers Violence 2015;30(17):3133–45.

52. The United States Department of Justice. Overview of Title IX of the Education Amendments of 1972, 20 U.S.C. A§ 1681 ET. SEQ. Available at: https://www.justice.gov/crt/overview-title-ix-education-amendments-1972-20-usc-1681-et-seq. 08/07/2015. Accessed August 19, 2019.

53. Fujiwara J. Sexual assault in the adolescent. Br Columbia Med J 2004;46:128–32.

54. National Institute of Justice. Overview of rape and sexual violence. Available at: https://nij.ojp.gov/topics/articles/overview-rape-and-sexual-violence. Accessed March 26, 2020.

55. Planty M, Langton L, Krebs C, et al. Female victims of sexual violence, 1994-2010. In: US Department of Justice, Office of Justice Programs, Bureau of Justice Statistics Special Report; March, 2013. Available at: https://www.bjs.gov/content/pub/pdf/fvsv9410.pdf. Accessed March 26, 2020.

APPENDIX 1: MANAGEMENT OF SEXUAL ASSAULT VICTIM RESOURCES

Statutes by State	https://www.childwelfare.gov/topics/systemwide/laws-policies/state/
Locate a child advocacy center	https://www.nationalcac.org/find-a-cac/
Physical examination	Publication of the American College of Emergency Physicians: https://www.acep.org/globalassets/new-pdfs/sexual-assault-e-book.pdf US Department of Justice Office on Violence Against Women, A National Protocol for Sexual Assault Medical Forensic Examinations Adults/Adolescents, 2013 NCJ 228119. Through the court room processes: https://cdn.ymaws.com/www.safeta.org/resource/

(continued on next page)

(continued)	
	resmgr/Protocol_documents/SAFE_PROTOCOL_2012-508.pdf.
Strangulation resources	Training Institute on Strangulation Prevention protocol for medical and radiographic evaluations and discharge instructions: https://www.strangulationtraininginstitute.com/medical-radiographic-imaging-recommendations/ https://www.familyjusticecenter.org/wp-content/uploads/2019/07/SS-Discharge-Information-v3.26.19.pdf
Locate a victim advocate	RAINN (Rape, Abuse & Incest National Network) resource for victims and health care providers: http://centers.rainn.org
Treatment guidelines	STD Guidelines: https://www.cdc.gov/std/tg2015/sexual-assault.htm The Centers for Disease Control and Prevention (CDC) Updated Guidelines for Antiretroviral Postexposure Prophylaxis After Sexual, Injection Drug Use, or Other Nonoccupational Exposure to HIV, 2016: https://www.cdc.gov/hiv/pdf/programresources/cdc-hiv-npep-guidelines.pdf. • Figure 2, nPEP considerations summary on page 45 • Table 2, recommended schedule of laboratory evaluations of source and exposed persons for providing nPEP with preferred regimens on page 27 The National Clinician's PEP Hotline:_ https://aidsetc.org/npep (888–448–4911)
Crime victim compensation fund	Compensation of funds and resources vary by state. Specific information regarding each state's resources is provided by the National Association of Crime Victim Compensation Boards: http://www.nacvcb.org/index.asp?sid=6
Mitigating adverse effects of sexual trauma	Jenny C, Crawford-Jakubiak JE. Committee on Child Abuse and Neglect. The evaluation of children in the primary care setting when sexual abuse is suspected. *Pediatrics* 2013;132(2):e558–e567; https://pediatrics.aappublications.org/content/132/2/e558
Mandatory reporter	RAINN State Law Data Base: https://apps.rainn.org/policy/?_ga=2.159887550.225882788.1556472416-1832397619.1556472416
Special population resources	Pachankis JE, Safren SA. Handbook of evidence-base mental health practice with sexual and gender minorities. Oxford University Press; 2019 Musicaro RM, Spinazzola J, Arvidson J, et al. The complexity of adaptation to childhood polyvictimization in youth and young adults: recommendations for multidisciplinary responders. Trauma Violence Abuse 2017;20(1):81-98
Thorough sexual assault resource lists	https://www.rainn.org/national-resources-sexual-assault-survivors-and-their-loved-ones https://www.acog.org/More-Info/SexualAssault
Quality improvement	Access to expert reviewers available through Midwest Regional Child Advocacy Center: myCasereview:

(continued on next page)

(*continued*)	
	http://www.mrcac.org/medical-academy/myCasereview/ Children's Minnesota offers QI projects to nurses and physicians: MyQIportal is attainable through: https://www.mrcac.org/medical-academy/myqiportal/
Prevention efforts	https://alteristic.org/services/green-dot/ STOP SV prevention strategies in a CDC technical package https://www.cdc.gov/ violenceprevention/pdf/sv-prevention-technical-package.pdf https://www.cdc.gov/violenceprevention/sexualviolence/ resources.html

APPENDIX 2: EDUCATIONAL OPPORTUNITIES

Online studies:	The New York Child Abuse Medical Provider Program online free "Evaluating Child Sexual Abuse" and "Adolescent Sexual Assault: Consent Issues" courses on https://champprogram.com/courses.asp Online self-paced twenty-seven hour Midwest Regional CAC's Medical Training Academy https://www.mrcac.org/elearning/mta/
Onsite preceptorship:	A 4-day intensive clinical experience, the Midwest Regional CAC's Medical Academy Preceptorship, https://www.mrcac.org/medical-academy/preceptorship/ is available in: TX, OR, MI, MO, PA
Webcasts on trauma sensitive topics:	The Wisconsin Child Abuse Network https://wichildabusenetwork.org/upcoming-webinars/ New York Child Abuse Medical Provider Program https://www.champprogram.com/webcasts.shtml National Child Advocacy Center Virtual Training Center https://www.nationalcac.org/online-training-catalog/

Human Immunodeficiency Virus in Adolescents
Risk, Prevention, Screening, and Treatment

Jennifer J. Chang, MD, AAHIVS[a],*, Amie M. Ashcraft, PhD, MPH[b]

KEYWORDS

• HIV • Adolescent • Risk • Prevention • Screening • Diagnosis • Treatment

KEY POINTS

• Adolescence is a time of marked change. Marginalized key populations, such as youth identifying with diverse sexual practices, injection drug use, and living in poverty, are at increased risk for human immunodeficiency virus (HIV) infection.

• HIV screening is underused in adolescent populations, and baseline HIV testing is recommended for all adolescents by the US Centers for Disease Control and Prevention (CDC).

• On diagnosis of HIV, treatment should be initiated as soon as safely possible, with expert guidance and consultation.

INTRODUCTION

Despite successes in the management of human immunodeficiency virus (HIV) infection with effective antiretroviral therapy (ART), adolescents and youth remain at risk for HIV infection because of physical, social, and economic factors, such engagement in risky behaviors; identification as lesbian, gay, bisexual, transgender, or queer (LGBTQ); and poverty. In 2017, youths aged 13 to 24 years constituted 21% of all new HIV diagnoses.[1] Key at-risk populations for acquired HIV infection include specific vulnerable populations: young men who have sex with men (MSM), transgender youth, injection drug users, and sex workers. In the United States, LGBTQ youth aged 13 to 24 years from black and Latinx subgroups disproportionately made up more than 75% of new infections among youth in 2017. Reaching key communities and age

[a] Department of Infectious Diseases, Kaiser Permanente Los Angeles Medical Center, 1505 North Edgemont Street, 2nd Floor, Los Angeles, CA 90027, USA; [b] Department of Family Medicine, West Virginia University, 1 Medical Center Drive, Box 9152, Morgantown, WV 26505, USA
* Corresponding author.
E-mail address: Jennifer.Jiwen.Chang@kp.org

Prim Care Clin Office Pract 47 (2020) 351–365
https://doi.org/10.1016/j.pop.2020.02.011
0095-4543/20/© 2020 Elsevier Inc. All rights reserved.
primarycare.theclinics.com

groups is critical in connecting youth infected with HIV to appropriate care, many of whom are not aware of their serostatus. Addressing barriers to treatment and engaging adolescents in routine care that results in durable viral suppression remains a great concern in the United States, where linkage to care is low at an estimated 25% to 75%[2] and the proportion of virally suppressed adolescents remains at 25%. This article provides an overview of the currently understood best practices associated with HIV risk, prevention, screening, and treatment of providers of adolescent health care within the context of adolescents' unique needs.

HUMAN IMMUNODEFICIENCY VIRUS RISK

Adolescents' brains are still developing well into their early 20s. The parts of the brain involved in experiencing emotions are sensitive and well developed, but the parts of the brain involved in regulating emotional responses and impulse control are still developing. This combination of heightened emotional response with immature behavioral control may lead to risky decisions and behavior and, ultimately, consequences affecting sexual health. Further, adolescents navigating the transition into sexual maturity experience developmental changes in their bodies, and in family and peer relationships, and may be affected by several factors that increase their risk of HIV infection. **Table 1** summarizes the major physical/behavioral, cognitive, social, and economic factors associated with this increased risk.

There are several ways adolescents can reduce their risk of HIV transmission, including:

- Engaging in less risky sexual or substance abuse–related behaviors, such as engaging in mutual masturbation or oral sex instead of penetrative intercourse (vaginal or anal sex), and using clean needles for injection drug use
- Getting tested and treated for other sexually transmitted infections (STIs)
- Using condoms and lubrication during sexual intercourse

HUMAN IMMUNODEFICIENCY VIRUS PREVENTION

In the United States, HIV is primarily acquired through sexual activity or injection drug use. Reducing transmission is challenging because of factors related to social context and (relatively private) behavior.[9] Risk factors and protective factors related to HIV transmission operate on multiple levels, including biological, interpersonal, community, and societal levels; therefore, prevention efforts for HIV must include a variety of strategies that are contextually appropriate for maximal relevance and effectiveness in the target population, especially adolescents. Although it is accepted that HIV prevention interventions take this integrated approach, there have been limited rigorous evaluations of preventive interventions specific to adolescents.

Currently available tools with demonstrated effectiveness for HIV prevention that can be integrated into combination prevention packages for adolescents include:

- Preexposure prophylaxis: the use of an antiretroviral medication to prevent HIV infection that is highly effective when used correctly; tenofovir-emtricitabine is US Food and Drug Administration approved for adolescents who weigh at least 35 kg.
- Postexposure prophylaxis: the use of antiretroviral drugs within 72 hours of possible exposure to HIV.
- Early HIV treatment: reduces HIV transmission by as much as 96% across diverse populations.[10–12]

Table 1
Factors associated with increased risk for human immunodeficiency virus infection in adolescents

Physical/Behavioral Factors	How Risk of HIV Infection Is Increased
Anatomy and physiology	Adolescent girls are particularly vulnerable to HIV infection because the cervix is still in development, with areas of exposed columnar epithelium and a thinner protective mucosa
Unprotected sexual activity	Adolescents engaging in vaginal, anal, and/or oral sex without a condom are at dramatically increased risk of HIV infection. Unprotected anal sex is the highest-risk sexual behavior[1]
Multiple sexual partners	Adolescents with multiple sexual partners are more likely to be exposed to an HIV and other STIs
Substance use/abuse; injection drug use	Alcohol and other drugs increase the likelihood of engaging in risky behaviors (eg, unprotected sexual activity and/or needle sharing)
Having another STI or women with yeast or bacterial vaginal infections	Ulceration or inflammation enables entry of HIV into vulnerable mucosal tissue
Cognitive Factors	**How Risk of HIV Infection Is Increased**
Lack of medically accurate information about HIV and sexual health	Adolescents may make sexual decisions based on misinformation or with incomplete information and inadvertently increase their risk[3]
Lack of understanding of relative risk	Most adolescents classify sexual behaviors as safe or unsafe and fail to appreciate that sexual behaviors represent a continuum from less risky to very risky,[3] leading them to underestimate the risk involved in sexual behaviors
Low literacy	Low levels of overall literacy and health literacy limit adolescents' ability to read, comprehend, and apply sexual health information
Perceived life expectancy	Youth who perceive themselves as having a shorter life expectancy may have more sexual partners and be less likely to use condoms[4]
Future orientation	Adolescents who consider the future and are willing to make sacrifices in the present (eg, delayed gratification) may be more likely to initiate sexual activity at a later age and have fewer sexual partners[5,6]
Failure or inability to prioritize health care and health screenings	Adolescents not getting their basic needs met (eg, food, shelter, safety) may be more concerned with survival than with making self-protective sexual choices and may engage in riskier behaviors as a result[4]

Social Factors	Description/Summary
LGBTQ identification	LGBTQ teens are at higher risk for HIV than heterosexual teens, in part because HIV rates are higher in these subpopulations.[7,8] In addition, LGBTQ teens are more likely to be homeless, to be injection drug users, to lack supportive adult relationships, and to engage in transactional/survival sex, all of which increase risk of HIV transmission
Race/ethnicity	Adolescents of color have a higher lifetime risk of HIV infection with associated risk factors of poverty, lack of health insurance, and reduced health care access
Early sexual initiation	Initiating sexual activity at younger ages is associated with higher levels of sexual risk taking, lower likelihood of using condoms, and more sexual partners
Lack of communication about sex and sexual health with parents or guardians	Parent-child communication about sex can have a powerful impact on adolescent sexual attitudes, behaviors, and health outcomes, with less communication associated with riskier sexual behaviors. The American Academy of Pediatrics recommends anticipatory guidance of adolescents in relation to sex beginning at 11 years of age
Lack of positive role models or supportive adult relationships	Youth without positive adult role models may be more likely to engage in risky sexual behaviors
Vulnerability to peer pressure	Adolescents are more likely to be sexually active if their friends are sexually active, if they perceive they will gain friends' respect by engaging in sexual activity
Older sexual partners	Adolescents with older sexual partners are more likely to engage in risky sexual behavior and to have unrecognized HIV infection
Lack of youth-friendly sexual and reproductive health information and care	If young people accessing health services feel embarrassed, stigmatized, or judgment from providers, they are less likely to be honest about their sexual partners and behavior, and they are more likely to avoid accessing sexual and reproductive health care altogether
Discrimination and inequality	These social factors in combination with poverty influence both local HIV prevalence as well as an individual's risk behaviors. Relationship instability caused by economic stress, discrimination, domestic violence migration, and incarceration can also increase risk[9]

Economic Factors	
Health care access	Limited health care access is associated with greater mistrust in health care systems and providers, engagement in fewer positive health behaviors (eg, getting tested for HIV), and increased sexual risk (including HIV transmission)
Insurance status	Insured adolescents visit health care providers twice as often as those who are uninsured. Uninsured adolescents are less likely to receive consistent medical care and are more likely to experience long wait times, be of low socioeconomic status, and/or be a person of color
Poverty	Adolescents living in poverty are disproportionately more likely to be infected with HIV
Rurality	Declines in formal sex education have been concentrated among young people residing in rural areas. For example, the share of rural adolescents who had received instruction about birth control declined from 71% to 48% among girls, and from 59% to 45% among boys
Homelessness or unstable housing	Adolescents with unstable housing are more likely to engage in unprotected sexual activity and sexual activity in exchange for money, drugs, or transitional housing, increasing risk of infection
Transactional or survival sex	Homeless or marginalized LGBTQ youth are at higher risk for engaging in survival or commercial sex work

Abbreviation: STI, sexually transmitted infection.

- Structural, biomedical, and behavioral interventions: should be used in combination to meet the HIV prevention needs of individuals and communities. Prevention interventions are in 3 major categories:
  - Structural interventions: seek to address the underlying social, economic, political, and environmental factors that make individuals and groups more vulnerable to HIV infection
  - Biomedical interventions: use a combination of clinical and medical approaches to prevent HIV; are typically used in combination with behavioral interventions
  - Behavioral interventions: seek to prevent HIV by attempting to change risky behaviors

Table 2 provides several suggested resources to use in HIV prevention with adolescents.

Table 2
Suggested resources for human immunodeficiency virus prevention with adolescents

Suggested Resource	Contents	Where to Access
A Guide for the Healthcare Professional: Discussing Sexual Health with Your Patients	• Tips for providers to guide discussions about sexual health with both adolescent and adult patients	https://www.cdc.gov/actagainstaids/pdf/campaigns/prescribe-hiv-prevention/aaa-php-discussing-sexual-health.pdf
Nonoccupational Postexposure Prophylaxis Toolkit	• A collaborative project from several organizations making up the AIDS Education and Training Center that provides up-to-date, step-by-step instructions online for the medical care of persons following possible HIV exposure	https://aidsetc.org/npep
Compendium of Evidence-based Interventions and Best Practices for HIV Prevention	• Structural approaches to HIV prevention that do not rely on individual behavior change to alter the environment • Interventions that improve linkage to, retention in, and reengagement with HIV care • Interventions that improve HIV medication adherence or viral load suppression among persons living with HIV • Interventions that show evidence of efficacy in changing sex or drug-injection behaviors that directly affect HIV transmission risk	https://www.cdc.gov/hiv/research/interventionresearch/compendium/index.html
Department of Health and Human Services Teen Pregnancy Prevention Evidence Review	• Programs that have been shown in at least 1 evaluation to have a positive impact on preventing teen pregnancies, STIs, and/or sexual risk behaviors	https://tppevidencereview.aspe.hhs.gov/

Abbreviation: AIDS, acquired immunodeficiency syndrome.

HUMAN IMMUNODEFICIENCY VIRUS SCREENING

The CDC recommends baseline HIV screening for all adolescents and adults 13 to 64 years of age at least once. For adolescents at high risk of infection, more frequent testing is indicated. This group includes MSM, sexual activity with HIV-positive (HIV+) partners, intravenous drug use, sex workers, history of STIs, pregnancy, or unknown HIV status of partners. For children and adolescents of mothers with HIV, screening should be offered if not already performed in infancy.

Recommended laboratory testing for HIV infection includes a combined antigen/antibody assay (HIV 1/2 Ag/Ab). HIV-1 antigen, otherwise referred to as p24

Table 3
Markers of human immunodeficiency virus infection and time to detection

Laboratory Marker	Mean (Range) Time from Infection to Detection (days)
HIV-1 RNA	5 (3–8)
p24 antigen	10 (7–14)
ELISA	14 (10–17)
Western blot, indeterminate	19 (15–23)
Western blot, positive, p31 antigen negative	89 (47–130)

Data from Fiebig EW, Dynamics of HIV viremia and antibody seroconversion in plasma donors: implications for diagnosis and staging of primary HIV infection. AIDS. 2003;17(13):1871-9.

antigen, is a viral core protein that is detectable transiently in early infection, before HIV-1 antibody is detectable. Advantages of the combination assay compared with prior HIV screening tests include the ability to detect p24 antigen following infection, and an improved window period from prior third-generation enzyme-linked immunosorbent assay (ELISA) assays for HIV-1 Ab or Western blot testing (**Table 3**).

Adolescents who show clinical signs of acute HIV infection (eg, influenzalike symptoms, fever, rash, and/or myalgia) may show falsely negative HIV 1/2 Ag/Ab testing. In contrast, during very early infection, the combination assay may be positive with a negative HIV Ab test. In these cases, HIV-1 RNA qualitative or quantitative polymerase chain reaction testing is helpful in distinguishing acute HIV infection from false-positive HIV screening tests in low-prevalence settings.

An estimated 50% of new cases of HIV are acquired through sex with persons with acute HIV infection.[13] Targeting those who are acutely infected with HIV is critical for reducing the incidence of new HIV infections and progress toward the goal of an acquired immunodeficiency syndrome (AIDS)–free generation.

PRESENTATION AND TREATMENT OF HUMAN IMMUNODEFICIENCY VIRUS INFECTION

Acute HIV infection may present as an influenzalike illness and frequently is misdiagnosed as mononucleosis or influenza. If infection is not detected in the early acute phase, there may not be symptoms for several years to prompt a patient to seek care, which again underscores the importance of universal screening for all adolescents, because patient histories may be unreliable.

Manifestations of chronic HIV infection may affect any organ system. Skin conditions, which may be typically self-limited (eg, eczema, seborrheic dermatitis, herpes simplex, or herpes zoster) may recur more frequently in chronic HIV infection. Overt symptoms of AIDS, such as wasting, cachexia, failure to thrive, and/or opportunistic infections (once cluster of differentiation [CD] 4+ lymphocyte counts have decreased to <200 cells/μL), may take years to develop.

General principles for the treatment of adolescents are similar to those for adult management, and data from adult trials are extrapolated to the adolescent population when guiding therapy decisions, particularly for perinatally infected youth with complex antiretroviral regimens or history of resistance. Expert consultation is strongly recommended in the initial diagnosis and clinical evaluation of HIV/AIDS before the initiation of ART. Competent providers may include infectious disease physicians with ongoing continuity and involvement in the care of people living with HIV, or primary care or advanced practice providers who have demonstrated competency in the management of HIV/AIDS by the American Academy of HIV Medicine or HIV Medical Association recommendations.

As early as safely possible to administer, ART should be offered to adolescents with normal hepatic and renal function who are willing and able to adhere to treatment. The benefits of early treatment have been clearly established in adults in the START[14] and TEMPRANO trials,[15] regardless of CD4 count. For patients presenting with longstanding, chronic infection or clinical syndromes of AIDS, careful clinical evaluation is necessary to identify other infections that take precedence for sequential treatment before HIV treatment. Failure to identify opportunistic infections and proceeding with treatment with ART may present undue risk of developing immune reconstitution syndrome, and increase risk for mortality.

Perinatally infected adolescents commonly show delayed growth and sexual maturity caused by HIV infection.[16] In addition, bone loss, metabolic complications, and cognitive and psychiatric comorbidities may be more prevalent in children with a history of ineffective therapy or adherence to therapy,[17,18] and considerations on initiating or restarting therapy for adolescents struggling with mental health or substance abuse disorders should be considered in choosing appropriate therapy. Drug resistance and complex dosing regimens in the treatment of adolescents with perinatal HIV infection underscore the need for behavioral strategies and partnerships with providers to preserve treatment options for the future.

Once HIV infection is confirmed, initial baseline testing is recommended (**Table 4**).

What to Start

Given potential challenges with adherence in the adolescent population, selection of a drug regimen should minimize the number and frequency of medications on a daily basis. After appropriate counseling and assessment of readiness in starting medications, initial treatment of HIV infection in adolescents should be individually tailored. An assessment of sexual maturity rating, or Tanner staging,[17] may guide dosing recommendations between pediatric versus adult dosing.

In the American context, guidelines for recommended therapy are continually updated by the US Department of Health and Human Services.[19] For sexual maturity rating (STM) stages 2 or less in children and adolescents greater than 25 kg, dolutegravir-based regimens with 2 nucleoside reverse transcriptase inhibitor (NRTI) drugs are recommended as first-line therapy.[20] For STM3 or more, the guidelines currently recommend a first-line regimen for adolescents with no childbearing potential to include an integrase strand inhibitor (INSTI; eg, raltegravir, elvitegravir, dolutegravir, or bictegravir), paired with 2 NRTI drugs. Because of preliminary data suggesting a possible association of dolutegravir with neural tube defects in infants born to mothers on dolutegravir-containing regimens,[21,22] dolutegravir should be avoided for all young women of childbearing age until further data are available. It is unclear at this time whether other INSTIs pose similar risks to neonates. Other recommended initial regimens include boosted protease inhibitors paired with 2 NRTIs, or NNRTI medications paired with 2 NRTIs.

Expert consultation is recommended before initiation of therapy if CD4 count or genotype resistance results are unknown, or if patients present with symptoms of profound immunosuppression or opportunistic infection, and ART should be delayed until identification and treatment of any potential underlying infection that could otherwise increase the risk of immune reconstitution inflammatory syndrome. Primary

Table 4
Initial baseline evaluation of adolescents with human immunodeficiency virus infection

Assay	Rationale
HIV Ag/Ab testing	Confirm HIV infection in cases where known HIV+ patient is establishing as a new patient in clinic and HIV RNA PCR is undetectable
Plasma HIV RNA, quantitative PCR (viral load)	Evaluate level of viremia
CD4 T-lymphocyte cell count	Assess stage of HIV infection
CBC	Evaluate for hematological abnormalities that may be present in chronic untreated HIV; eg, HIV-associated idiopathic thrombocytopenic purpura, normocytic anemia, pancytopenia
Serum electrolytes	Evaluate for concomitant metabolic or respiratory abnormalities
Liver function tests	Evaluate hepatic function before initiation of potentially hepatotoxic ARVs
BUN/creatinine, urinalysis	Evaluate renal function before initiation of potentially nephrotoxic ARVs
HIV genotype resistance testing	Evaluate for potential transmitted resistance
Hepatitis A IgG	Immunize if there is no evidence of immunity against hepatitis A
HBsAg HBcAb HBsAb	Concomitant HBV infection or history of infection affects treatment decisions. Immunize if no evidence of immunity against HBV and no active HBV disease
Hepatitis B quantitative viral load (conditional)	Recommended if evidence of prior infection without immunity (HBcAb+ with HBsAg- and HBsAb-) or active HBV infection
HCV antibody	Assess for HCV coinfection
Fasting blood glucose or hemoglobin A1c	Some ARVs are associated with metabolic syndrome and may increase risk of diabetes
Fasting serum lipids	ARVs may cause dyslipidemia
Syphilis, gonorrhea, chlamydia evaluation	Assess for concomitant STIs and offer NAAT swab testing of oral and rectal sites where appropriate
Other Tests	
Tuberculosis screening (TST or interferon-gamma release assay)	Treat latent tuberculosis infection to prevent progression to active TB
HLA-B*5701	If considering abacavir for regimen, presence of this variant increases risk for drug hypersensitivity and/or Stevens-Johnsons syndrome and is not recommended
Pregnancy test	Identify risk for perinatal transmission
G6PD deficiency (conditional)	Order if dapsone is indicated

Conditional: to be ordered if prior laboratory values abnormal, or if planning specific therapy for the future.

See AIDSinfo guidelines for tables regarding frequency of testing.

Abbreviations: ARVs, antiretroviral medications; BUN, blood urea nitrogen; CBC, complete blood count; G6PD, glucose-6-phosphate-dehydrogenase; HBcAb, hepatitis B core antibody; HBsAb, hepatitis B surface antibody; HBsAg, hepatitis B surface antigen; HBV, hepatitis B virus; HCV, hepatitis C virus; Ig, immunoglobulin; NAAT, nucleic acid amplification test; PCR, polymerase chain reaction; TB, tuberculosis; TST, tuberculin skin test.

Adapted from AIDSinfo, Laboratory Testing Schedule for Monitoring Patients with HIV Before and After Initiation of Antiretroviral Therapy, https://aidsinfo.nih.gov/guidelines/htmltables/1/6341.

Table 5
Primary prophylaxis of opportunistic infections among adolescents

Opportunistic Infections	Indication	Preferred Regimen	Alternative Regimen
TB (latent TB infection)	+ Interferon-gamma release assay or TST for patients with HIV independent of CD4 count Active TB has been excluded	INH 300 mg + pyridoxine 25–50 mg PO daily for 9 mo, or INH 900 mg PO BIW by direct supervision + pyridoxine 25–50 mg PO daily for 9 mo	Rifampin 600 mg PO daily for 4 mo, or Rifabutin for 4 mo (dose adjusted based on ART regimen), or Rifapentine (weight dependent)[a] PO + INH 900 mg PO + pyridoxine 50 mg once weekly for 12 wk The potential for drug-drug interactions with rifamycins and ART is high.[1–3] Before initiating, compatibility should be assessed because rifamycins are known to accelerate the metabolism of several ARTs
Coccidioidomycosis	+ IgM or IgG serologic testing among patients with CD4 counts <250 cells/μL living in endemic regions Screening usually performed annually for patients with CD4 counts <250 cells/μL	Fluconazole 400 mg PO daily Therapy is discontinued in patients receiving ART once CD4 counts >250 cells/μL for at least 6 mo	—

	Indication	Preferred	Alternative
Pneumocystis carinii	CD4 counts <200 cells/μL, or CD4 counts >200 cells/μL but <250 cells/μL and monitoring CD4 cell count every 3 mo not feasible	TMP-SMX 1 DS PO daily, or TMP-SMX 1 SS PO daily Therapy may be discontinued when ART results in CD4 counts >200 cells/μL for >3 mo. Therapy can also be discontinued in patients with CD4 counts 100–200 cells/μL if on ART and have had an undetectable viral load for at least 6 mo	TMP-SMX 1DS PO 3 times weekly, or Dapsone 100 mg PO daily or 50 mg PO BID, or Dapsone 50 mg PO daily + (pyrimethamine 50 mg + leucovorin 25 mg) PO weekly, or Dapsone 200 mg + pyrimethamine 75 mg + leucovorin 25 mg PO weekly, or Aerosolized pentamidine 300 mg via Respigard nebulizer every month, or Atovaquone 1500 mg PO daily, or Atovaquone 1500 mg + pyrimethamine 25 mg + leucovorin 10 mg PO daily
Histoplasmosis	Endemic regions with >10 cases/100 patient-years) or at an increased occupational risk and CD4 count ≤150 cells/μL should receive therapy. Antifungal usually not administered because there is limited evidence supporting efficacy of prophylaxis[4]	Itraconazole 200 mg PO daily Therapy can be discontinued once CD4 count >150 cells/μL for more than 6 mo after the initiation of ART[4]	—
Toxoplasmosis	+ IgG serology in patients with a CD4 count ≤100 cells/μL	TMP-SMX DS PO daily Among patients receiving ART, therapy may be discontinued when CD4 count >200 cells/μL for at least 3 mc	TMP-SMX 1DS PO 3 times weekly, or TMP-SMX 1 SS PO daily, or Dapsone 100 mg PO daily or 50 mg PO BID, or Dapsone 50 mg PO daily + (pyrimethamine 50 mg + leucovorin 25 mg) PO weekly, or Dapsone 200 mg + pyrimethamine 75 mg + leucovorin 25 mg PO weekly, or Atovaquone 1500 mg PO daily, or Atovaquone 1500 mg + pyrimethamine 25 mg + leucovorin 10 mg PO daily

(continued on next page)

Table 5
(continued)

Opportunistic Infections	Indication	Preferred Regimen	Alternative Regimen
MAC	If CD4 count <50 cells/μL and initiating ART, routine antimicrobial prophylaxis not indicated If CD4 count <50 cells/μL and not on ART, antimicrobial prophylaxis should be initiated and continued until ART is started, after ruling out active disseminated MAC	Azithromycin 1200 mg PO once weekly, or Azithromycin 600 mg PO twice weekly, or Clarithromycin 500 mg PO BID	Rifabutin 300 mg PO daily Active TB must be ruled out before starting this therapy Dose may need to be adjusted based on ART therapy

Abbreviations: BID, twice daily; BIW, twice weekly; DS, double strength; INH, isoniazid; MAC, *Mycobacterium avium* complex; PO, by mouth; TMP/SMX, trimethoprim/sulfamethoxazole.
[a] 32.1 to 49.9 kg, 750 mg; greater than 49.9 kg, 900 mg.

Table 6
Recommended vaccinations for adolescents infected with human immunodeficiency virus

	Age			CD4 Cell Count (Cells/μL)	
Vaccine	13–15 y	16 y	17–18 y	<15% and Total CD4 <200/mm3	>15% and CD4 ≥200/mm3
Hepatitis A	2 doses	2 doses	2, 3, or 4 doses[a]	2, 3, or 4 doses[a]	
Hepatitis B	2 or 3 doses	3 doses	2, 3, or 4 doses[b]	2, 3, or doses[b]	
Tdap	1 dose Tdap, then Td booster every 10 y			1 dose Tdap, then Td booster every 10 y	
Hib	1 dose[c]			1 dose[c]	
PCV13	1 dose			1 dose	
PPSV23	2 doses[d]			2 doses[d]	
Influenza	1 dose annually			1 dose annually; LAIV contraindicated	
MMR	2 doses			Contraindicated	2 doses
Varicella	2 doses			Contraindicated	2 doses
MenACWY	2 doses, at least 8 wk apart[e,f]			2 doses, at least 8 wk apart[e]	
MenB	2 or 3 doses depending on vaccine			2 or 3 doses depending on vaccine	
HPV	3 doses			3 doses	

Abbreviations: HPV, human papilloma virus; MMR, measles, mumps, rubella.

[a] Adolescents 18 years of age and older may receive the combined HepA and HepB vaccine, Hep A/Hep B combination, as a 3-dose series or 4-dose series.

[b] Adolescents aged 11 to 15 years may use an alternative 2-dose schedule with at least 4 months between doses (adult formulation Recombivax HB). Adolescents 18 years of age and older may receive a 2-dose series (Heplisav-B).

[c] Adolescents 18 years of age and older may receive the combined HepA and HepB vaccine, Twinrx, as a 3-dose series or 4-dose series.

[d] Unvaccinated (less than routine series through 14 months or no doses 14 months or older) persons aged 5 to 18 years.

[e] PPSV23 should be administered 8 weeks after the most recent dose of PCV13 and dose 2 of PPSV23 administered at least 5 years after dose 1 of PPSV23.

[f] If using Menactra, it must be administered at least 4 weeks after completion of the PCV13 series.

Adapted from Advisory Committee on Immunizations Practices (ACIP), 2017. Updated with immunization recommendations from CDC Guidelines. Available at: https://www.cdc.gov/vaccines/schedules/hcp/schedule changes.html

prevention of opportunistic infections is also critical, particularly for patients who may not be consistently adherent to ART (**Table 5**).

Immunizations

Immunizations for adolescents and youth infected with HIV are inclusive of recommendations for HIV-negative youth, with additional recommendations regarding pneumococcal, hepatitis A, hepatitis B, meningitis, and Haemophilus influenzae type B vaccines (**Table 6**). Exceptions include instances where CD4 level is less than 200 cells/μL and where immunization either may result in ineffective antibody production or pose complications related to administration of live vaccine in severely immunocompromised youthWhere CD4 levels are less than 200 cells/microliter, immunization may be result in ineffective antibody production or pose complications related to administration of live vaccine in severely immunocompromised youth. For this reason, MMR (measles, mumps, rubella) and varicella vaccinations are contraindicated for adolescents with CD4 count less than 200 cells/μL.

SUMMARY

Adolescents are at risk for HIV infection because of a multitude of factors. At-risk youth present great potential for lasting, positive changes in sexual behavior and attitudes toward sexual health with appropriate counseling and education. Several behavioral and biochemical modalities for prevention are available to reduce risk. For adolescents who are not infected with HIV, baseline screening for HIV infection is strongly recommended. For young adults newly diagnosed with HIV infection, expert consultation is advised for positive HIV test results in order to start treatment as soon as safely possible. In the modern era, the advent of effective ART has allowed HIV+ youth to live normal lifespans, although challenges remain in engaging and retaining patients in care.

ACKNOWLEDGMENTS

The authors wish to thank Janelle Rodriguez, MD for her contributions to **Tables 5** and **6.**

DISCLOSURE

The authors have nothing to disclose.

REFERENCES

1. CDC. HIV surveillance: adolescents and young adults. 2017 slideset from the NCHHSTP. Washington, DC: 2018. Available at: https://www.cdc.gov/hiv/pdf/library/slidesets/cdc-hiv-surveillance-adolescents-young-adults-2017.pdf.
2. Zanoni BC, Mayer KH. The adolescent and young adult HIV cascade of care in the United States: exaggerated health disparities. AIDS Patient Care STDS 2014;28(3):128–35.
3. Downs JS. Prescriptive scientific narratives for communicating useable science. PNAS 2014;111(suppl 4):13627–33.
4. Scott-Sheldon LA, Carey MP, Vanable PA, et al. Subjective life expectancy and health behaviors among STD clinic patients. Am J Public Health 2010;34(3):349–61.
5. Rothspan S, Read SJ. Present versus future time perspective and HIV risk among heterosexual college students. Health Psychol 1996;15(2):131–4.
6. Polgar M, Auslander W. HIV prevention for youths in foster care: understanding future orientation and intended risk behaviors. J HIV AIDS Soc Serv 2009;8(4):397–413.
7. CDC. Gay and bisexual teen males no more likely than heterosexual teen males to engage in several sexual risk behaviors; still at substantially higher risk of HIV infection. Newsroom release from the National Center for HIV/AIDS, viral hepatitis, STD, and TB prevention (NCHHSTP). Washington, DC: 2016.
8. Vogel DL, Heimerdinger-Edwards SR, Hammer JH, et al. "Boys don't cry": examination of the links between endorsement of masculine norms, self-stigma, and help-seeking attitudes for men from diverse backgrounds. J Couns Psychol 2011;58(3):368–82.
9. Pellowski JA, Kalichman SC, Matthews KA, et al. A pandemic of the poor: social disadvantage and the US HIV epidemic. Am Psychol 2013;68(4):197–209.
10. Cohen MS, Chen YQ, McCauley M, et al. Antiretroviral therapy for the prevention of HIV-1 transmission. N Engl J Med 2016;375(9):830–9.

11. Eisinger RW, Diffenbach CW, Fauci AS. HIV viral load and transmissibility of HIV infection: undetectable equals untransmittable. J Am Med Assoc 2019;321(5): 451–2.

12. CDC. Diagnoses of HIV infection in the United States and dependent areas, 2017. HIV Surveillance Report 2018;29:14–5.

13. Brenner BG, Roger M, Routy JP, et al, Quebec Primary HIV Infection Study Group. High rates of forward transmission events after acute/early HIV-1 infection. J Infect Dis 2007;195(7):951–9.

14. INSIGHT START Study Group, Lundgren JD, Babiker AG, Gordin F, et al. Initiation of antiretroviral therapy in early asymptomatic HIV infection. N Engl J Med 2015; 373(9):795–807.

15. TEMPRANO ANRS Study Group, Danel C, Moh R, Gabillard D, et al. A trial of early antiretrovirals and isoniazid preventive therapy in Africa. N Engl J Med 2015; 373(9):808–22. Available at: http://www.ncbi.nlm.nih.gov/pubmed/26193126.

16. Chantry CJ, Byrd RS, Englund JA, et al, Pediatric AIDS Clinical Trials Group Protocol 152 Study Team. Growth, survival and viral load in symptomatic childhood human immunodeficiency virus infection. Pediatr Infect Dis J 2003;22(12): 1033–9.

17. Cruz ML, Cardoso CA. Perinatally infected adolescents living with human immunodeficiency virus (perinatally human immunodeficiency virus) World J Virol 2015;4(3):277–84.

18. Tanner JM. Growth at adolescence. Oxford: Blackwell Scientific Publications; 1962.

19. Panel on Antiretroviral Guidelines for Adults and Adolescents. Guidelines for the use of antiretroviral agents in adults and adolescents with HIV. Department of Health and Human Services. Available at: http://aidsinfo.nih.gov/contentfiles/lvguidelines/AdultandAdolescentGL.pdf. Accessed March 26,2020.

20. Panel on Antiretroviral Therapy and Medical Management of Children Living with HIV. Guidelines for the Use of Antiretroviral Agents in Pediatric HIV Infection. Available at: http://aidsinfo.nih.gov/contentfiles/lvguidelines/pediatricguidelines.pdf. Accessed March 16,2020.

21. Zash R, Holmes L, Makhema J, et al. Surveillance for neural tube defects following antiretroviral exposure from conception. Presented at: 22nd International AIDS Conference; July 23-27. Amsterdam, 2018.

22. Zash R, Makhema J, Shapiro RL. Neural-tube defects with dolutegravir treatment from the time of conception. N Engl J Med 2018;379(10):979–81. Available at: https://www.ncbi.nlm.nih.gov/pubmed/30037297.

Adolescent Sexual Health

Identity, Risk, and Screening for Sexually Transmitted Infections

Roanna Kessler, MD[a], B. Tate Hinkle, MD, MPH[b,c],
Amy Moyers, MD[d], Benjamin Silverberg, MD, MSc[d,e,f],*

KEYWORDS

- Sexual health • SOGIE • Minority populations • Risk • Screening
- Asymptomatic infection • Sexually transmitted infections (diseases)

KEY POINTS

- Development of sexual orientation and gender identity and expression (SOGIE) is an integral part of adolescent physical and mental health.
- The United States has the highest rate of sexually transmitted infections (STIs) in the industrialized world, and approximately half of these infections occur in individuals aged 15 to 24 years.
- Human papilloma virus infection of the genital tissue is the most common STI in the United States and worldwide.
- The incidence of syphilis is once again increasing in the US, and men who have sex with men (MSM) are disproportionately affected.
- The US Centers for Disease Control and Prevention recommend that sexually active women under 25 years old be screened for gonorrhea and chlamydia annually.

INTRODUCTION

Adolescence, the transition from childhood to adulthood, begins with the onset of puberty and is characterized by individuals' struggle to define themselves and develop

[a] Johns Hopkins University Student Health and Wellness Center, Homewood Student Affairs, 1 East 31st Street, N200, Baltimore, MD 21218, USA; [b] Total Healthcare at Russell Medical Center, 3504 Highway 280, Alexander City, AL 35010, USA; [c] Department of Family Medicine, UAB Huntsville Regional Medical Campus, 301 Governors Drive SW, Huntsville, AL 35801, USA; [d] Department of Family Medicine, WVU Medicine, 6040 University Town Center Drive, Morgantown, WV 26501, USA; [e] Department of Emergency Medicine, WVU Medicine, 1 Medical Center Drive, Box 9149, Morgantown, WV 26506, USA; [f] Division of Physician Assistant Studies, Department of Human Performance, West Virginia University School of Medicine, 64 Medical Center Drive, Box 9226, Morgantown, WV 26506, USA
* Corresponding author. WVU Student Health, 390 Birch Street, Morgantown, WV 26506, USA
E-mail address: benjamin.silverberg@hsc.wvu.edu

Prim Care Clin Office Pract 47 (2020) 367–382
https://doi.org/10.1016/j.pop.2020.02.012
0095-4543/20/© 2020 Elsevier Inc. All rights reserved.

primarycare.theclinics.com

autonomy while adhering to cultural expectations (or not). This population is prone to objectively risky behaviors, such as unprotected intercourse, so it is imperative that clinicians engage adolescents in candid, nonjudgmental conversation about sexual activity to mitigate adverse outcomes.

Per the 2017 Youth Risk Behavior Surveillance Survey (YRBS),[1] 52.2% of high school students had had sexual contact at least once in their lives before being polled and 47.8% had not. Further, 28.7% had had sexual intercourse with at least 1 other person in the preceding 3 months (defined as currently sexually active). Of these, 53.8% used a condom during their last sexual encounter. Of students who had sexual contact with the same sex or with both sexes, 20.1% nonetheless identified as heterosexual and 11.4% were still uncertain of their sexual identity. Overall, 85.4% identified as heterosexual, 2.4% identified as gay/lesbian, 8% identified as bisexual, and 4.2% were not yet sure of their sexual identity.

Most reported cases of *Neisseria gonorrhoeae* (GC) and *Chlamydia trachomatis* (CT) in the United States occur in adolescents and young adults (AYAs). Oral sex, which some adolescents do not consider to be sex, is also common in this age group. Consequently, there is a higher prevalence of pharyngeal gonorrhea in this population.[2] Risk factors for sexually transmitted infections (STIs) include early sexual debut, multiple concurrent sex partners, inconsistent/incorrect use of barrier devices (eg, condoms), and barriers to accessing health care.[3] Lesbian, gay, bisexual, and transgender (LGBT) youth are more likely to be currently sexually active, have earlier sexual debut, and have multiple sexual partners. In addition, they are less likely to use condoms compared with heterosexual youth.[4]

SEXUAL ORIENTATION AND GENDER IDENTITY AND EXPRESSION

The development of SOGIE (sexual orientation and gender identity and expression) adds to the soul searching that adolescents are already doing. Every individual goes through SOGIE. It is not unique to LGBT people, but because of heteronormativity (the assumption that everyone is heterosexual and thereby heterosexuality is superior), they tend to struggle more with it. Heteronormativity causes invisibility and stigmatization of other sexualities and may reinforce gender stereotypes (ie, masculine men and feminine women).

Sexual orientation refers to the romantic (emotional) and/or sexual (physical) attraction to men, women, both, or neither. However, it is often conflated with sexual identity (eg, straight, gay, lesbian, bisexual, pansexual, asexual, same-gender-loving [SGL]) and sexual behavior (eg, men who have sex with men [MSM], women who have sex with men [WSM]). Sexual feelings are a spectrum, and attraction and intimacy are not just about intercourse. **Fig. 1** simplifies the different dimensions of sex and gender by presenting multiple lines, but it is limited by a visual binary.

In this context, sex is the biological, binary assignment to the male or female category at birth, based on genetics (XX or XY) and/or external genitalia. This assignment, too, is often conflated with the culturally driven concept of gender. Gender identity is a person's inner sense of self being a girl/woman, a boy/man, both, neither, or something else (eg, genderfluid). It is not determined by assigned sex; sex and gender are distinct categories. In contrast, gender expression is how individuals express their sense of self and is typically influenced by their assigned sex at birth, sexual orientation, and/or gender identity.

Remember:

- Gender identity/expression do not necessarily indicate sexual orientation/ practice.

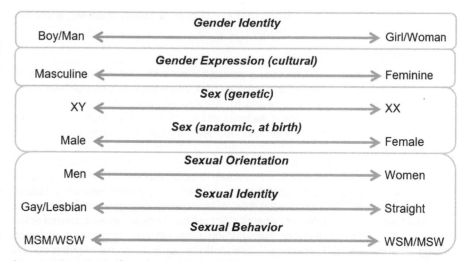

Fig. 1. Key terms as related to SOGIE. MSM, men who have sex with men; MSW, men who have sex with women; WSM, women who have sex with men; WSW, women who have sex with women.

- Orientation does not necessarily reflect practice (eg, a person may identify as gay but remain a virgin, another may identify as straight but consent to same-sex sexual contact in exchange for financial gain).
- Sexual practice may change over time. As such, it is reasonable to repeat related questions in future clinical encounters.
- One risk does not necessarily beget another. However, one STI may.[5]

ELICITING A SEXUAL HISTORY

In many societies, people are conditioned to find sex to be an awkward (or potentially even "dirty") topic to talk about, especially with a close family member, let alone a stranger. The plethora of slang words that can be used to describe certain anatomy or sexual activities does not make this easier; the vernacular may even lead to miscommunication and misunderstanding. To this end, clinicians, whose job it is to mitigate health risks, are often left with the burden of broaching the topic of sexual health. Consequently, the first principle of taking an adolescent sexual history is for health care providers to be comfortable starting the conversation. If they are uncomfortable raising the question, then the patient is likely to pick up on that disquiet, offering curt or incomplete responses.[6] One observational study found that, in a third of annual adolescent visits, there was no discussion of sexuality issues, and, when conversation did occur, the duration was brief, around 30 seconds.[7] Thus, when working with adolescent patients, clinicians should consider meeting the patient "where they are" in relation to language and cognitive ability. This requirement may mean a departure from technically correct but sterile medical terminology and instead echoing the words used by the patient. When faced with a patient who is new to the provider, casual, innocuous conversation before this can be used to ascertain the individual's level of maturity and diction.[8,9] Because adolescents are not always aware of their own feelings, it may be prudent for clinicians to ask them what they think about a particular issue, rather than how they feel about it.[9] In addition, because the examination room may be the only place where patients can safely ask questions, medically accurate, evidence-based information that is inclusive of LGBT, disabled, and other minority populations should be offered.[10]

Issues Surrounding Confidentiality

An important consideration in discussing sexual history with adolescents is confidentiality. One randomized controlled trial showed that, when providers guaranteed confidentiality, adolescents were more willing to disclose sensitive information and seek follow-up health care.[11] In a recent national study, 12.7% of sexually active AYAs on a parent's health insurance plan did not seek sexual and reproductive health care because they were worried their parents might find out. Spending time alone with the health care provider improved the odds of getting a sexual risk assessment and undergoing chlamydia testing.[12] Providers should also keep in mind that confidentiality can potentially be breached through billing and health insurance claims, and they may want to offer confidential, free, or low-cost testing options.[13] Exceptions to confidentiality vary by state but generally include child abuse/neglect, sexual activity between an adult and a minor, suicidal/homicidal ideation or attempt, gunshot/stabbing wounds, and STI reporting.[14] The Guttmacher Institute maintains a current listing of state laws and policies as they relate to teen sexual health and confidentiality (https://www.guttmacher.org/state-policy/explore/minors-access-sti-services).

Effective Ways to Elicit Information

Patients are more comfortable disclosing personal information when the provider asks open-ended questions.[15] It can also be helpful to make normative statements (taking the onus off the patient), use understandable terminology, and set a nonjudgmental tone for the conversation. Because gender identity and sexual orientation can be fluid, it is helpful to ask directly what behaviors are practiced with partners; for instance, touching and oral, vaginal, or anal sex.[16]

The Five P's Framework

The US Centers for Disease Control and Prevention (CDC)'s Five P's strategy for obtaining a sexual history,[17] listed in **Box 1**, is a helpful way to organize a sexual history. Other clinicians have suggested expanding this list to also ask about preferences, pleasure, and intimate partner violence.[18]

Opportunity to Screen for Assault and Abuse

Taking a sexual history also creates an opportunity to screen for sexual abuse or assault. Many adolescents do not disclose that they have been forced or pressured to have sex, even when they have visited a primary care physician in the past year.[19] One study of urban adolescent clinics showed that intimate partner violence (IPV) was common among female patients regardless of reason for visit, but screening by providers was low. Patients who report poor overall health and have forgone medical care are even more likely to have experienced IPV.[20]

Use of Previsit Forms

There is some evidence to suggest that using previsit questionnaires may be a helpful adjunct in obtaining sensitive information. One study using a standardized Safe Times Questionnaire (which included questions about sexuality, abuse, family, development, immunizations, nutrition, education, employment, and safety) showed that using the form could decrease visit time and obtain more accurate information.[21] In a more recent study, a pediatric emergency department created a computerized questionnaire with an embedded decision tree that would generate recommendations and

---

Box 1
Five P's framework by the Centers for Disease Control and Prevention

1. Partners
   ○ Gender and number of partners (eg, "How many new partners have you had since your last screening?")

2. Practices
   ○ Oral, vaginal, and anal sex; use of sex toys (eg, "The type of testing we recommend depends on your sexual practices. Which body parts do you use for sex?")
   ○ Other risks (eg, "Have you or any of your partners exchanged sex for money or drugs?")

3. Protection from STIs
   ○ Condom usage (eg, "Did you use a condom during your last sexual encounter? Is that what you do typically?")

4. Past history of STIs
   ○ Last STI screening, if ever (eg, "Have you ever had an STI in the past?")
   ○ Known exposures to STIs

5. Pregnancy
   ○ Attitudes toward pregnancy (eg, "Are you currently intending to get pregnant? If not, what are you doing to avoid it?")

---

resources based on patient responses. Both providers and patients preferred using the computerized system rather than face-to-face interviews, and nearly all adolescents (95%) reported that it was easy to complete the questionnaire and understand the questions.[22]

Sample Previsit Questionnaire

Box 2 offers an example questionnaire that incorporates the concepts of normalizing, assuring confidentiality, open-ended questions, the Five P's, and screening for assault.

Validity of Self-Report

One caveat is the reliability of self-report. In a survey of adolescent men, more than 90% of respondents who ever reported a history of an STI recanted their reports over time.[23] In another study of adolescent girls, 17% of participants with a laboratory-confirmed STI had either self-reported lifetime abstinence, or recent abstinence from vaginal sex.[24] Thus, it is important to keep in mind that adolescents may underreport their past medical history and behaviors when deciding on screening tests.

BURDEN OF DISEASE

According to the World Health Organization (WHO), more than 1 million STIs are acquired daily worldwide.[25] The United States has the highest rate of STIs in the industrialized world: approximately 20 million new cases annually, costing the health care system $16 billion each year.[2,26] The CDC estimates the prevalence of STIs at around 110 million cases.[5,27] Half of all new infections occur in individuals aged 15 to 24 years,[2,3,5] a notable statistic because this demographic represents only 25% of the sexually active population.[3] Other investigators report that 1 in 4 adolescents acquires an STI annually.[28] The true incidence of STIs is hard to know, because some infections are asymptomatic[27] and some (eg, herpes simplex virus [HSV], human papilloma virus [HPV], and trichomonas) are not reportable.[5] Best estimates of the burden of these diseases are as follows:

Box 2
Example previsit questionnaire

The following questions are about your sexual health. We ask these questions of all patients regardless of age or relationship status. Everything you tell us is confidential unless we are required to report it by law. This information will not be discussed with anyone without your permission.

When was the last time you were tested for STIs?	Approximate date:
Have you ever been diagnosed with an STI?	Yes/no
Have you had sexual contact in the last 60 days?	Yes/no
Do you use a condom or barrier?	Always/most of the time/sometimes/rarely/never
Have you had sexual contact with men, women, or both?	Men/women/both men and women
The type of testing we recommend depends on your sexual behaviors. Which of the following apply to you:	No sexual activity/oral sex (giving)/oral sex (receiving)/vaginal sex/anal sex bottom (receptive)/anal sex top (insertive)
Have you ever used a needle to inject drugs?	Yes/no
Have you ever had sexual contact with someone who injected drugs (eg, heroin)?	Yes/no/uncertain
Have you ever had sexual contact with someone who has human immunodeficiency virus (HIV)?	Yes/no/uncertain
Have you completed your human papilloma virus (HPV) vaccine series?	Yes/no/uncertain
If you are currently in a relationship, do you feel safe?	Yes/no/not in relationship/uncertain/prefer not to answer
Has anyone ever forced you to perform sexual acts without your consent?	Yes/no/uncertain/prefer not to answer

---

- HPV is the most common STI in the United States and worldwide,[2] with 14.1 million new cases annually and 79.1 million total cases.[26,29] Approximately 50% of new infections occur in adolescents.

- Chlamydia, the second most common STI in the United States, had a reported incidence of more than 1.7 million in 2017[25] (up >100,000 cases from the year before[8]), costing the health care system approximately $632.3 million.[30] Between 2003 and 2017, there was a 95% increase in cases of chlamydia in the United States.[30] Women aged 15 to 24 years have the highest rates of chlamydia infection in the United States. (Rates for men are much lower, but highest among men 20–24 years old.[3]) AYAs account for 65% of reported cases of chlamydia in the United States.[2] The WHO estimates 131 million people are infected annually worldwide.[31]

- There were 555,608 reported cases of gonorrhea in the United States in 2017,[25] with a total cost of $198.4 million.[30] Between 2003 and 2017, there was a 66% increase in cases of gonorrhea in the United States.[30] Although the highest rates of gonorrhea infection are seen in the southeastern states, rates are climbing in the west.[30] Again, rates are highest among AYAs,[3] accounting for 53% of reported cases of gonorrhea in the United States.[2] Approximately 78 million people are infected annually worldwide.[31] In a 2013 report, the CDC warned that increasing resistance of *Neisseria gonorrhoeae* to antibiotics posed an urgent threat,[2] and, in 2018, the United Kingdom saw its first cases of multidrug-resistant gonorrhea infection (in heterosexual women).

- In 2017, there were 30,644 reported cases of primary and secondary syphilis in the United States,[25] costing the health care system an estimated $45 million.[30] Men accounted for more than 88% (26,885) of these cases. In addition, there were 918 cases of congenital syphilis,[25] which leads to infant death in up to 40% of cases.[30] Approximately 5.6 million people worldwide are infected with syphilis annually.[31] In 2012, mother-to-child transmission of syphilis resulted in an estimated 143,000 early fetal deaths/stillbirths, 44,000 babies being born preterm or low birthweight, and 102,000 infected neonates.[31]
- Approximately 1.2 million individuals with human immunodeficiency virus (HIV) are living in the United States. More than half are more than 50 years of age. There are an estimated 40,000 new HIV infections annually, with the greatest proportion (>35% of cases) occurring in persons 20 to 29 years old.[8] However, 26% of new infections occur in AYA aged 13 to 24 years.[3,4]
- Although the incidence of acute hepatitis A infections in the United States decreased steadily between 2001 and 2011, recent outbreaks have been linked to contaminated imported foods. The ongoing outbreak in central Appalachia, which began in late 2017, has made more than 10,754 Kentuckians, West Virginians, and Ohioans sick and has claimed at least 100 lives.[32]
- An estimated 2.2 million people in the United States have chronic hepatitis B. The greatest number of infections come from foreign-born individuals from Africa, Asia, and the Pacific Islands. There are 21,000 new infections annually as well.[27]
- By comparison, 3 million people in the United States have chronic hepatitis C, although effective antiviral treatments may have reduced that number. There are 41,000 new infections annually,[27] which are associated with illicit drug use and coinfection with HIV.[2]
- HSV is prevalent in the United States: more than half of adult Americans have HSV-1 (which can afflict the mouth or genitals) and an estimated 12% to 22% are seropositive for HSV-2 (which typically only causes genital infections).[3,4,27]
- There were an estimated 3.7 million total cases of trichomoniasis in the United States in 2008,[8] with 1.09 million being new cases.[26]
- *Mycoplasma genitalium*, which was first isolated in 1981, is more common than gonorrhea but less common than chlamydia. In young adults, it was found in 15% to 30% of cases of urethritis and 10% to 30% of cases of cervicitis.[2]

SCREENING RECOMMENDATIONS

Not all STIs are symptomatic, and sometimes acute symptoms resolve, even though the infection has not. Consequently, the 2015 CDC guidelines recommend routine screening for sexually active adolescents. Examination and testing should be based on the patient's anatomy.[6]

- Sexually active women less than 25 years old should be screened annually for gonorrhea and chlamydia. Screening is conducted using nucleic acid amplification test (NAAT) because of its high sensitivity and specificity. Either first-catch (so-called dirty) urine or mucous membrane swabs of the vagina, urethra, or endocervix can be used for NAAT; however, rectal and pharyngeal swabs are not FDA-approved for testing via NAAT.[33]
- Based on efficacy and cost-effectiveness, routine screening for GC/CT is not currently recommended for young men but should definitely be considered for populations with high prevalence of infection (eg, correctional facilities, sexual health clinics, adolescent clinics, MSM).

- HIV screening should be discussed and offered to all adolescents. The CDC and United States Preventive Services Task Force (USPSTF) recommend that all adults be screened at least once in their lifetime for HIV. The frequency of repeat testing depends on individual risk. For example, seronegative individuals with HIV-positive partners should be tested routinely. In addition, those on HIV preexposure prophylaxis (PrEP) should be screened for HIV and other STIs every 3 to 6 months as part of appropriate medication management.
- The USPSTF recently expanded its recommendation on screening for hepatitis C: as with HIV, all adults should be tested at least once.[34]
- Screening for syphilis in asymptomatic individuals is limited to MSM and pregnant women. The rapid plasma reagin (RPR) and Venereal Disease Research Laboratory (VDRL) tests have high false-positive rates so any positive should be followed up with a confirmatory fluorescent treponemal antibody-absorbed (FTA-Abs) test or *Treponema pallidum* particle agglutination (TP-PA).[3]
- Cervical cancer screening by Pap smear (cytology) begins at age 21 years, regardless of sexual debut. Because of the high prevalence and spontaneous clearance of HPV in younger populations, testing for HPV is not recommended until age 30 years.[3]
- Screening for trichomonas, bacterial vaginosis (BV), HSV, hepatitis A, and other STIs in asymptomatic adolescents is not recommended.

The USPSTF recommendations vary slightly from the CDC and are listed in **Table 1**. Clinicians are not following these guidelines, though. One study showed that only 47% of sexually active women less than 24 years of age with commercial health insurance had been screened for chlamydia. Similar young women with Medicaid fared only slightly better, with 54.6% having been screened.[27] Another study revealed that, of the 7,300 American physicians surveyed, less than one-third routinely screened their patients for STIs. Only slightly more than half were reporting diagnoses of syphilis and HIV, and even fewer were reporting cases of gonorrhea and chlamydia.[26] Per the 2017 YRBS, only 9.3% of high school students reported ever having been tested for HIV.[1]

Hunter and colleagues[26] recommend that, in addition to reviewing professional and national guidelines, "clinicians should consult with local public health officials and use available local epidemiologic data to tailor screening programs based on the community and populations served."

SPECIAL POPULATIONS

Although anyone who is sexually active is at risk of acquiring an STI, young people (aged 15–24 years), gay/bisexual men, and pregnant women may be more affected by STIs than other groups.[8] Gay, bisexual, and other MSM accounted for 68% (17,736) of all cases of STIs in the United States in 2017.[25] Racial and ethnic minorities are also disproportionately affected by STIs. African Americans have the highest STI prevalence rates in the United States. (By comparison, Asian Americans have the lowest.) Therefore, it is not surprising that young MSM of color have had high rates of HIV and syphilis in their communities.[2] In addition, incarcerated individuals are at higher risk for HIV and hepatitis C, potentially caused by involvement in the sex and/or drug trades. Note that minors cannot legally consent to sexual activity, regardless of their own willingness, which makes any involvement in the sex trade (sex trafficking and so-called survival sex) illegal.

Pregnancy

Pregnant adolescents are significantly more likely to not use condoms during sexual intercourse compared with nonpregnant adolescents.[35] STIs in pregnancy can have

Table 1
Sexually transmitted infection screening recommendations by the United States Preventive Services Task Force

Concern	Population	Recommendation	Grade	Release Date
BV	Low-risk asymptomatic pregnant women	Do not screen in asymptomatic pregnant women at low risk for preterm delivery	D	February 2008[a]
	High-risk asymptomatic pregnant women	Insufficient evidence to recommend for or against screening of asymptomatic pregnant women at high risk for preterm delivery	I	February 2008[a]
CT	Sexually active women	Screen all sexually active women aged ≤24 y and older at increased risk for infection	B	September 2014[a]
	Sexually active men	Insufficient evidence to recommend for or against screening of sexually active men of any age	I	September 2014[a]
GC	Sexually active women	Screen all sexually active women aged ≤24 y and older at increased risk for infection	B	September 2014[a]
	Sexually active men	Insufficient evidence to recommend for or against screening of sexually active men of any age	I	September 2014[a]
HBV	Pregnant women	Screen pregnant women at their first prenatal visit	A	July 2019
	Individuals at high risk for infection	Screen individuals at high risk for infection	B	May 2014[a]
HCV	Adolescents and adults aged 18–79 y	Screen all individuals aged 18–79 y and younger adolescents and older adults at increased risk of infection	B	March 2020
HSV	Asymptomatic adolescents and adults (including pregnant women)	Do not perform routine serologic screening	D	Nov 2016

(continued on next page)

Table 1
(continued)

Concern	Population	Recommendation	Grade	Release Date
HIV	Adolescents and adults aged 15–65 y	Screen all individuals aged 15–65 y and younger adolescents and older adults at increased risk of infection	A	June 2019
	Pregnant women	Screen all pregnant women, including those who present in labor or at delivery with unknown HIV status	A	June 2019
	Individuals at high risk for infection	Offer preexposure prophylaxis with antiretroviral therapy to individuals who are at high risk for infection	A	June 2019
HPV	Women aged 21–65 y	Cervical cytology should be performed every 3 y in women aged 21–29 y; women aged 30–65 y should have cytology every 3 y or high-risk HPV testing ± cytology every 5 y	A	Aug 2018
	Women aged <21 y	Do not screen women aged <21 y	D	Aug 2018
Syphilis	Asymptomatic adolescents and adults (except pregnant women) at increased risk for infection	Screen individuals at high risk for infection	A	June 2016
	Pregnant women	Screen all pregnant women early	A	September 2018
Behavioral counseling	Sexually active adolescents and adults	Intensive behavioral counseling recommended for all sexually active adolescents and adults at increased risk for STIs	B	September 2014[a]

[a] Recommendation being updated at time of publication.
Data from U.S. Preventive Services Task Force. Available at: https://www.uspreventiveservicestaskforce.org/Search. Accessed March 14, 2020.

detrimental effects on women, their partners, and their fetuses. All pregnant women and their partners should be counseled regarding STIs. During the first prenatal visit, women should be tested for HIV, syphilis, Hepatitis B virus (HBV), Hepatitis C virus (HCV) and GC/CT. As with nonpregnant adolescents, routine screening for trichomonas, BV, and HSV are not recommended unless the patient is symptomatic.[36]

Persons with Developmental Disabilities

Developmental disabilities can predispose adolescents to sexual abuse and sexual dysfunction. Comprehensive sexuality education and screening is important for all youth, including those with developmental disabilities.[37] Adolescents with disabilities are less likely than their peers to receive information on contraceptive options, STIs, and screening for cervical cancer. One study showed that students in special education, particularly young women with intellectual disabilities, were at increased risk for having an STI. Disabled adolescents are often systematically excluded from sex education, which may increase their risk for poor health outcomes. Providers should aim to provide developmentally appropriate information and promote healthy sexuality among AYAs with developmental disabilities.[38]

Correctional Facilities

Multiple studies have shown high rates of STIs in incarcerated populations, including HIV, viral hepatitis, syphilis, GC/CT, and trichomonas. This population shows increased risk behaviors, such as using drugs and alcohol, engaging in commercial or coerced sex, having unprotected sex, and having multiple sexual partners. Many persons in correctional facilities also have a history of limited access to medical care.[39] A large multicenter analysis of chlamydia prevalence in correctional facilities in the United States showed a high chlamydia rate in women in both juvenile and adult facilities (14.3% and 7.5%), supporting a screening policy in incarcerated populations.[40] The CDC recommends that women 35 years old and under, and men younger than 30 years old in correctional facilities should be screened for GC/CT at intake. Syphilis screening should also be considered if there is a high local prevalence rate of syphilis.[17]

Men Who Have Sex with Men

Some MSM are at higher risk for HIV and other STIs because they engage in anal sex and the rectal mucosa is particularly susceptible to certain pathogens. From the 1980s through the mid-1990s, the frequency of unprotected sex, bacterial STIs, and HIV declined significantly in MSM. However, since that time, unsafe sexual practices among MSM have increased in the United States and many other countries, leading to higher rates of syphilis, gonorrhea, and chlamydia. About two-thirds of the cases of primary and secondary syphilis are diagnosed in MSM.[39] Gay and bisexual adolescents are often at a disadvantage with regard to sexual education as well: instruction tends to focus on penetrative penile-vaginal intercourse, usually to the exclusion of discussion of anal and oral sex and other forms of sexual contact.

The CDC recommends the following screening tests for MSM at least annually:

- HIV
- Syphilis
- Urine NAAT for GC/CT in men who have insertive anal intercourse
- Rectal NAAT for GC/CT in men who have receptive anal intercourse
- Pharyngeal NAAT for GC in men who have receptive oral intercourse

Other tests and vaccines to consider:

- HBV surface antigen to detect chronic hepatitis B infection
- HCV screening among past or current drug users and persons with HIV
- Anal cytology to detect HPV infection and associated conditions, such as anogenital warts or anal squamous intraepithelial lesions (data are insufficient to recommend this screening routinely)
- Vaccination against hepatitis A, hepatitis B, and HPV[17]

Women Who Have Sex with Women

WSW have a wide diversity of sexual practices, including oral-genital sex, digital-genital sex, and penetrative sex toys; however, use of barrier protection (eg, condoms, gloves, dental dams) is infrequent.[41] Common infections among WSW include HPV, trichomonas, and BV. Providers should not assume that WSW are at low risk for STIs, and should proceed with STI and cervical cancer screening according to general guidelines for women. In this population, it is particularly important to obtain a comprehensive sexual history to determine which tests are indicated.[17]

Transgender Persons

There are high national and international rates of HIV in transgender women.[42] The few studies of HIV prevalence in transgender men suggest that HIV infection is less frequent than in transgender women.[43] When deciding on screening, providers should

Table 2
Recommended[a] reportable sexually transmitted infections to the Centers for Disease Control and Prevention's National Notifiable Diseases Surveillance System

Infectious Agent	Diagnosis	Years Notifiable
C trachomatis	Any infection	2010–present
	Genital infections	1995–2009
	Lymphogranuloma venereum	1941–1994
N gonorrhoeae	Any infection	1944–present
T pallidum	Any infection	1944–present
	Syphilitic stillbirth	1941–present
Haemophilus ducreyi	Chancroid	1944–present
Hepatitis A	Acute infection	1966–present
Hepatitis B	Acute infection	1966–present
	Chronic infection	2003–present
	Perinatal infection	1995–present
Hepatitis C	Acute infection	1994–present
	Chronic infection	2010, 2016–present
	Past or present infection	2003–2009, 2011–2015
	Perinatal infection	2018–present
HIV	Any infection (AIDS reclassified as HIV stage III)	2009–present
	AIDS	2000–2008
Zika virus	Any infection or disease	2016–present

Abbreviation: AIDS, acquired immunodeficiency syndrome.
[a] Reportable conditions vary by state.
Data from Centers for Disease Control and Prevention. National Notifiable Diseases Surveillance System (NNDSS). Available at: https://wwwn.cdc.gov/nndss/conditions/notifiable/2018/infectious-diseases/. Accessed June 29, 2019.

consider the diversity of anatomy among transgender men and women, because many have not undergone gender-affirming surgery.[44] Again, a thorough sexual history is paramount, because the STI risk for transgender patients is based on current anatomy and sexual behaviors.[45]

REPORTING INFECTIONS

The Council of State and Territorial Epidemiologists (CSTE) recommends that "while the list of reportable conditions varies by state … state health departments [are encouraged to] report cases of selected diseases to the CDC's National Notifiable Diseases Surveillance System (NNDSS)."[46] In some states, both confirmed and probable cases should be reported. **Table 2** summarizes current recommendations.

According to one study, nearly two-thirds of high-risk, private sector patients had untreated partners.[26] Assistance in notifying these partners is more likely with possible syphilis or HIV infection, and uncommon with GC/CT.[26] However, almost all of these individuals preferred to inform their partners of the potential need for testing and treatment, and a slightly smaller number were willing to deliver the treatment themselves.[26] As of June 2019, expedited partner therapy (EPT), which facilitates treatment of partners of patients diagnosed with gonorrhea or chlamydia, is permissible or potentially allowable in all American states and territories except for South Carolina.[47]

On diagnosis with an STI, all sexual partners from the previous 60 days, or the last sexual contact if more than 60 days have elapsed before symptoms or diagnosis, should be evaluated.[2] In the case of syphilis, sexual partners from the last 3 to 12 months should be notified, depending on the stage of syphilis at diagnosis.[22]

SUMMARY

Adolescence is a time burgeoning self-expression and identity, which can, at times, lead to behaviors that put AYAs at risk for STIs. By starting an open-ended, nonjudgmental conversation about SOGIE, as well as learning about STI disease burden and screening in special populations, health care professionals can serve to mitigate this risk.

ACKNOWLEDGMENTS

The authors wish to thank Carrie Pratt, Rene Dobranski, and Kimberly Quedado for their thoughtful feedback on this article.

DISCLOSURE

The authors have nothing to disclose.

REFERENCES

1. Kann L, McManus T, Harris WA, et al. Youth risk behavior surveillance – United States, 2017. MMWR Surveill Summ 2018;67(8):1–114.

2. Wangu Z, Burstein GR. Adolescent sexuality: updates to the sexually transmitted infection guidelines. Pediatr Clin North Am 2017;64:389–411.

3. Gibson EJ, Bell DL, Powerful SA. Common sexually transmitted infections in adolescents. Prim Care Clin Office Pract 2014;41:631–50.

4. Wood SM, Salas-Humara C, Dowshen NL. Human immunodeficiency virus, other sexually transmitted infections, and sexual and reproductive health in lesbian, gay, bisexual, transgender youth. Pediatr Clin North Am 2016;63:1027–55.
5. Jennings PR, Flenner RW. Sexually transmitted infections: a medical update. Physician Assist Clin 2017;2:207–18.
6. Phoenix J. "Caring for the transgender client" (chapter 11). In: Quallich SA, Lajiness M, Mitchell K, editors. Manual of men's health: primary care guidelines for APRNs & PAs. New York: Springer; 2019. p. 117–27.
7. Alexander SC, Fortenberry JD, Pollak KI, et al. Sexuality talk during adolescent health maintenance visits. JAMA Pediatr 2014;168(2):163–9.
8. Prosser R. "The itchy, scratchy, bumpy, and burning truths about sex, and pre-exposure prophylaxis (PrEP)" (chapter 17). In: Quallich SA, Lajiness M, Mitchell K, editors. Manual of men's health: primary care guidelines for APRNs & PAs. New York: Springer; 2019. p. 231–41.
9. McGarry ML. "Male adolescent health: addressing a critical need" (chapter 5). In: Quallich SA, Lajiness M, Mitchell K, editors. Manual of men's health: primary care guidelines for APRNs & PAs. New York: Springer; 2019. p. 45–55.
10. American Academy of Family Physicians – Adolescent Health Care, Sexuality, and Contraception. Available at: https://www.aafp.org/about/policies/all/adolescent-sexuality.html. Accessed September 5, 2019.
11. Ford CA, Millstein SG, Halpern-Felsher BL, et al. Influence of physician confidentiality assurances on adolescents' willingness to disclose information and seek future health care. A randomized controlled trial. JAMA 1997;278(12):1029–34.
12. Leichliter JS, Copen C, Dittus PJ. Confidentiality issues and use of sexually transmitted disease services among sexually experienced persons aged 15–25 years — United States, 2013–2015. MMWR Morb Mortal Wkly Rep 2017;66:237–41.
13. The Society for Adolescent Health and Medicine, American Academy of Pediatrics. Confidentiality protections for adolescents and young adults in the health care billing and insurance claims process. J Adolesc Health 2016;58(3):374–7.
14. Ford C, English A, Sigman G. Confidential Health Care for Adolescents: position paper for the society for adolescent medicine. J Adolesc Health 2004;35(2): 160–7.
15. Lewis CC, Matheson DH, Brimacombe CA. Factors influencing patient disclosure to physicians in birth control clinics: an application of the communication privacy management theory. Health Commun 2011;26(6):502–11.
16. Marcell AV, Burstein GR, Committee on Adolescence. Sexual and reproductive health care services in the pediatric setting. Pediatrics 2017;140(5).
17. Workowski KA, Bolan GA. Sexually transmitted diseases treatment guidelines, 2015. MMWR Recomm Rep 2015;64(3):1–137.
18. Cavanaugh T. Sexual health history: talking sex with gender non-conforming and trans patients. Available at: https://fenwayhealth.org/wpcontent/uploads/Taking-a-Sexual-Health-History-Cavanaugh-1.pdf. Accessed January 29, 2020.
19. Wilson KM, Klein JD. Opportunities for appropriate care: health care and contraceptive use among adolescents reporting unwanted sexual intercourse. Arch Pediatr Adolesc Med 2002;156(4):341–4.
20. Miller E, Decker MR, Raj A, et al. Intimate partner violence and health care-seeking patterns among female users of urban adolescent clinics. Matern Child Health J 2010;14(6):910–7.
21. Schubiner H, Tzelepis A, Wright K, et al. The clinical utility of the Safe Times Questionnaire. J Adolesc Health 1994;15(5):374–82.

22. Miller MK, Mollen C, Behr K, et al. Development of a novel computerized clinical decision support system to improve adolescent sexual health care provision. Aced Emerg Med 2019;26(4):420–33.

23. Dariotis JK, Pleck JH, Sonenstein FL, et al. What are the consequences of relying upon self-reports of sexually transmitted diseases? Lessons learned about recanting in a longitudinal study. J Adolesc Health 2009;45(2):187–92.

24. Brown JL, Sales JM, DiClemente RJ, et al. Predicting discordance between self-reports of sexual behavior and incident sexually transmitted infections with African American female adolescents: results from a 4-city study. AIDS Behav 2012;16(6):1491–500.

25. Centers for Disease Control and Prevention – Reported STDs in the United States, 2017. Available at: https://www.cdc.gov/nchhstp/newsroom/docs/factsheets/std-trends-508.pdf. Accessed June 29, 2019.

26. Hunter P, Dalby J, Marks J, et al. Screening and prevention of sexually transmitted infections. Prim Care Clin Office Pract 2014;41:215–37.

27. Levy SB, Gunta J, Edemekong P. Screening for sexually transmitted diseases. Prim Care Clin Office Pract 2019;46:157–73.

28. Vermillion ST, Holmes MM, Soper DE. Adolescents and sexually transmissible diseases. Obstet Gynecol Clin North Am 2000;27(1):163–79.

29. American Sexual Health Association – Fast facts. Available at: http://www.ashasexualhealth.org/stdsstis/hpv/fast-facts/. Accessed September 15, 2019.

30. National Coalition of STD Directors – Chlamydia, gonorrhea, and syphilis: STDs on the rise. Available at: http://www.ncsddc.org/wp-content/uploads/2018/09/STD-101_NCSD-STD-Handout-1.3-DIGITAL-1.pdf. Accessed February 5, 2019.

31. WHO launches new treatment guidelines for chlamydia, gonorrhea, and syphilis. Available at: https://www.who.int/reproductivehealth/topics/rtis/stis-new-treatment-guidelines/en/. Accessed February 5, 2019.

32. Centers for Disease Control and Prevention – Widespread person-to-person outbreaks of hepatitis A across the United States. Available at: https://www.cdc.gov/hepatitis/outbreaks/2017March-HepatitisA.htm. Accessed September 19, 2019.

33. Committee on Adolescence and Society for Adolescent Health and Medicine. Screening for nonviral sexually transmitted infections in adolescents and young adults. Pediatrics 2014;134(1):e302–11. Available at: http://pediatrics.aappublications.org/content/134/1/e302. Accessed May 20, 2019.

34. American Academy of Family Physicians – USPSTF: Screen Adults 18-79 for Hepatitis C Infection. Available at: https://www.aafp.org/news/health-of-the-public/20190904uspstf-hepc.html. Accessed September 5, 2019.

35. Niccolai LM, Ethier KA, Kershaw TS, et al. Pregnant adolescents at risk: sexual behaviors and sexually transmitted disease prevalence. Am J Obstet Gynecol 2003;188(1):63–70.

36. American Academy of Pediatrics, American College of Obstetricians and Gynecologists. Guidelines for perinatal care. 6th edition. Washington, DC: American College of Obstetricians and Gynecologists; 2007.

37. Greydanus DE, Omar HA. Sexuality issues and gynecologic care of adolescents with developmental disabilities. Pediatr Clin North Am 2008;55(6):1315.

38. Walters FP, Gray SH. Addressing sexual and reproductive health in adolescents and young adults with intellectual and developmental disabilities. Curr Opin Pediatr 2018;30(4):451–8.

39. CDC. Sexually transmitted disease surveillance 2013. Atlanta (GA): US Department of Health and Human Services; 2014.

40. Joesoef MR, Weinstock HS, Kent CK, et al. Corrections STD Prevalence Monitoring Group. Sex and age correlates of Chlamydia prevalence in adolescents and adults entering correctional facilities, 2005: implications for screening policy. Sex Transm Dis 2009;36(2 Suppl):S67–71.
41. Fethers K, Marks C, Mindel A, et al. Sexually transmitted infections and risk behaviours in women who have sex with women. Sex Transm Infect 2000;76:345–9.
42. Operario D, Soma T, Underhill K. Sex work and HIV status among transgender women: systematic review and meta-analysis. J Acquir Immune Defic Syndr 2008;48:97–103.
43. Sevelius J. "There's no pamphlet for the kind of sex I have": HIV-related risk factors and protective behaviors among transgender men who have sex with nontransgender men. J Assoc Nurses AIDS Care 2009;20:398–410.
44. Reisner SL, Perkovich B, Mimiaga MJ. A mixed methods study of the sexual health needs of New England transmen who have sex with nontransgender men. AIDS Patient Care STDS 2010;24:501–13.
45. Catallozzi M, Rudy BJ. Lesbian, gay, bisexual, transgendered, and questioning youth: the importance of a sensitive and confidential sexual history in identifying the risk and implementing treatment for sexually transmitted infections. Adolesc Med Clin 2004;15(2):353–67.
46. National Notifiable Diseases Surveillance System (NNDSS) – Data collection and reporting. Available at: https://wwwn.cdc.gov/nndss/case-definitions.html. Accessed June 29, 2019.
47. Centers for Disease Control and Prevention – Legal Status of Expedited Partner Therapy (EPT). Available at: https://www.cdc.gov/std/ept/legal/. Accessed September 29, 2019.

Adolescent Substance Abuse

Mark Garofoli, PharmD, MBA, BCGP, CPE

KEYWORDS

- Addiction • Substance use disorder • Substance abuse • Opioids • Vaping
- Marijuana • Alcohol • Stimulants

KEY POINTS

- Adolescent substance abuse is America's top public health problem, as people are most likely to begin abusing drugs (including tobacco, alcohol, prescription drugs, and other illicit substances) during adolescence and young adulthood.
- The CRAFFT and DAST questionnaires are brief, reliable tools for adolescent substance abuse screening.
- The vast majority (90%) of cigarette smokers smoke their first cigarette by the age of 18 years, yet more adolescents use alcohol than cigarettes.
- Despite the changing state marijuana laws across the country in recent years, past-year use of marijuana for high school students reached its lowest levels in more than 2 decades in 2016 and has since remained stable.
- Opioid availability and abuse continues to decline in the United States, with approximately 1 in 3 adolescent students reporting opioids available in their environment, whereas stimulant availability and use is much higher with 2 in 3 adolescent students reporting stimulants being available in their environment.

INTRODUCTION

The National Center on Addiction and Substance Abuse at Columbia University has explicitly stated that adolescent substance abuse is America's #1 public health problem.[1] There is no more evident need for action and understanding than in the present, especially considering that the harm does not stop at the mere substance abuse, which is associated with an increased risk of motor vehicle crashes, emergency department admissions, and suicide. In addition, approximately 75% of adolescents with substance use disorder also having a comorbid mental illness.[2]

EPIDEMIOLOGY

People are most likely to begin abusing drugs (including tobacco, alcohol, prescription drugs, and other illicit substances) during adolescence and young adulthood.[3] By the time they are senior students, almost 70% of high school students will have tried

West Virginia University (WVU) School of Pharmacy, WVU Medicine Center for Integrative Pain Management, 1120-B Health Sciences North, Morgantown, WV 26506, USA
E-mail address: mkgarofoli@hsc.wvu.edu

Prim Care Clin Office Pract 47 (2020) 383–394
https://doi.org/10.1016/j.pop.2020.02.013
0095-4543/20/© 2020 Elsevier Inc. All rights reserved.
primarycare.theclinics.com

alcohol, 50% will have taken an illegal drug, nearly 40% will have smoked a cigarette, and more than 20% will have misused a prescription drug for a nonmedical purpose.[4]

One in eight high school students has a substance use disorder (ie, addiction) involving nicotine, alcohol, or other drugs. Of note, substance abuse can be a repetitive or continued misuse of substances or a single instance, whereas substance use disorder is a chronic medical condition whereby the brain's physiologic responses actually change, among other differences, in addition to the continued misuse of substances despite negative consequences. Generally speaking, 90% of people with substance use disorder began smoking, drinking, or using other drugs before they turned 18 years of age. Furthermore, 25% of those who started using these substances before turning 18 years become addicted, as compared with 4% for those who first started using at age 21 years or later. Drug use at an early age is clearly an important predictor of development of a substance use disorder later in life. Most of those who have a substance use disorder started using before age 18 years and developed their disorder by age 20 years.[5] The likelihood of developing a substance use disorder is greatest for those who begin use in their early teens. For example, 15% of people who start drinking by age 14 years eventually develop alcohol abuse or dependence (as compared with just 2% of those who wait until they are 21 years or older).[6] Considering that approximately half of all high school students (more than 6 million students) currently use cigarette, alcohol, marijuana, or cocaine (not even factoring in those in juvenile incarceration nor those who dropped out of high school), it becomes more apparent how substance use and addiction is the leading cause of preventable death and disability in the United States.[1]

Substance use costs America almost $500 billion dollars annually, which boils down to approximately $1500 per capita. The high cost of substance use in America stems from, among other things, accidents, infectious diseases (eg, human immunodeficiency virus [HIV], hepatitis C, etc.), crimes, child neglect and abuse, unplanned pregnancies, homelessness, and unemployment. Undoubtedly that amount of money could easily and effectively be spent elsewhere on substance abuse prevention and countless other societal efforts.[1]

PHYSIOLOGY

The adolescent brain is often likened to a car with a fully functioning gas pedal (the dopamine reward system) but weak brakes (the prefrontal cortex). Teenagers are highly motivated to pursue pleasurable rewards and avoid pain, but their judgment and decision-making skills are still developing and limited, which affects their ability to weigh risks accurately and make sound decisions, including decisions about using drugs. For these reasons, adolescents are a major target for prevention messages promoting healthy, drug-free behavior and giving young people encouragement and skills to avoid the temptations of experimenting with drugs.[7]

The prefrontal cortex region of the brain functions in decision-making, judgment, and impulse control. The nucleus accumbens region of the brain functions in motivation and memory. Neither are fully developed in teenagers (or actually anyone younger than 25 years), which makes them more prone than adults to originally taking risks (such as illicit substance utilization) in the first place. In addition, addictive substances (ie, controlled substances or illicit substances) physically alter the brain's structure and function more intensely than an adult's brain, which further impairs judgment to increase the risk of substance use disorder.[1]

Different substances affect the brain differently, but a common factor is that they all increase the level of the chemical *dopamine* in brain circuits that control reward and pleasure. Unfortunately, drugs of abuse are able to hijack this process. The "high" produced by drugs of abuse represents a flooding of the brain's reward circuits with much more dopamine than natural rewards generate. Not all young people are equally at risk for developing an addiction. Various factors including inherited genetic predispositions and adverse experiences in early life make trying drugs and developing a substance use disorder more likely.[8]

SCREENINGS

Often times, adolescents will "act out" with behavioral changes including aggression, impulsivity, hyperactivity, or depression, which will eventually affect academic performance, social integration, or other facets of life. Parents, community leaders, or teachers may end up referring these adolescents to a doctor for evaluation, as these mood changes may even stem from substance abuse.[2]

Drug abuse screenings are reviewed further in this discussion. However, when any respective drug abuse screening results in the possibility of substance use and/or abuse, the natural next step is to conduct a more in-depth evaluation and/or to refer the patient to an addiction specialist, with particular attention paid to evaluating the adolescent for co-occurring other mental illness. As is included in most drug abuse screenings, a thorough review of a respective adolescent's family history of substance use and psychiatric disorders should be conducted. One of the intentions of these patient-provider conversations is to build trust in order to attain all pertinent information needed in order to best help an adolescent patient. Then subsequent conversations regarding the bigger picture consequences of drug abuse or substance use disorder including school performance, social and psychological functioning, peer attitudes, and ultimately the willingness for treatment can proceed more smoothly and with greater impact.[2]

Even though almost everyone has been advised of the consequences of drug abuse at some point, health care professionals should always make at least an attempt to remind and perhaps reframe the direct consequences, perhaps in a personalized manner to maximize the impact for a given adolescent patient. There are multiple strategies for facilitating actual change for adolescent patients in these situations. Motivational interviewing is suggested as a way to open an exchange with the adolescent and strive for positive change. At the very least, one can use interviewing domains such as assessment and feedback, negotiation and goal setting, behavioral modification techniques, self-help directions, and follow-up and reinforcement. Examples of the deployment of these strategies include conversations on what a respective adolescent patient and their respective friends do for fun, diving deeper into whether or not any illicit substances are involved or if they feel pressure from their peers to experiment with illicit substances. Conversely, an adolescent may be asked what they already know about alcohol and/or drugs, followed up by an invitation to discuss further and asking if they have any questions.[2]

Whether a 2-minute conversation or a 1-hour "all-hands-on-deck" conversation, interventions can, in fact, make a positive difference, which is particularly important to remember given that the longer adolescents defer experimentation, the less likely they are to develop long-term drug abuse problems.[2]

CRAFFT Questionnaire

The CRAFFT questionnaire is a brief, reliable tool for adolescent substance abuse screening.[9] This screening includes 2 parts—Part A and Part B—and the probability of diagnosis is shown in **Fig. 1**. If a respondent answers no to all 3 of the Part A

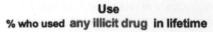

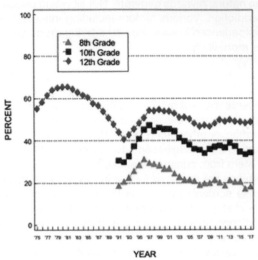

Fig. 1. Lifetime illicits. (*From* Johnston LD, Miech RA, O'Malley PM, et al. 2017 overview: Key findings on adolescent drug use. Monitoring the Future, Institute for Social Research, The University of Michigan. Available at: http://www.monitoringthefuture.org/pubs/monographs/mtf-overview2017.pdf.)

questions, then he or she is only asked one Part B question pertaining to being in a car with someone else who has ingested substances. If, however, the respondent answers yes to any of the 3 questions in Part A, then he or she is asked the 6 questions included in Part B. The title of the screening stems from the first letter of each of the Part B question topics, including Car, Relax, Alone, Forget, Family/Friends, and Trouble.

DAST

The DAST was originally published in 1982 by Dr. Harvey Skinner and was modified from the Michigan Alcoholism Screening Test (MAST). The DAST is available in 3 versions (DAST-28, DAST-20, and DAST-10) varying in the amount of questions therein and each being a successive update to the prior while reducing the question burden. There is no great difference in validity nor utility among the 3 versions (nor the adolescent version DAST-A), other than that the DAST-10 includes the most recently revised question wording and fewest number of questions. Scores greater than 12 on the DAST-28 tool indicate a definitive substance abuse problem. Scores greater than 5 on the DAST-10 tool indicate a substantial/severe level of drug abuse.[10]

SUBSTANCES OF ABUSE

Over the past 2 decades, the use of illicit substances by the adolescent population in the United States has remained stagnant. Approximately 50% of 12th grade students report having used an illicit substance at least once in their respective lifetime (**Fig. 2**). Of note, from the 8th grade, gradually to the 12th grade, illicit substance use at some point in one's lifetime more than doubles.[11] These trends suggest that the prime

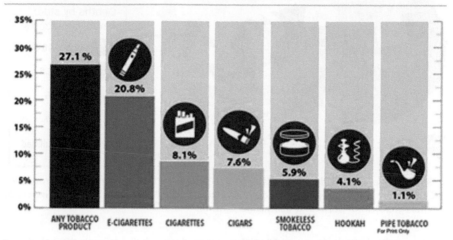

Fig. 2. Tobacco use in students. (*From* Centers for Disease Control and Prevention (CDC). Smoking and tobacco use fact sheet. Revised February 2019. Available at: https://www. cdc.gov/tobacco/data_statistics/fact_sheets/youth_data/tobacco_use/index.htm.)

opportunity to reach the adolescent youth population with prevention efforts is during the high school years.

More specifically, alcohol and tobacco (nicotine) are the substances most commonly abused by adolescents, followed by marijuana. The next most popular substances differ between age groups. Young adolescents tend to favor inhalant substances, whereas older teens are more likely to use synthetic marijuana, prescription opioids, and stimulant medications.[1]

Nicotine

In the United States, the use of tobacco products is primarily established during the adolescence years. Alarmingly, 90% of cigarette smokers had their first cigarette by the age of 18 years, whereas 98% started smoking by the age of 26 years. In addition, every single day approximately 2000 youth younger than 18 years smoke their first cigarette, with 300 youth moving onward to becoming daily cigarette smokers. The overall utilization of nicotine products in the United States in 2018 by type of nicotine products is shown in **Fig. 3**.[12]

In a survey conducted by the University of Michigan via National Institutes of Health/ National Institute on Drug Abuse in 2018, it was found that approximately 18% of 8th grade students, 32% of 10th grade students, and 37% of 12th grade students reported vaping within the past year. From 2017 to 2018, merely 1 year, the vaping within the last year rates increased by approximately one-third for high school students, to approximately 18% of 8th grade students, 30% of 10th grade students, and 37% of 12th grade students. Most concerning is that, after alcohol, vaping has become the second most common form of substance use for high school students. Multiple factors contribute to the increased utilization; indeed, more school students reported that vaping devices and e-liquids containing nicotine are "easy" or "very easy" to obtain in 2018 than in 2017.[13]

The Juul devices are leading the pack in terms of e-cigarette and vaping market share across the United States, with increasing sales of ~700% from 2016 to 2017

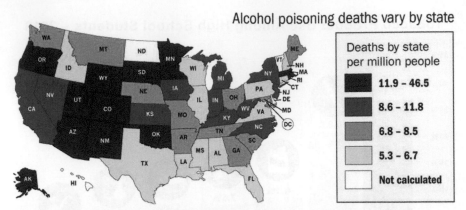

Fig. 3. Alcohol poisoning deaths by state. (*From* Centers for Disease Control and Prevention (CDC) Vital Signs: alcohol poisoning deaths. January, 2015. Available at: https://www.cdc.gov/vitalsigns/alcohol-poisoning-deaths/index.html.)

(2 million e-cigarette devices and 16 million vaping devices).[14] Juuling is the act of vaping from a Juul"pod." Juul pods contain e-liquid/juice—relatively large nicotine doses along with intriguing flavorings—and are heated in a device that resembles a USB thumb drive (and can actually be recharged via USB). This method of administration provides a quick and powerful dose of nicotine. Vaporized nicotine from e-cigarettes travels through the body and past the blood brain barrier to cause a dopamine surge within approximately 5 seconds of inhaling. Tolerance typically develops quickly causing more frequent puffing and/or higher concentrations to be used.

Juul pods are available in 3% and 5% strength (0.7 mL nicotine), with the 5% Juul pods containing approximately 40 mg nicotine, and the 3% Juul pods containing approximately 23 mg nicotine, a "very high" nicotine dose. In general, a Juul pod contains the equivalent amount of nicotine to one pack of tobacco cigarettes.[15] The amount of nicotine in any respective e-cigarette, vaping device, or other formulation is extremely important to consider, given both the addictive properties of nicotine and the long-term, high-risk cardiovascular concerns for the substance. One must always consider the amount of nicotine within any respective nicotine product in order to ensure a relative level of safety between various nicotine products, with particular attention to interchangeability.

In addition, 2.4% of middle school students and approximately 11% high school students reported current use of 2 or more tobacco products in the past 30 days in 2018.[11] Given that the utilization of even one form of nicotine/tobacco is concerning, the fact that adolescents are using multiple forms is truly worrisome.

Marijuana

Marijuana and cannabis, whether illicit, recreational, or "medical," is at a pivotal point in American history for both legislation and perception. However, the fundamental properties of the core substances within the various types of plants have not necessarily changed much over the past centuries. Although there are many harmful substances (eg, carcinogens) in any type of marijuana plant, there is always a high concentration of the 2 most widely known components, tetrahydrocannabinol (THC) and cannabidiol (CBD). The balance of the two has varying effects on cognition and function. THC utilization typically leads to euphoric and hunger, whereas CBD has shown promise in small studies on inflammation and other therapeutic areas. The challenge is being able to definitively state which substance and how much of it is in any given product because they lack monitoring similar to that of the Food and Drug Administration on prescription medications. Without a "watchdog" approach to the regulation of marijuana and cannabis products, perceptions of the effects of these products continue to fluctuate.

The perceptions of harm and disapproval of marijuana use have trended downward in recent years for high school students. Approximately 1 in 16 high school seniors report daily use of marijuana. Despite the changing state marijuana laws across the country in recent years, past-year use of marijuana for high school students reached its lowest levels in more than 2 decades in 2016 and has since remained stable.[6]

High school students reporting personal use of synthetic cannabinoids or synthetic marijuana (eg, K2, Spice, etc.) within the preceding 12 months has dropped significantly over recent years, from approximately 11% (2011) to 4% (2018).[6] Nonetheless, every day, more than 3000 teens use marijuana for the very first time.[16] Health care professionals need to aim to reduce the number of new marijuana utilizers, and less long-term utilizers for that matter, to prevent long-term direct complications from the numerous substances within marijuana (carcinogens similar to, if not worse than, tobacco leaves) along with the countless indirect complications such as increased utilization of other substances of abuse. Marijuana use is linked with lower academic performance, being less likely to graduate from high school, and a lower likelihood of enrolling in higher education, all leading to earning a lower income (or even be unemployed) and thus explaining lower life satisfaction ratings associated with marijuana use.[16]

In general, as the perception of harm from marijuana use decreases, the utilization of marijuana increases.[16] Conversely, if perhaps society concentrates on correcting the falsely low perception of harm from marijuana use to a more realistic long-term level, the use of marijuana could justifiably decrease. In fact, one could extrapolate this mantra to the utilization of any and all substances of abuse, let alone those discussed here.

Alcohol

From 2013 to 2018, both daily alcohol use and binge drinking (defined as consuming ≥ 5 drinks at one period of time within the preceding 2 weeks) decreased significantly among high school students.[6] Adults who began to use alcohol before age 15 years are 5 times more likely to report previous-year alcohol dependence or abuse than those who began alcohol use at age 21 years or older.[2] Remarkably, more adolescents use alcohol than cigarettes.[17]

In the United States, a standard drink contains approximately 14 g of ethyl alcohol. This amount is typically found in approximately 12 oz of beer (assuming 5% alcohol content), 5 oz of wine (assuming 12% alcohol content), or 1.5 oz liquor (assuming 40% alcohol content).[13] Young adults need to be educated on these numbers in order to prevent unintentional intoxication (or even death) from the consumption of varying amounts of different forms of alcohol. Perhaps this concept could even be incorporated into the mathematical curricula of middle and high schools across the country, not only to avoid negative health outcomes but also to apply such learning to quotidian concerns.

Adolescence is a maturing period, which includes considerable changes in life—in particular one's behavior. Although they are an expected part of the growth and maturation process, these changes can also indicate a problem with alcohol (or other substances). Parents, teachers, friends, family, and community members need to remain vigilant for the following warning signs that may indicate underage drinking: changes in mood (eg, anger); declining academic performance; rebellion; changing groups of friends; low energy; less interest in activities, hobbies, or appearance; and slurred speech, coordination problems, or even finding alcohol products among one's belongings.[13]

Alcohol poisoning death rates vary by gender and geographic location. Based on 2015 data, there is a higher rate of alcohol poisoning deaths in the western portion of the United States (**Fig. 4**), whereas there is a much higher rate of alcohol poisoning deaths in men compared with women.[18]

Binge drinking is the consumption of a large quantity of drinks on occasion and differs in quantity for men and women (≥4 drinks for women and ≥5 drinks for men). Medication misuse is a term commonly used synonymously with abuse or diversion, but the term misuse is specific to 2 activities: either use without a prescription or use only for the feeling euphoria. Over the course of 2012 to 2014, more than half of the 4 million Americans who misused prescription opioids also engaged in binge drinking. In addition, people who binge drank were twice as likely to misuse prescription opioids as compared with nondrinkers, regardless of age and sex.[19]

Opioids

Americans constitute less than 5% of the world's population but consume 80% of the world's opioid supply (99% of the hydrocodone supply) and 66% of the world's illegal drugs.[20] Roughly 21% to 29% of patients prescribed opioids for chronic pain misuse them, in other words, approximately 1 out of every 4 patients.[21] Furthermore, approximately 2,000,000 Americans struggle with opioid use disorder, with approximately 25% being addicted to heroin. Each day, approximately 120 people in the United States die from an opioid overdose—one death every 12 minutes.[22–24] Further, approximately every 25 minutes, a baby is born dependent on opioids due to its mother's use of opioids during pregnancy.[25] Increased injection drug use, another aspect of the epidemic, greatly contributes to the spread of infectious diseases such as HIV and hepatitis C.[26]

Approximately 75% of those who first become addicted to prescription narcotics eventually turn to heroin, which is often cheaper and more readily available.[27] This fact alone cuts to the main issue facing our nation in the "opioid crisis": What drives

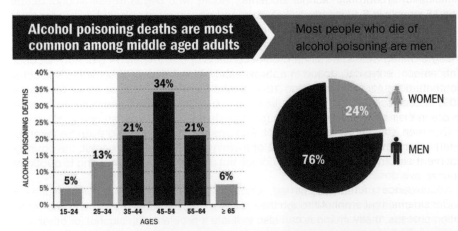

Fig. 4. Alcohol poisoning deaths by age and sex. (*From* Centers for Disease Control and Prevention (CDC) Vital Signs: alcohol poisoning deaths. January, 2015. Available at: https://www.cdc.gov/vitalsigns/alcohol-poisoning-deaths/index.html.)

one to use an opioid in the first place? Many factors contribute to one's use of illicit substances (such as heroin) including facets of life such as genetic predispositions; job security and availability; and the feelings of hope, belonging, and/or safety, among many others. However, one must also realize that even though approximately 75% of those addicted to heroin began their general opioid utilization with prescription opioids, the actual source of those prescription opioids may not necessarily be a legal avenue, such as a health care setting. In fact, most of those describing the source of their respective prescription opioid medications admit family, friends, street dealers, or any combination thereof, whether paying or sharing, were their own respective source of prescription opioids.[28]

As with any substances of abuse, one must keep in mind the source of any respective substance of abuse and also analyze dynamic substance use/abuse trends across the country and regionally. Over recent years, illicit heroin has been found to be adulterated (or "laced") with various other substances including diltiazem, diphenhydramine, and fentanyl or fentanyl derivatives (eg, carfentanyl). For additional perspective, one can consider that heroin is generally 3 times more potent than morphine (the gold standard of opioid potency measurement), whereas fentanyl is 100 times as potent, and carfentanyl is an impressive 10,000 times as potent. A mere speck of carfentanyl, the size of a grain of salt, can kill a human being if ingested. Thousands of people die annually due to heroin overdoses across the United States, and more and more of those drug overdose deaths are due to heroin mixed with these adulterants.[29]

Despite the staggering statistics that illustrate the number of opioid overdose deaths continues to increase across the country, the misuse of prescription opioids has dropped significantly in 12th grade students over the past 5 years. In fact, approximately 30% of 12th grade students stated that prescription opioids were easily available in the 2018 survey, compared with more than 50% in 2010.[6] Similar to society's overall increasing drug overdose deaths due to some type of opioid, the drug overdose deaths due to stimulants (primarily methamphetamine) are on the increase as well. The following section discusses adolescent stimulants use.

Stimulants

Although drug overdose deaths are continually on the increase, the actual percentage of adolescents in the United States who have stated using an amphetamine stimulant in the past year is less than 10%.[11] This relatively low statistic does not necessarily align with the typical stereotypes across the country of students using stimulants—primarily amphetamines and other attention deficit hyperactivity disorder (ADHD) medications—to enhance academic performance. However, the actual supply of amphetamines for adolescents in the United States is staggering, with approximately 60% of adolescents stating that amphetamines are readily available for their own purchase in their daily environment.

Common stimulants reported to be used by adolescents include amphetamine, methylphenidate, and, in general, those prescription medications used for the management and treatment of ADHD.[11] Conversely, the most of the stimulants involved in drug overdose deaths across the United States for decades has been one single illicit substance: meth(amphetamine).[21]

Considering that amphetamine stimulants are readily available in typical adolescent environments, relatively few adolescents report actually using the stimulants (<10%), perhaps the trend in drug use for adolescent youths in the United States is improving and not as rampant as it is stereotyped to be.[11] Furthermore, given that most of the drug overdoses in the United States involve adults, not adolescents, and even though the substances are readily available, perhaps the United States adult population can reflect on the decisions of our youth population resulting in lower drug overdose rates. These significant positive changes in adolescent drug use beg one to wonder if perhaps adolescents no longer aim for absolute avoidance without any consideration, or a "Just Say No" approach, but instead have steadfastly avoided high-risk scenarios and substances with a "Just Say *Know*" mentality.

SUMMARY

Only 35% of adolescents reported discussing substance use with their primary care physicians, although 65% of the sample said they wanted to.[2] This underscores perhaps the most important effort that health care professionals can make related to adolescent substance abuse: conversations. One must overcome inertia to consistently and customarily ask the questions that net the greatest yield, which are also some of the most basic. In fact, whether an adolescent or an adult, all patients deserve to be asked if they have used *any* illicit substance *ever* for the sake of consistency, implementation, and for the bettering of overall patient care, perhaps at the same time of asking what over-the-counter, supplement, and prescription medications have ever been used. After all, people respect what you inspect, not what you expect.

DISCLOSURE

The author has nothing to disclose.

REFERENCES

1. The CASA National Advisory Commission on Substance Use among America's High School Age Teens. Adolescent substance abuse: America's #1 public health problem. New York: That National Center on Addiction and Substance Abuse at Columbia University; 2011.
2. Griswold K, Aronoff H, Kernan J, et al. Adolescent Substance Use and Abuse: Recognition and Management. American Family Physician 2008;77(3):331–6.
3. NIDA. Principles of adolescent substance use disorder treatment: a research-based guide. National Institute on Drug Abuse website. 2014. Available at:https://www.drugabuse.gov/publications/principles-adolescent-substance-use-disorder-treatment-research-based-guide. Accessed January 24, 2019.
4. Johnston LD. Monitoring the Future National Results on Adolescent Drug Use: Overview of Key Findings, 2013. Bethesda, MD: National Institute on Drug Abuse; 2013.
5. Dennis M, Babor T, Roebuck M, et al. Changing the focus: the case for recognizing and treating cannabis use disorders. Addiction 2002;97(s1):4–15.
6. Substance Abuse and Mental Health Services Administration. Results from the 2012 national survey on drug use and health: summary of national findings. Rockville (MD): Substance Abuse and Mental Health Services Administration; 2013. NSDUH Series H-46, HHS Publication No. (SMA) 13-4795.
7. Robertson EB, David SL, Rao SA. Preventing Drug Use among Children and Adolescents: A Research-Based Guide for Parents, Educators, and Community Leaders, 2nd ed. Bethesda, Maryland: National Institutes of Health (NIH) Publication No. 04-4212(A); 1997.
8. Bethesda, MD: National Institute on Drug Abuse, 2003. Available at: www.drugabuse.gov/pdf/prevention/RedBook.pdf. Accessed March 14, 2019.

9. Knight JR, Shrier LA, Bravender TD, et al. A new brief screen for adolescent substance abuse. Arch PediatrAdolesc Med 1999;153(6):591–6. Available at: https://www.integration.samhsa.gov/clinical-practice/sbirt/CRAFFT_Screening_interview.pdf.

10. Yudko E, Lozhkina O, Fouts A. A comprehensive review of the psychometric properties of the Drug Abuse Screening Test. J Subst Abuse Treat 2007;32(2): 189–98.

11. Johnston LD, Miech RA, O'Malley PM. Monitoring the Future national survey results on drug use: 1975-2017: overview, key findings on adolescent drug use. Ann Arbor (MI): Institute for Social Research, The University of Michigan; 2018.

12. Centers for Disease Control and Prevention (CDC). Smoking and tobacco use fact sheet. 2019. Available at:https://www.cdc.gov/tobacco/data_statistics/fact_sheets/youth_data/tobacco_use/index.htm. Accessed March 14, 2019.

13. National Institute of Health: National Institute on Drug Abuse, Drug Facts. 2018. Available at: https://www.drugabuse.gov/publications/drugfacts/monitoring-future-survey-high-school-youth-trends. Accessed March 14, 2019.

14. NIH New Release. Available at: https://www.nih.gov/news-events/news-releases/teens-using-vaping-devices-record-numbers. Accessed March 14, 2019.

15. Juul Website. Available at: https://www.juul.com/. Accessed April 4, 2019.

16. Available at: https://www.drugabuse.gov/sites/default/files/marijuanauseinfo.pdf. Accessed March 14, 2019.

17. National Institute on Alcohol Abuse and Alcoholism. Underage drinking fact sheet. 2017. Available at:https://www.niaaa.nih.gov/publications/brochures-and-fact-sheets/underage-drinking. Accessed March 14, 2019.

18. Centers for Disease Control and Prevention (CDC) vital signs: alcohol poisoning deaths, 2015. Available at: https://www.cdc.gov/vitalsigns/alcohol-poisoning-deaths/index.html. Accessed March 14, 2019.

19. Esser MB, Guy GP, Zhang K, et al. Binge drinking and prescription opioid misuse in the US 2012-2014. Am J Prev Med 2019;57(2):197–208.

20. Machikanti L, Fellows B, Ailinani H, et al. Therapeutic use, abuse, and nonmedical use of opioids: a ten-year perspective. Pain Physician 2010;13:401–35. Available at:http://www.painphysicianjournal.com/current/pdf?article=MTM4Mg%3D%3D&journal=57.

21. Vowles KE, McEntee ML, Julnes PS, et al. Rates of opioid misue, abuse, and addiction in chronic pain: a systematic review and data synthesis. Pain 2015; 156(4):569–76. Available at:https://journals.lww.com/pain/Abstract/2015/04000/Rates_of_opioid_misuse_abuse_and_addiction_in.3.aspx.

22. German Lopez, In one year, drug overdoses killed more Americans than the entire Vietnam War did, Vox (June 8, 2017), https://www.vox.com/policy-and-politics/2017/6/6/15743986/opioid-epidemic-overdose-deaths-2016. Accessed March 15, 2019.

23. Centers for Disease Control and Prevention (CDC). Vital signs: overdoses of prescription opioid pain relievers – United States, 1999-2008. MMWR Morb Mortal Wkly Rep 2011;60:1487–92. Available at:https://www.cdc.gov/mmwr/preview/mmwrhtml/mm6043a4.htm.

24. Jones CM, Mack KA, Paulozzi LJ. Pharmaceutical overdose deaths, United States, 2010. JAMA 2013;309:657–9. Available at: https://jamanetwork.com/journals/jama/fullarticle/1653518.

25. Tolia VN, Patrick SW, Bennett MM, et al. Increasing incidence of the neonatal abstinence syndrome in U.S. neonatal ICUs. N Engl J Med 2015;372:2118–26. Available at:https://www.nejm.org/doi/full/10.1056/NEJMsa1500439.

26. National Institute on Drug Abuse, West Virginia Opioid Summary, NIH (Feb. 2018), Available at: https://www.drugabuse.gov/drugs-abuse/opioids/opioid-summaries-by-state/west-virginia-opioid-summary. Accessed March 15, 2019.

27. Substance Abuse and Mental Health Services Administration, Results from the 2013 National Survey on Drug Use and Health: Summary of National Findings, U.S. Dept. of Health & Human Servs., NSDUH Series H-48, HHS Publication No. (SMA) 14-4863 (Sept. 2014), Available at: https://www.samhsa.gov/data/sites/default/files/NSDUHresultsPDFWHTML2013/Web/NSDUHresults2013.htm. Accessed March 15, 2019.

28. 2017 DEA National Drug Threat Assessment. Available at: https://www.dea.gov/docs/DIR-040-17_2017-NDTA.pdf. Accessed March 14, 2019.

29. DEA 2018 National Drug Threat Assessment (NDTA). Available at: https://www.dea.gov/documents/2018/10/02/2018-national-drug-threat-assessment-ndta. Accessed March 14, 2019.

Moving?

Make sure your subscription moves with you!

To notify us of your new address, find your **Clinics Account Number** (located on your mailing label above your name), and contact customer service at:

Email: journalscustomerservice-usa@elsevier.com

800-654-2452 (subscribers in the U.S. & Canada)
314-447-8871 (subscribers outside of the U.S. & Canada)

Fax number: 314-447-8029

Elsevier Health Sciences Division
Subscription Customer Service
3251 Riverport Lane
Maryland Heights, MO 63043

*To ensure uninterrupted delivery of your subscription, please notify us at least 4 weeks in advance of move.

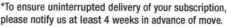

Printed and bound by CPI Group (UK) Ltd, Croydon, CR0 4YY

03/10/2024

01040405-0001